TESTING OF COMMUNICATING SYSTEMS XIV

IFIP - The International Federation for Information Processing

IFIP was founded in 1960 under the auspices of UNESCO, following the First World Computer Congress held in Paris the previous year. An umbrella organization for societies working in information processing, IFIP's aim is two-fold: to support information processing within its member countries and to encourage technology transfer to developing nations. As its mission statement clearly states,

IFIP's mission is to be the leading, truly international, apolitical organization which encourages and assists in the development, exploitation and application of information technology for the benefit of all people.

IFIP is a non-profitmaking organization, run almost solely by 2500 volunteers. It operates through a number of technical committees, which organize events and publications. IFIP's events range from an international congress to local seminars, but the most important are:

- The IFIP World Computer Congress, held every second year;
- open conferences;
- working conferences.

The flagship event is the IFIP World Computer Congress, at which both invited and contributed papers are presented. Contributed papers are rigorously refereed and the rejection rate is high.

As with the Congress, participation in the open conferences is open to all and papers may be invited or submitted. Again, submitted papers are stringently refereed.

The working conferences are structured differently. They are usually run by a working group and attendance is small and by invitation only. Their purpose is to create an atmosphere conducive to innovation and development. Refereeing is less rigorous and papers are subjected to extensive group discussion.

Publications arising from IFIP events vary. The papers presented at the IFIP World Computer Congress and at open conferences are published as conference proceedings, while the results of the working conferences are often published as collections of selected and edited papers.

Any national society whose primary activity is in information may apply to become a full member of IFIP, although full membership is restricted to one society per country. Full members are entitled to vote at the annual General Assembly, National societies preferring a less committed involvement may apply for associate or corresponding membership. Associate members enjoy the same benefits as full members, but without voting rights. Corresponding members are not represented in IFIP bodies. Affiliated membership is open to non-national societies, and individual and honorary membership schemes are also offered.

TESTING OF COMMUNICATING SYSTEMS XIV

Application to Internet Technologies and Services

IFIP TC6 / WG6.1 Fourteenth International Conference on Testing of Communicating Systems (TestCom 2002)
March 19–22, 2002, Berlin, Germany

Edited by

Ina Schieferdecker
Fraunhofer FOKUS Berlin
Germany

Hartmut König
Brandenburg University of Technology at Cottbus
Germany

Adam Wolisz
Technical University of Berlin
Germany

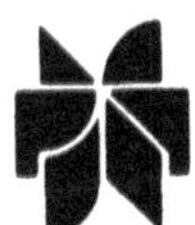

SPRINGER SCIENCE+BUSINESS MEDIA, LLC

Library of Congress Cataloging-in-Publication Data

IFIP TC6/WG6.1 International Conference on Testing of Communicating Systems (14th: 2002 Berlin, Germany)

Testing of communicating systems XIV : application to Internet technologies and services : IFIP TC6/WG6.1 International Conference on Testing of Communicating Systems (TestCom 2002), March 19-22, 2002, Berlin, Germany) / edited by Ina Schieferdecker, Hartmut König, Adam Wolisz.

p. ; cm. — (International Federation for Information Processing ; 82)

Includes bibliographical references and index.

DOI 10.1007/978-0-387-35497-2

1. Telecommunication systems—Testing—Congresses. I. Schieferdecker, Ina. II. König, Hartmut, Prof. Dr.-Ing. habil. III. Wolisz, Adam. IV. Title. V. International Federation for Information Processing (Series) ; 82.

TK5101.A1 I337 2002
621.382—dc21 2002019553

Printed on acid-free paper.
www.springer.com/mycopy

Contents

Preface ix

Conference Committees xi

Keynote Speech I - Abstract

Testing of IP Services & Applications in a Service Provider Environment 17
Andreas Gehring

Session I Testing TCP/IP

A TCP Test System Specifying only Exceptional Packet Sequences 21
Tomohiko Ogishi, Toru Hasegawa, Toshihiko Kato, Kenji Suzuki

Verifying IP Meters from Sampled Measurements 39
Carlos Veciana-Nogués, Albert Cabellos-Aparicio, Jordi Domingo-Pascual, Josep Solé-Pareta

Testing IP Differentiated Services Implementations 55
Carlos Parada, Jorge Carapinha, Francisco Fontes, Solange Lima, Paulo Carvalho

Invited Talk I - Abstract

Achieving High Reliability for Ubiquitous Information Technology 75
Robert V. Binder

Session II Testing Internet Systems

An Automated, Flexible Testing Environment for UMTS 79
Jan Bredereke, Bernd-Holger Schlingloff

Testing Mobile Agents 95
Mikael Marche, Yves-Marie Quemener, Roland Groz

Testing Access to External Information Sources in a Mediator Environment 111
Zoltán Ádám Mann, Jacques Calmet, Peter Kullmann

Session III Industrial Session I

Compliance of Wireless Application Protocols 129
Ousmane Koné

A Flexible Traffic Generator for Testing PABX and Call Center Performance 139
Georg Rößler, Thomas Steinert

Session IV Interoperability Testing

Interoperability Test Generation for Communication Protocols based on Multiple Stimuli Principle 151
Soonuk Seol, Myungchul Kim, Samuel T. Chanson

Automated Generation of Interoperability Tests 169
Cédric Besse, Ana Cavalli, Myungchul Kim, Fatiha Zadi

Keynote Speech II – Abstract

Applying Formal Methods in Mobile Protocol Testing 187
Ari Ahtiainen

Session V Industrial Session II

Experiences of TTCN-3 Test Executor Development 191
János Zoltán Szabó

Position Statement: Making TTCN-3 testing a success 201
Wolfgang Sachse

Position Statement: Testing Automation with Computer Aided Test Case Generation 209
Tapio Heikkilä, Petri Tenno, Jarmo Väänänen

Session VI Test Automation

Automated Testing in Practice: The Highway Tolling System 219
René G. de Vries, Axel Belinfante, Jan Feenstra

Ad-hoc Protocol Modelling, Validation and Automated Test Suite Generation 235
Endre Horváth

Session VII Test Generation and Selection

Generate Certified Test Cases by Combining Theorem Proving and Reachability Analysis 249
Richard Castanet, Davy Rouillard

Test Selection, Trace Distance and Heuristics 267
Loe M. G. Feijs, Nicolae Goga, Sjouke Mauw, Jan Tretmans

Formulation of the Interaction Test Coverage Problem as an Integer Program 283
Alan W. Williams, Robert L. Probert

Session VIII Testing Distributed Systems

Principles of Distributed Test Synthesis based on True-concurrency Models 301
Claude Jard

Fault Detection within a Component of a System of Communicating FSMs 317
Ana Cavalli, Svetlana Prokopenko, Nina Yevtushenko

Invited Talk II

Hardware/Software Integration Testing for the new Airbus Aircraft Families 335
Jan Peleska

Session IX FSM-based Testing

Test Generation for CEFSM Combining Specification and Fault Coverage 355
Sergiy Boroday, Alex Petrenko, Roland Groz, Yves-Marie Quemener

FSM-based Re-Testing Methods 373
Khaled El-Fakih, Nina Yevtushenko, Gregor v. Bochmann

A New Approach To Checking Sequence Generation for Finite State Machines 391
Burak Serdar, Kuo-Chung Tai

Session X TTCN-3

Timed TTCN-3 - A Real-Time Extension for TTCN-3 407
Zhen Ru Dai, Jens Grabowski, Helmut Neukirchen

Implementation of TTCN-3 Test Systems using the TRI 425
Stephan Schulz, Theofanis Vassiliou-Gioles

A Definition and Utilisation of OMG IDL to TTCN-3 Mappings 443
Michael Ebner, Aihong Yin, Mang Li

Author Index 459

Partners of TestCom 2002 461

Preface

This volume contains the proceedings of TestCom 2002, the IFIP TC 6 / WG 6.1 International Conference on Testing Communicating Systems, held in Berlin, Germany, on March, 19th through 22nd, 2002. TestCom denotes a series of international working conferences on testing communicating systems in the data and telecommunication domain. The conference provides a forum for researchers, vendors and users to review, discuss and learn about new approaches, concepts and experiences in the field of testing of communicating systems. This conference in particular focuses on the exchange and discussion of concepts and practices in testing Internet related systems, services and protocols.

TestCom 2002 is the fourteenth in a series of annual meetings sponsored by IFIP TC 6 / WG 6.1. The thirteen previous meetings were held in Vancouver, Canada (1988), Berlin, Germany (1989), Mclean, U.S.A. (1990), Leidschendam, the Netherlands (1991), Montreal, Canada (1992), Pau, France (1993), Tokyo, Japan (1994), Evry, France (1995), Darmstadt, Germany (1996), Cheju Island, Korea (1997), Tomsk, Russia (1998), Budapest, Hungary (1999), and Ottawa, Canada (2000).

The scope of the papers presented at TestCom 2002 covers the testing of internet services, of TCP/IP, and of wireless applications, the interoperability test, test automation, test generation and selection, the testing of distributed systems, FSM-based testing, TTCN-3, and industrial experience in testing communication systems.

The TestCom 2002 program consisted of 8 sessions, 2 industrial sessions, and a working session. Two invited talks and two keynote speeches gave an overview on actual trends in the telecommunication area and formulated requirements to the testing process. The conference was preceded by 3 half-day tutorials. The proceedings contain the 21 regular and 3 short papers accepted and presented at the conference. They were selected from 54 submitted papers in a careful selection procedure based on the assessment of three referees for each paper. The proceedings also include the text of the invited talk by Jan Peleska as well as the abstracts of the invited talk by Robert V. Binder, and of the keynote speeches by Andreas Gehring (T-Systems Nova) and by Ari Ahtiainen (Nokia). In addition, two position statements presented in the industrial session belong to this volume.

TestCom 2002 was organized under the auspices of IFIP TC 6 by FOKUS Berlin, the Fraunhofer Institute for Open Communication Systems, and by BTU Cottbus, the Brandenburg University of Technology at Cottbus. It was supported by a number of partners including Danet, the German Research Society (DFN), the German Society of Informatics (GI), Nokia, Telelogic, Testing Technologies, Tektronix, and T-Systems.

We would like to express our gratitude to the numerous people who have contributed to the success of TestCom 2002. The reviewing process was one of the major efforts during the preparation of the conference. It was completed by experts from around the world. The reviewers are listed in this proceedings. We also thank Mrs. Yana Lambert of Kluwer for her constructive support when editing these proceedings. Finally we would like to thank the local organizers for the excellent running of the conference, especially Birgit Benner, Gudrun Quandel, Temenuga Veleva, Guergana Vladova, Daniel Dietterle, and Niels Bischof. Our special thanks goes to Mrs. Katrin Willhöft for the final formatting of the proceedings.

Ina Schieferdecker, Hartmut König, Adam Wolisz

Conference Committees

Conference Chairmen

Ina Schieferdecker
Fraunhofer FOKUS Berlin

Hartmut König
Brandenburg University of Technology at Cottbus

Adam Wolisz
Technical University of Berlin

Steering Committee

S. T. Chanson, *Hong Kong University of Science and Technology, China*
R. Groz, *France Telecom, France*
G. Leduc, Chairman, *University of Liege, Belgium*
A. Petrenko, *CRIM, Canada*

Technical Programme Committee

B. Baumgarten, GMD SIT, Germany
G. v. Bochmann, University of Ottawa, Canada
S. Budkowski, INT, France
A. R. Cavalli, INT, France

G. Csopaki, Budapest University, Hungary
S. Dibuz, Ericsson, Hungary
R. Dssouli, Concordia University of Montreal, Canada
J. Grabowski, University of Lübeck, Germany
T. Higashino, Osaka University, Japan
D. Hogrefe, University of Lübeck, Germany
C. Jard, IRISA, France
M. Kim, ICU University, Korea
R. Lai, La Trobe University, Australia
D. Lee, Bell Labs Research, USA.
J. Maldonado, University of Sao Paulo, Brazil
J. de Meer, Condat AG, Germany
O. Monkewich, Nortel Networks, Canada
R. L. Probert, University of Ottawa, Canada
K. Stöttinger, Deutsche Telekom, Germany
K. Suzuki, Advanced Communication, Japan
K. Tarnay, Nokia, Hungary
J. Tretmans, University of Twente, The Netherlands
A. Ulrich, Siemens, Germany
H. Ural, University of Ottawa, Canada
M. U. Uyar, City University of New York, USA
A. Wiles, ETSI, France
C. Willcock, Nokia, Germany
J. Wu, Tsinghua University, China
N. Yevtushenko, Tomsk State University, Russia

Additional Reviewers

A. Belifante, University of Twente, The Netherlands
M. van der Bijl, University of Twente, The Netherlands
M. Blake, condat AG Berlin, Germany
S. Boroday, CRIM, Canada
R. H. Carlucci Santana, University of Sao Paulo, Brazil
D. Chen, Tsinghua University, China
P. Deussen, GMD FOKUS Berlin, Germany
M. Ebner, University of Lübeck, Germany
K. El-Khatib, University of Ottawa, Canada
A. Ennouaary, Concordia University of Montreal, Canada
J. Feenstra, University of Twente, The Netherlands
R. Gecse, Ericsson, Hungary
T. Hasegawa, KDDI R&D Labs, Japan

O. Henniger, Fraunhofer SIT, Darmstadt, Germany
M. Higuchi, Osaka University, Japan
R. Horvath, Nokia, Hungary
T. Horvath, Nokia, Hungary
I. Hwang, INT Evry, France
A. Idoue, KDDI R&D Labs, Japan
S. Kang, ICU University, Korea
T. Kasza, Budapest University, Hungary
T. Kato, KDDI R&D Labs, Japan
F. Khendek, Concordia University of Montreal, Canada
I. Koufareva, Tomsk State University, Russia
G. Kovacs, Budapest University, Hungary
S. Leppanen, Nokia NRC,
Z. Li, Tsinghua University, China
W. Lopes de Souza, University of San Marcos, Brazil
S. Maag, INT Evry, France
A. Nakata, Osaka University, Japan
H. Neukirchen, University of Lübeck, Germany
T. Ogishi, KDDI R&D Labs, Japan
Z. Pap, Budapest University, Hungary
S. Prokopenko, Tomsk State University, Russia
Z. Rethati, Budapest University, Hungary
C. Rinderknecht, ICU University, Korea
Z. Ru Dai, University of Lübeck, Germany
M. J. Santana, University of Sao Paulo, Brazil
M. Schmitt, University of Lübeck, Germany
M. Söderlund, Nokia NRC, Germany
J. Z. Szabó, Ericsson, Hungary
S. Tobies, Nokia NRC, Germany
C. Viho, IRISA, France
R. de Vries, University of Twente, The Netherlands
K. Yasumoto, Osaka University, Japan
X. Yin, Tsinghua University, China
X. Yu, Tsinghua University, China
F. Zaidi, INT Evry, France
Y. Zhao, Tsinghua University, China
T. Zseby, GMD FOKUS Berlin, Germany

Organisation Committee

B. Benner, FOKUS Berlin, Germany
T. Veleva, FOKUS Berlin, Germany
G. Quandel FOKUS Berlin, Germany
N. Bischof, BTU Cottbus, Germany
D. Dietterle, BTU Cottbus, Germany
K. Willhöft BTU Cottbus, Germany

KEYNOTE SPEECH I - ABSTRACT

TESTING OF IP SERVICES & APPLICATIONS IN A SERVICE PROVIDER ENVIRONMENT

Andreas Gehring
T-Systems Nova, Technologiezentrum, Germany

Abstract A service providers (SP) environment requires several stages and types of testing and quality assurance (QA) before a new service or application can be launched in the network environment. The test procedures cover the whole range from evaluation of single network and server platform components to end-2-end testing depending on the type of application or product. This includes as well technical parameters like QoS in the network and availability of the service as user oriented parameters like usability and user friendliness. This keynote introduces categories of services & applications and gives an overview of the principle testing methods for the single service categories. It describes the stages of a product roll-out of a SP and the tests which are applied to the service components in each phase.

SESSION I

TESTING TCP/IP

A TCP TEST SYSTEM SPECIFYING ONLY EXCEPTIONAL PACKET SEQUENCES

Tomohiko Ogishi, Toru Hasegawa, Toshihiko Kato and Kenji Suzuki
KDDI R&D Laboratories, Inc., Japan

Abstract Although TCP is widely used in Internet, new specifications are still proposed and implemented. In the circumstance above, it is highly possible that some errors are detected on the communication between new and old implementations. Several test tools were developed so far. However, they do not have enough function to customize test sequence or need significant effort to specify the sequence. We developed a TCP test system which specifies only exceptional packet sequence in the test scenario. The system performs exceptional packet sequence only when the condition specified in the test scenario is satisfied. Otherwise, it performs ordinary TCP behavior. The system is implemented by modifying TCP module of NetBSD with SACK code developed by Pittsburgh Supercomputing Center. We also evaluated SACK implementation as an example of recent specification using the test system.

Keywords: TCP, exceptional packet sequence, test scenario, congestion control, selective acknowledgment

1. INTRODUCTION

TCP [1] is widely used as a protocol to provide reliable transfer from the dawn of Internet. The TCP protocol functions and implementations have been modified and extended in the long history of TCP. Currently, the TCP implementations in widely spread PCs and workstations are fairly stable and the users seldom feel inconvenience at TCP communications. However, there are several implementation errors as reported in [2]. Due to those errors, TCP communications in specific situations, such as a long haul TCP communication, suffer from problems like serious throughput degradation. Those well-known errors have been fixed in the higher version of implementations, but, still now, new functions, such as a new congestion control mechanism in NewReno [3] and the selective acknowledgment (SACK) [4], are proposed and integrated into available TCP implementations. It is highly possible that not detected errors related to conventional functions [5] and errors related to new functions [3,4] bring new problems in TCP communications.

In order to detect such errors, some tools for testing TCP implementation are required. So far, various tools have been developed [6], which are classified into two groups, monitors and testers. The monitors collect packet data exchanged between end systems and analyzes TCP protocol behaviors. TCPAnaly [7] and the Intelligent TCP Analyzer [8] are categorized in this group. However, the monitors cannot control packet sequences in the testing, and it is not easy to detect errors in TCP implementations by monitors.

On the other hand, the testers can generate packets suitable for a specific testing purpose. But, the testers developed so far [9-11] have some issues to perform the TCP implementation testing. Among them, TBIT [9] and Nmap [10] use some predefined test sequences. The purpose of TBIT is to check the compliance and used parameter values of TCP implementations, and that of Nmap is to estimate the version of operating systems from the TCP behaviors. That is, those systems do not allow test operators to use test sequences specific to their test purposes. On the other hand, [11] proposes a TCP test system which can generate test sequences based on test scenario specification written in TTCN [12]. This system allows test operators to use suited test sequences. However, the task to generate a test sequence will be a hard job for test operators because it is required to specify all input and output events used in the sequence.

Considering these issues, it is important to reduce the burden for test operators to specify a test sequence. When a test operator tries to test a normal behavior of TCP module in a system under test, it is possible to use an ordinary TCP module as a tester. A specially ordered mechanism is used only when a test operator tries to test an exceptional behavior of TCP. Therefore, we propose a TCP test system which uses an ordinary TCP module for testing normal TCP behaviors and which allows test operators to specify a test sequence only for testing exceptional TCP sequences. By using our TCP test system, a test operator can perform exceptional test sequence, such as sending SYN segment in ESTABLISHED state, sending ACK segment with smaller acknowledgment number, and sending SACK options with the first and the second SACK blocks misordered. A test operator does not need to specify normal sequences but describe exceptional part in a test scenario. The TCP module in the test system behaves normally if the condition on a test scenario is not satisfied. If the condition is satisfied, it runs the actions specified in the test scenario. It also saves a communication log which is examined after the test run is over.

In this paper, we describe the requirements, design and implementation of the TCP test system. We also describe the evaluation result of SACK implementation by using the system. In Section 2, we describe the requirement and the design principles of our test system. Sections 3 and 4 show the detailed design and the implementation, respectively. Section 5 gives an evaluation of SACK implementation by using the test system. Finally, Section 6 makes a conclusion.

2. REQUIREMENTS AND DESIGN PRINCIPLES

As described above, the following is required for the TCP test system.

- The test system should provide a convenient method to specify a test scenario in order to reduce the burden for test operator.
- The essential functions of TCP such as connection establishment have been tested sufficiently so far, and are used without any problem. However, in some recent specifications, there are some additional functions which rely on implementers' decision. For example, SACK specifies the format of SACK blocks, but, it does not specify the retransmission manner when a packet with SACK option is received. Therefore, it is such an additional function that should be tested by the TCP test system.
- In the test of additional functions, it is expected that a test operator will examine the test result in detail, estimate the reasons for the result by emulating the TCP behaviors of the system under test, and give the verdict for the test. In order to reduce the burden for the test result analysis, the TCP test system should generate enough information on the communication in the test logs.

Based on these requirements, we have adopted the following design principles in order to develop the TCP test system.

1. The test system is composed by *test execution part* and *test analysis part.* The test execution part communicates with system under test using some TCP application program for testing. It performs exceptional behaviors specified in a test scenario while communicating by normal behavior. It collects the communication log for later analysis. The test analysis part analyzes the communication log in an offline manner.
2. Only the exceptional sequences are described in a test scenario. This means that the TCP test system communicates with system under test

according to the normal TCP procedure, while it is not directed to follow exceptional sequence. Once it is directed, it sends segments with the parameter values and with the order which are specified in the test scenario.

3. In order to develop the test execution part, we use TCP application program and in-kernel TCP module. We use public software such as *ftp* or *ttcp* as a TCP application program. We modify the in-kernel TCP module in order to realize the test scenario execution and the communication log collection. We believe that this implementation scheme requires less amount of work compared with the implementation of the test execution part from the scratch, although our scheme requires the kernel modification.
4. A test scenario is composed by a set of rows, each of which specifies a *condition* and an *action*. A condition specifies whether to trigger the corresponding action. We use three types of conditions; the parameter values of received segments, the parameter values of segments going to be sent and the expiration of user-defined timers. The action specifies whether to send segments if the condition is satisfied. We use two type of actions; a sending of a segments with the specific parameter values, and the discard of a segment which is sent by the original TCP module.

3. DETAILED DESIGN

3.1 Structure

Figure 1 shows the functional structure of the TCP test system. The test system is composed by test execution part and test analysis part as described in the previous section. The test execution part includes *scenario loader*, TCP application program, in-kernel TCP module and network interface. In the in-kernel TCP module, *scenario interpreter* and *log collector* are implemented. Scenario loader provides the operator to configure the test environment. It selects the test scenario performed at scenario interpreter and whether the communication log is collected or not. TCP application program actually sends or receives user data on TCP by communicating with server or client program running on system under test. Scenario interpreter reads the test scenario and decides whether the action in the test scenario is executed or not. When the action is executed, it directly sends the packets described in the action to network interface through log collector. The interpreter maintains the scenario counter indicating the line of test scenario. Log collector is placed on the network interface and monitors the segments received from or sent to network interface, and collects a communication log related to the test. It also refers to the scenario counter when a segment is added to the communication log. *Log analyzer* in the test analysis part provides the operator to analyze the communication log.

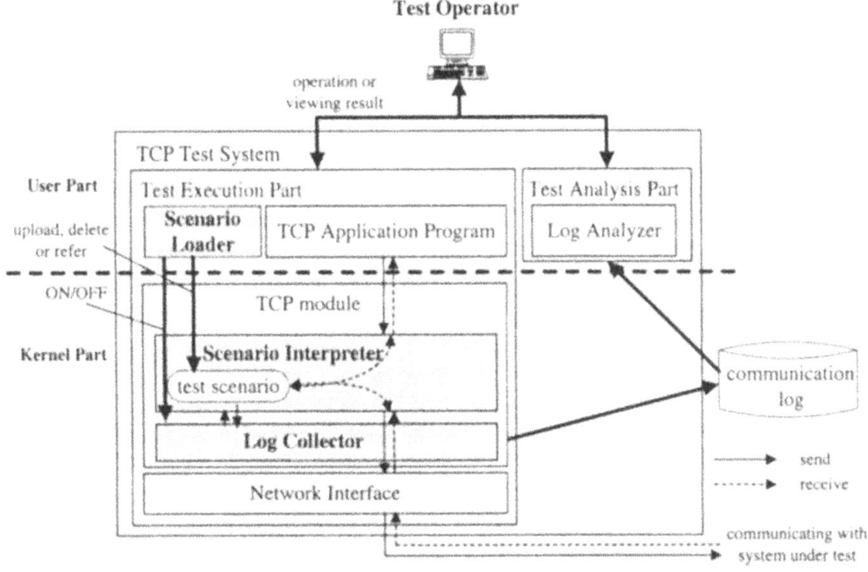

Figure 1. Structure of TCP Test System.

3.2 Test Scenario

Figure 2 shows an example of test scenario. The test scenario consists of *header* and *content parts*. In the header part, IP addresses and port numbers for source and destination, which indicate TCP connections under test. For example, if 20 is specified as source port number, the TCP behavior of FTP data connections becomes the target. In this case, TCP connections with other source port number such as FTP control connection or WWW client behaves without any influence of test scenario. In other words, the system can protect other application programs from being affected by the test scenario. In the header part, TCP options used at connection establishment and the parameter value of each option are also specified by using *syn-opt* key. When the key is specified, the specified options are forced to be used in SYN or SYN+ACK segment without negotiating with peer end system. In the example of Fig. 2, TCP options are sent with maximum segment size

(MSS) option set 10 bytes, sack permitted option, timestamp option and window scale factor (WSF) option set 0.

In the content part, the behaviors after establishing TCP connection are specified. In the each line of content part, the condition and the action are specified by being separated with semi-colon. In the condition, a trigger event and its parameter values are specified. There are three types of trigger events, *recv*, *send* and *wait*, which mean received packet, sending packet and timer expiration, as described above. In the case of *recv* and *send* events, several expressions such as “=”, “<=”, “>=”, “>” and “<” can be used with a compared value. If *any* is specified as the value, the condition always becomes true as far as the parameter exists. At the end of the condition, *var-upd* which means whether internal variables related to the received packet such as *rcv_nxt* are updated or not is also specified. If *var-upd* is OFF at *recv* event, it becomes the same situation that the received packet is lost at network. In the action, a packet to be sent with its parameter values at a true condition is specified. All of the parameter values in the TCP header except urgent pointer and checksum should be specified in the action. TCP options such as MSS and SACK are specified with parameter values if the options are included in the sent packet. At the end of the condition, *var-upd* which means whether internal variables related to the sent packet such as *snd_nxt* are updated or not is also specified. If no packet is desired to be sent, *ignore* is specified as action. If multiple packets are desired to be sent at a time, the second and later actions are specified without conditions.

Each line of content part in Figure 2 is interpreted as the following way:

line 1: If a packet with its sequence number (*seq*) equal to 1 is received, update the internal variables for the received packet, send a packet with its *seq* set 1, acknowledgment number (*ack*) set 11, flag bit (flag) set ack flag and window size (*win*) set 20 bytes and update the internal variables for the sent packet. Here, the value specified in *seq* or *ack* is relative one to the initial send sequence number or initial receive sequence number.

line 2: If a packet with *seq* equal to 11 is received, ignore the received packet without updating the internal variables.

line 3: If a packet with *seq* equal to 1 and *ack* equal to 11 is going to be sent, stop the packet being sent while updating the internal variables for the packet.

line 4: Wait one time slot (considered 500 millisecond) and send a packet with *seq* set 1, *ack* set 11, *flag* set ack flag and *win* set 30 bytes without updating internal variables for the packet.

line 5: If a packet with *seq* equal to 11 is received, ignore the received packet while updating the internal variables.

line 6: If a packet with *seq* equal to 21 is received, ignore the received packet without updating the internal variables.

line 7-10: If a packet with *seq* equal to 31 is received, update the internal variables for the received packet, send 4 duplicate packets with its *seq* set 1, *ack* set 11, the blocks for selective acknowledgment (*sack*) set 31-41, *flag* set ack flag and *win* set 30 bytes and update the internal variables for every sent packet.

line 11: If a packet with *seq* greater than 70 is received, update the internal variables for the received packet, send a packet with its *seq* set 1, *flag* set rst flag and *win* set 30 bytes and update the internal variables for the sent packet.

```
       <header>
       src-addr=192.168.0.1
       dst-addr=192.168.0.2
       src-port=20
       syn-opt=mss(10), sack, timestamp, wsf(0)

       <content>
line 1 recv seq=1 var-upd=ON      ; send seq=1 ack=11 flag=(ack) win=20 var-upd=ON
     2 recv seq=11 var-upd=OFF    ; ignore
     3 send seq=1 ack=11 var-upd=yes ; ignore
     4 wait 1                     ; send seq=1 ack=11 flag=(ack) win=30 var-upd=OFF
     5 recv seq=11 var-upd=ON     ; ignore
     6 recv seq=21 var-upd=OFF    ; ignore
     7 recv seq=31 var-upd=ON     ; send seq=1 ack=21 sack=(31-41) flag=(ack) win=30 var-upd=ON
     8                            ; send seq=1 ack=21 sack=(31-41) flag=(ack) win=30 var-upd=ON
     9                            ; send seq=1 ack=21 sack=(31-41) flag=(ack) win=30 var-upd=ON
    10                            ; send seq=1 ack=21 sack=(31-41) flag=(ack) win=30 var-upd=ON
    11 recv seq>70 var-upd=ON     ; send seq=1 flag=(rst) win=30 var-upd=ON
```

Figure 2. Example of Test Scenario.

3.3 Scenario Interpreter

The flow chart presenting how scenario interpreter works is illustrated in Fig. 3. Scenario interpreter maintains a test scenario loaded to the test system. It examines all packets which are received or going to be sent and checks whether the TCP connection of the packet is under test or not. If the connection is under test, the interpreter checks whether the TCP state is ESTABLISHED or not. If not, the packet is dealt as a normal TCP behavior. Only if *syn-opt* is specified in the header part of the test scenario and SYN or SYN+ACK segments is going to be sent, the TCP options for the sent packet are modified as what specified at *syn-opt* before sending it. If the state is ESTABLISHED, the interpreter maintains the *scenario counter*, which indicates the line executed currently. The counter starts at the first line of the content part when the TCP state enters ESTABLISHED and is incremented only when the condition at the counter is satisfied and the action is executed. If the counter reaches to the end, further events are dealt as normal TCP behavior. If the trigger event is *wait*, a timer is invoked. The expired time is set to the number of time slots specified in the condition. While the timer is working, the following sent or received events obey to normal TCP behavior. When the timer is expired, the action for the *wait* is executed and the scenario counter is incremented. Even if the counter reaches to the end, the communication under test does not finish at the time. It continues by normal TCP behavior.

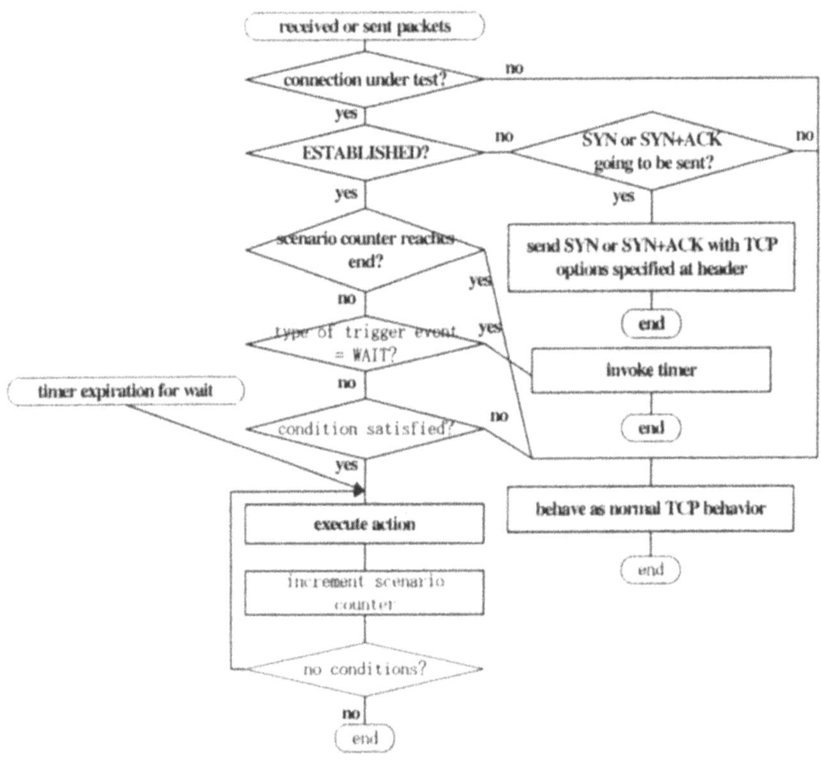

Figure 3. Flow Chart for Scenario Interpreter.

Figure 4 illustrates the sequence of communication when the test scenario in Fig. 2 is performed. The test causes the system under test (SUT) retransmit by timeout and fast retransmit. The scenario was written with a knowledge that SUT performs slow start with initial congestion window set 1. Therefore, SUT cannot send any packet after sending the first DATA segment of its *seq* 21, which causes retransmit by timeout. The test system sends 4 duplicate ACK segments illegally, which causes fast retransmit at SUT. The sequence includes a part behaving normally. In the part, DATA segments from 21 to 70 are sent and acknowledged. The test system does not need to specify this part in the test scenario.

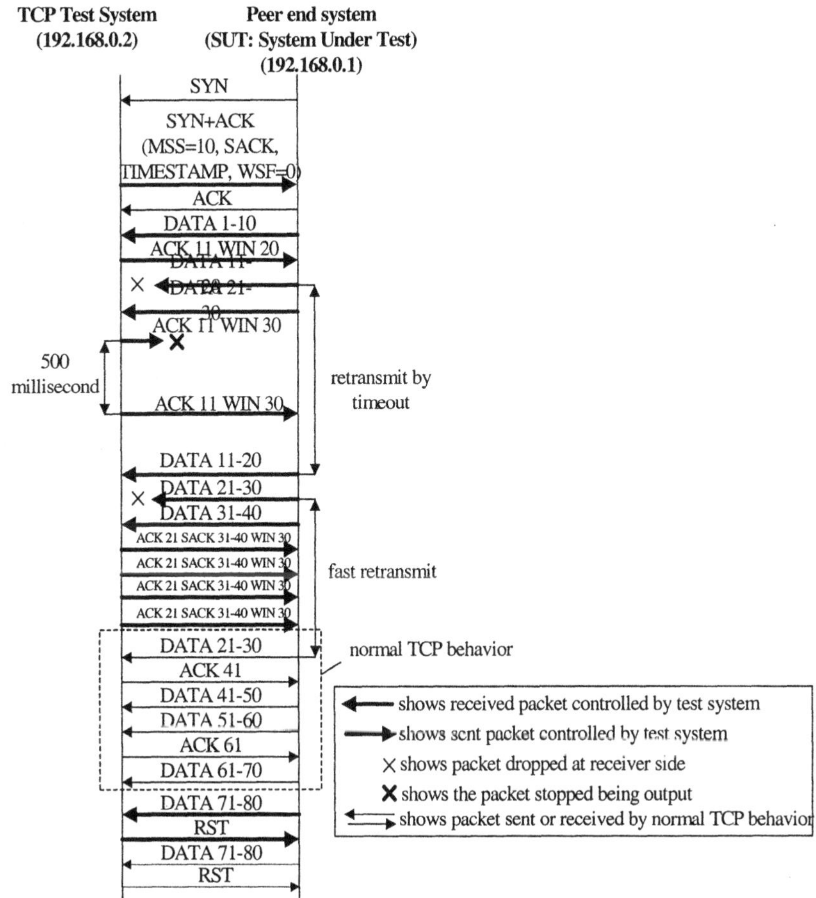

Figure 4. Example of Exceptional Packet Sequences.

3.4 Log Collector

Log collector saves a packet received or going to be sent to the communication log if the TCP connection of the packet is under test and the function is set on. Figure 5 shows a communication log collected at the test of Fig. 2. The output format is almost same as that of *tcpdump* [14]. The differences are as follows:

- The communication log shows the scenario counter on the top of line for each event.
- The communication log can show the packets which are not actually sent or received at TCP of the test system using parenthesis such as line 2 and line 3.
- The communication log shows whether internal variables are updated or not. If updated, (var-upd) is added to the line.

```
0: 0.000000    SYN seq=3,325,424 win=32,768 mss=1,460 sack-permitted timestamp wsf=0
0: 0.000128 SYN+ACK seq=1,783,630 ack=1 win=32,768 mss=10 sack-permitted timestatmp wsf=0
0: 0.000233    ACK seq=1 ack=1 win=32,768 (var-upd)
1: 0.001733    DATA seq=1 ack=1 win=32,768 len=10 (var-upd)
1: 0.001855    ACK seq=1 ack=11 win=20
2: 0.001934    (DATA seq=11 ack=1 win=32,768 len=10)
3: 0.002018 (ACK seq=1 ack=11 win=8,760) (var-upd)
4: 0.478445 ACK seq=1 ack=11 win=30
5: 3.712842    DATA seq=11 ack=1 win=32,768 len=10 (var-upd)
6: 3.712932    (DATA seq=21 ack=1 win=32,768 len=10)
7: 3.713015    DATA seq=31 ack=1 win=32,768 len=10 (var-upd)
7: 3.713099 ACK seq=1 ack=21 sack=(31-41) win=30 (var-upd)
8: 3.713131 ACK seq=1 ack=21 sack=(31-41) win=30 (var-upd)
9: 3.713148 ACK seq=1 ack=21 sack=(31-41) win=30 (var-upd)
10: 3.713166 ACK seq=1 ack=21 sack=(31-41) win=30 (var-upd)
11: 3.713275    DATA seq=21 ack=1 win=32,768 len=10
11: 3.713383 ACK seq=1 ack=41 win=8,760
11: 3.713425    DATA seq=41 ack=1 win=32,768 len=10
11: 3.713499    DATA seq=51 ack=1 win=32,768 len=10
11: 3.713548 ACK seq=1 ack=61 win=8,760
11: 3.713552    DATA seq=61 ack=1 win=32,768 len=10
11: 3.713631    DATA seq=71 ack=1 win=32,768 len=10
11: 3.713693 RST seq=1 win=30 (var-upd)
end:3.713755    DATA seq=81 ack=1 win=32,768 len=10
end:3.713830 RST seq=1 win=8,760
```

Figure 5. Example of Communication Log.

4. IMPLEMENTATION

We implemented the TCP test system based on NetBSD 1.3.2 with SACK developed by Pittsburgh Supercomputing Center (PSC) [15] by modifying its source code. Scenario loader was implemented as a user program. Scenario interpreter and log collector were implemented in the kernel by modifying PSC's TCP module. For the interface for scenario loader to control the in-kernel module, we used *setsockopt()* function. The test scenario is loaded to TCP module through this function. The test scenario in the TCP module is deleted or referred to though the function. The test scenario is maintained as a global variable in the TCP module and copied to *tcpcb* structure [16] when *connect()* or *accept()* is invoked at a TCP connection under test. We modified the source codes related to TCP module in the following way in order to handle scenario interpretation and realize exceptional packet sequences:

- The source code for interpretation is newly added to the TCP module.
- In order to send exceptional packets specified in the test scenario, the packet in the action is constructed before tcp_output() is called.
- In order to interrupt the receiving and sending processes when the condition specified in the test scenario is satisfied, the codes for checking the condition is added to the top parts of tcp_input() and tcp_output().
- In order to avoid internal variables for updating when var-upd is OFF, tcp_input() and tcp_output() include the codes to skip the update.
- The wait function is realized in the same way as the system timer used for detecting retransmission timeout.

Through the implementation of the test system in the TCP module, it was difficult to stop all of disagreeable packets such as ACK for window update. The difficulty comes from the situation that the window update ACK is sent spontaneously. Actually, the window update ACK is sent when an application program reads received data. Therefore, the test system cannot avoid sending window update ACKs independently of test scenario. To cope with this situation, we provided following solutions:

- If we found a disagreeable window update ACK through the communication log after executing a test scenario, we added one line to the current test scenario which ignores the sent the ACK as described in Paragraph 3.2. Our test system is designed to facilitate such an incremental modification of test scenario because we need to specify only exceptional behavior.
- We provided another mode for the behavior of scenario interpreter, which does not output any packets as far as a packet is not described in the test scenario as an action. Therefore, this mode does not produce any window update ACK.

As a TCP application program, public tools such as *ftp* and *ttcp* can be used. Only the total size of data and the direction should be controlled by the test operator. As log analyzer, a simple text viewer is used. To realize the log collector, a system function *syslog* is used. The code to write the *syslog* is added to in-kernel TCP module.

4.1 evaluation of SACK implementation

We evaluated SACK implementations in various operating systems using the implemented TCP test system. Figure 6 shows the network configuration of this test. We attached a network simulator between the test system and the system under test, and inserted one-second round trip delay in order to examine how the congestion control works. We used *ftp* as application program and created a file of 16 Kilobytes at the system under test and sent the file to the test system. We tested the sender's behavior when ACK segments with SACK options (which we call SACK segments) are received. The operating systems we tested are SPARC Solaris 2.6 with SACK patch (which we call Solaris 2.6), Intel Solaris 8 (which we call Solaris 8), Linux kernel 2.4.2 (which we call Linux), NetBSD 1.3.2 with SACK code developed by PSC (which we call NetBSD), and Windows 98 Second Edition (which we call Windows 98). We performed three different tests described in the following subsections.

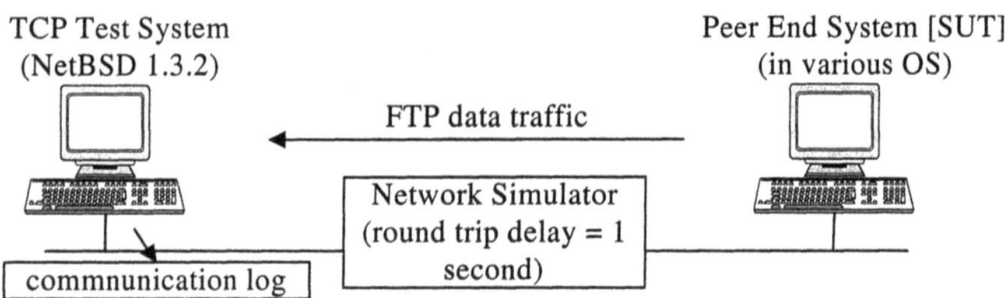

Figure 6. Network Configuration for SACK Testing.

4.2 Multiple Drops in a Window

SACK function notifies the sender with a range of dropped packets accurately, which is the same as that maintained by the receiver. If the sender implements the retransmission algorithm effectively, it can theoretically send all dropped packets in a window in one round trip time (RTT). Therefore, SACK function is effective between end systems over a link with long RTT such as satellite link. An approach to realize sender's behavior is proposed by [17] as pipe algorithm. We tested retransmission algorithm using the test scenario depicted in Fig. 7. This test scenario is very simple. It sets MSS as 100 bytes and emulates drops at network of every other packet after congestion window extends enough. Since the actions for received packets such as the packet with its *seq* 3501, the test system sends SACK segments against each packet received in this RTT.

```
       <header>
       src-addr=192.168.0.1
       dst-addr=192.168.0.2
       src-port=20
       syn-opt=mss(100),sack
       <content>
line 1 recv seq=3401 var-upd=OFF; ignore;
     2 recv seq=3601 var-upd=OFF; ignore;
     3 recv seq=3801 var-upd=OFF; ignore;
     4 recv seq=4001 var-upd=OFF; ignore;
     5 recv seq=4201 var-upd=OFF; ignore;
     6 recv seq=4401 var-upd=OFF; ignore;
```

Figure 7. Test Scenario for Multiple Drops in a Window.

Table 1. Result for Multiple Drops in a Window

OS	Total Time (second)	Initial Congestion Window	number of ACK	RTT
Solaris 2.6	15.1	2	23	1
Solaris 8	14.1	4	23	2
Linux	15.2	2	24	1
NetBSD	16.1	2	23	1
Windows 98	17.3	2	24	3

Table 1 shows the result of the test. Each column represents the operating system (OS), total elapsed time to transmit 16 Kilobytes, initial congestion window (ICW) used at slow start, number of ACK segments the SUT received before receiving duplicate ACK and RTT taken for retransmitting 6 dropped packets. Through this test, we found following facts and problems:

- All implementations deal with SACK options to retransmit dropped packets. If the retransmission algorithm for SACK were not implemented, it might take six RTTs to retransmit all of the dropped packets.
- Solaris 8 took two RTTs and Windows 98 took three RTTs to recover from dropped packets. However, we can not say the retransmission algorithms of these operating systems were worse than those of others. For example, when we set the ICW of Solaris 8 to 2, the RTT becomes one like others. From another test which drops 1501, 1701 and 1901, Linux took two RTTs while Solaris 2.6 and NetBSD took one. We think RTT taken to recover from multiple drops is highly related to ICW and

number of ACK because these values decide the value of congestion window when the congestion occurs.

- We found typical implementations, which are inconsistent with [13], on Linux, Solaris 2.6 and Window 98. All of them seem to inflate window before receiving three duplicate ACK segments. In addition, Linux retransmits faster (by one duplicate ACK in this test) than other implementations when it receives SACK segments. Since Windows 98 sent only 96 bytes when it retransmitted the packet with its seq 4001, it took another one RTT to retransmit the rest of 4 bytes.

4.3 Delay and Loss of SACK

SACK segments may not be arrived in correct order to the sender. This situation is possible according to the network condition. Figure 8 shows the test for the sender's behavior when SACK segments are delayed and lost in network. In this figure, SACK segments for DATA with *seq* 3501 and 3901 are lost shown in line 2 and 6, and 3701 is delayed shown in line 4 and 9.

```
       <header>
       src-addr=192.168.0.1
       dst-addr=192.168.0.2
       src-port=20
       syn-opt=mss(100),sack
       <content>
line 1 recv seq=3401 var-upd=no; ignore;
     2 send ack=any var-upd=no; ignore;
     3 recv seq=3601 var-upd=no; ignore;
     4 send ack=any var-upd=no; ignore;
     5 recv seq=3801 var-upd=no; ignore;
     6 send ack=any var-upd=no; ignore;
     7 recv seq=4001 var-upd=no; ignore;
     8 send ack=any var-upd=no; send tcp seq=1 ack=3401 flag=(ack) sack=(4101-4201,3901-
       4001,3701-3801,3501-3601) win=16400 var-upd=no;
     9 ; send tcp seq=1 ack=3401 flag=(ack) sack=(3701-3801,3501-3601) win=16400 var-upd=no;
    10 send ack=any var-upd=no; send tcp seq=1 ack=3401 flag=(ack) sack=(4101-4301)
       win=16400 var-upd=no;
    11 send ack=any var-upd=no; send tcp seq=1 ack=3401 flag=(ack) sack=(4101-4401)
       win=16400 var-upd=no;
     :                    :
    17 send ack=any var-upd=no; send tcp seq=1 ack=3401 flag=(ack) sack=(4101-5001)
       win=16400 var-upd=no;
       <end>
```

any is used when the condition is true on all value

Figure 8. Test Scenario for Delay and Loss of SACK Segments.

All implementations behaved well for these situations. The lost packets were retransmitted in one RTT in sequential order. We can estimate that current SACK implementations do not consider the order of arrival from this result.

4.4 Duplicate and Identical SACK

The third test we performed was sender's behavior to multiple duplicate ACK segments with duplicate and identical SACK. The literature [18] describes that a duplicate SACK segment is sent when the receiver receives a segment including the range of sequence number previously received. The format of duplicate SACK is the same as *normal* SACK specified in [4] except it uses older ranges of sequence number in SACK block relative to the acknowledgement number. Since the use of duplicate SACK was recently specified, it seems there were few implementations to support this. It is mentioned that Linux supports it. The duplicate ACK segment with the same SACK blocks, which we call *identical* SACK, should not be occurred as far as it is not duplicated in network in the current specifications. However, we think the sender should deal well the receipt of identical SACK. Figure 9 shows the test scenario for duplicate SACK.

```
        <header>
        src-addr=192.168.0.1
        dst-addr=192.168.0.2
        src-port=20
        syn-opt=mss(100),sack
        <content>
line 1  recv seq=3401 var-upd=no; ignore;
     2  send ack=any var-upd=no; send tcp seq=1 ack=3401 flag=(ack) sack=(3501-3601) win=16400 var-
        upd=no;
     3  send ack=any var-upd=no; send tcp seq=1 ack=3401 flag=(ack) sack=(3501-3701) win=16400 var-
        upd=no;
     :                                  :
    11  send ack=any var-upd=no; send tcp seq=1 ack=3401 flag=(ack) sack=(3501-4501) win=16400 var-
        upd=no;
    12  ; send tcp seq=1 ack=3401 flag=(ack) sack=(1001-1101,3501-4501) win=16400 var-upd=no;
    13  ; send tcp seq=1 ack=3401 flag=(ack) sack=(1101-1201,3501-4501) win=16400 var-upd=no;
     :                                  :
    22  ; send tcp seq=1 ack=3401 flag=(ack) sack=(2001-2101,3501-4501) win=16400 var-upd=no;
    23  send ack=any var-upd=no; send tcp seq=1 ack=3401 flag=(ack) sack=(3501-4601,2001,2101)
        win=16400 var-upd=no;
    24  send ack=any var-upd=no; send tcp seq=1 ack=3401 flag=(ack) sack=(3501-4701,2001,2101)
        win=16400 var-upd=no;
     :                                  :
    36  send ack=any var-upd=no; send tcp seq=1 ack=3401 flag=(ack) sack=(3501,5901,2001,2101)
        win=16400 var-upd=no;
        <end>
```

Figure 9. Test Scenario for Duplicate SACK.

The implementations other than Linux seem to inflate window when it receives duplicate or identical SACK. The behavior is not agreeable from the theory in the pipe algorithm. NetBSD decrements *pipe* value every time when it receives duplicate ACK without referring the values in SACK block by referring its source code. Solaris 2.6, Solaris 8 and Windows 98 seem to implement in the same way since the result in the communication log was the same. On the other hand, Linux did not inflate window to duplicate SACK. It maintains the bytes of unacknowledged segments instead of *pipe* value by referring the source code. The result for identical SACK was also the same as above.

5. CONCLUSION

In this paper, we described the design, implementation and experimental result of a TCP test system. The system is designed to reduce the burden of test operator by specifying only exceptional behaviors which the operator wishes to test in the test scenario among a complete communication. The system supports a variety of description of the test scenario. It provides three types of trigger events as the condition to cause the exceptional behavior, which are received packet, sending packet and timer expiration. The condition is described using parameters in the packet. As the action for an event, a packet with any parameter values can be produced. It is also possible not to send any packet for an action. The function above is useful for testing congestion control, which is one of the most important functions in TCP.

The scenario interpreter selects the action to each event by the condition described in the test scenario. If the condition is satisfied, the action described in the test scenario is executed. If not, the action is determined by the behavior of original TCP module.

The scenario interpreter and the log collector of the test system are implemented into the TCP module by modifying the module itself. It is implemented on NetBSD with SACK code developed by PSC. The test scenario is uploaded to the TCP module before it is executed. This implementation facilitates the combination of normal TCP behavior and scenario-oriented TCP behavior in a communication.

For the experimental usage of the system, we described the evaluation of SACK implementations on several operating systems. We selected test cases which can happen in actual environment. We found several facts and problems in SACK implementations in some operating systems. It is considered that the test system is effective on testing of TCP through this experiment.

This research is funded by TAO (Telecommunications Advancement Organization of Japan).

REFERENCES

[1] W. Stevens, "TCP/IP Illustrated, Vol. 1: The Protocols," Addison Wesley, 1994.
[2] V. Paxson, M. Allman, S.Dawson, W.Fenner, J. Griner, I. Heavens, K. Lahey, J. Semke and B. Volz, "Known TCP Implementation Problems," RFC 2525, Mar. 1999.
[3] S. Floyd and T. Henderson, "The NewReno Modification to TCP's Fast Recovery Algorithm," RFC2582, Apr. 1999.
[4] M. Mathis, J.Mahdavi, S.Floyd, and A. Romanow, "TCP Selective Acknowledgment Option," RFC 2018, Oct. 1996.
[5] S. Savage, N. Cardwell, D. Wetherall and T. Anderson, "TCP Congestion Control with a Misbehaving Receiver, " Proc. of SIGCOMM 1999, Aug. 1999.
[6] S. Parker and C. Schmechel, "Some Testing Tools for TCP Implementors," RFC 2398, Aug. 1998.
[7] V. Paxon, "Automated Packet Trace Analysis of TCP Implementations," in Proc. of SIGCOMM '97, Aug. 1997.
[8] T. Kato, T. Ogishi, A. Idoue and K. Suzuki, "Design of Protocol Monitor Emulating Behaviors of TCP/IP Protocols," in Proc. of IWTCS '97, Sep. 1997.
[9] J. Padhye and S. Floyd, "On Inferring TCP Behavior," in Proc. of SIGCOMM '2001, Aug. 2001.
[10] Fyodor, "Remote OS Detection via TCP/IP Stack Fingerprinting," http://www.insecure.org/nmap/nmap-fingerprinting-article.html, Dec. 1998.
[11] R. Gecse and P. Krémer, "Automated Test of TCP Congestion Control Algorithm," in Proc. of IWTCS '99, Sep. 1999.
[12] "OSI - Open System Interconnection, Conformance testing methodology and framework," ISO/IEC 9646, 1997
[13] M. Allman, V. Paxson and W. Stevens, "TCP Congestion Control," RFC 2581, Apr. 1999.
[14] "tcpdump/libpcap Homepage," http://www.tcpdump.org.
[15] "Pittsburgh Supercomputing Center (PSC) Homepage," http://www.psc.edu/networking/tcp.html
[16] G. Wright and W. Stevens, "TCP/IP Illustrated, Vol. 2: The Implementation," Addison Wesley, Jan. 1995.
[17] K. Fall and S. Floyd, "Simulation-based Comparisons of Tahoe, Reno, and SACK TCP," SIGCOMM CCR, Jul. 1996.
[18] S. Floyd, J. Mahdavi, M. Mathis and M. Podolsky, "An Extension to the Selective Acknowledgement (SACK) Option for TCP," RFC 2883, Jul. 2000.

VERIFYING IP METERS FROM SAMPLED MEASUREMENTS

Carlos Veciana-Nogués, Albert Cabellos-Aparicio, Jordi Domingo-Pascual, Josep Solé-Pareta
Centre de Comunicacions Avançades de Banda Ampla (CCABA)
Departament d'Arquitectura de Computadors
Universitat Politècnica de Catalunya (UPC)
Jordi Girona, 1-3, 08034 Barcelona, Catalunya (Spain)
Phone: + 34 934017182
Fax: + 34 934017055
{carlosv,acabello,jordid,pareta}@ac.upc.es

Abstract Traffic measurement and analysis is nowadays a very critical task and requires complex and high-cost traffic analysis equipment and infrastructure. The difficulty increases when high bandwidth connections are to be monitored. Network topology, the network technology used, applications and user behavior influence the overall traffic on the network. For network planning and provisioning is crucial to know the trends of the traffic behavior, that is why the analysis of protocol application is very useful. Most recent low-cost monitoring platforms for high-speed links rely on samples of the whole traffic. The purpose of the measurements range from monitoring and traffic characterization, to charging and billing. It is a must to know the statistical validity of the sampled data and the consequent detailed results obtained by classifying the traffic according to different categories. This fact is even more important when it is intended to be used for charging or cost sharing. In this paper we propose an approach to validate the statistical capture of our system. We compare full traffic measurements which contain all the traffic with sampled traffic measurements, in order to know what is the threshold of a sampled traffic to estimate the real traffic with a certain degree of confidence. Results are presented using traffic from a real network environment and comparing our capture platform results with results derived from the real traffic.

Key words: Passive IP traffic analysis, ATM, statistic validation

1. INTRODUCTION

New transmission technologies and new applications change the patterns of the traffic in the network. Moreover, new users with different profiles can change the patterns of the traffic. The knowledge of the Internet traffic characteristics is necessary to optimize resources, to plan the growth of the network, and to know the usage of the resources.

New trends in charging and billing proposals are based on traffic classification[1]. This classification could be made based on traffic volumes besides of the usage time or a fixed cost for renting links or access connections. The traffic classification for high-speed links is a high-cost and difficult management issue. The complexity of the traffic analysis for a network is related to the amount of traffic carried on, the topology of the network, the number of users, and the degree of detail desired to the reports.

Traffic characterization could be made at different levels. A first approach is to characterize the traffic based on network parameters (i.e. delay, losses, throughput, jitter, etc.) to study the network behavior. Another approach may characterize the traffic based on protocol parameters (i.e. number of flows, session duration, application types, etc.). Finally, any cross-related characterization or traffic analysis can be made based on any parameter at any level of the communication stack.

There are some projects working on IP traffic measurement on high-speed networks. CAIDA [2][3] consortium is making traffic analysis based on statistical measurements. SPRINT [4] labs makes traffic analysis based on the analysis of a complete (full) traffic capture during given periods. While the former can report very useful data about trends in the network behavior, the latter can report very detailed information about network parameters for a short period of time, including IP flows analysis and network QoS parameters across network nodes.

Several projects, CASTBA [5], MEHARI [6] and MIRA [7] projects, are our contribution to the traffic analysis in the Spanish NRN RedIRIS[8]. The main difference between our projects and the other traffic analysis initiatives has been the need of a full packet capture to perform traffic analysis at application header level. This means a lower capture ratio than if capturing only the IP and the TCP/UDP Transport headers.

We assume that the characteristics of the traffic change along the time, but they are more or less stable for short time periods (weeks or months) [5]. Our methodology consists on long-term traffic analysis based on samples using a low-cost hardware. The traffic is periodically validated with short-term full traffic analysis performed with high-cost equipment. As the load of the link under analysis increases, the sample corresponds to a smaller percentage of the total traffic. Then the main concern in this paper is how significant may be the conclusions derived from the sampled captures.

In the next Section we describe a generic architecture for the capture and analysis platform and our implemented system is presented. Section 3 describes the validation approach and Section 4 the application to the MIRA platform is presented. Section 5 discusses the results for MIRA analysis. Finally, Section 6 presents some conclusions and the ongoing work.

2. PLATFORM DESCRIPTION

A generic traffic analysis platform may be divided into two subsystems: the Traffic Capture Subsystem (TCS) and the Traffic Analysis Subsystem (TAS).

The TCS is a hardware platform that collects samples of the whole traffic in a high-speed link. The traffic capture is passive (usually with optical splitters), without interfering the performance of the network. Each packet of the network is labeled with a time stamp for further calculations and time estimations. The amount of traffic captured into each sample is bounded by the size of the buffers in the traffic capture equipment.

The Traffic Analysis Subsystem (TAS) is divided into several subsystems in order to improve the performance during the analysis (Figure 1). Some different modules may be defined in the TAS architecture: the preprocessing modules (PM), and the analysis modules (AM) -which can run in parallel on different machines-. The PM acts as a collector [9], reading all the samples, and extracting all the significant parameters of the traffic. This reduces the amount of data to be processed by the AM. The AM reorganize the data, add new attributes with queries to external databases, and producc reports about the captured traffic. The number of samples analyzed depends on the complexity and computation requirements of the PM and AM. An overflow control protocol is defined between PM and TCS to avoid data overflow. While PM is reading data, TCS is stopped and waits for a signal to continue capturing.

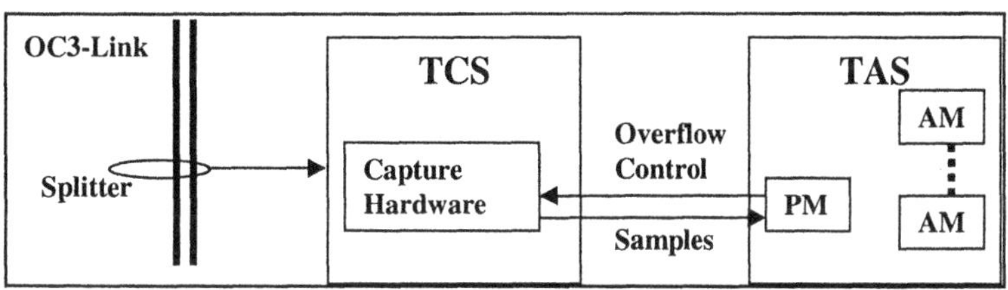

Figure1. Capture and Analysis Modular Architecture.

As it has been explained, the TCS provides the TAS with samples. Then, the confidence of the final reports depends on the percentage of the whole traffic that the traffic samples represent.

The Spanish National Research Network [8] backbone was designed as a star. The core was settled in Madrid. There are 17 links, each one connecting a Comunidad Autonoma[1] (CA) to the central interconnection point. In the early stage of our project, about 1997, the bandwidth assigned to our CA was 10/8Mbps (in/out). Input traffic means traffic coming from the central interconnection point to our CA, and the output traffic is the reverse one. This allowed us to capture between the 10% and the 20% of the whole traffic, fair enough to make estimations about the whole traffic with a great level of confidence. Nowadays, the bandwidth assigned to the Catalunya link is 155Mbps (in/out) with a mean load about 64Mbps, while the size of the TCS buffers is the same. The percentage of the traffic captured is clearly lower now. In the near future, the link will be upgraded to 622Mbps. This fact places a real challenge for our traffic analysis platform because as the percentage of captured traffic diminishes we must validate the confidence of the results derived from it. The current low-cost traffic capture platforms have known limitations for full traffic capture at speeds over 622Mbps. Then a validation of a sampling method is need for the future short-term.

Figure 2 shows the current deployment of analysis points in the Spanish NRN. In this paper, we focus on the study of the TCS in one CA, the one located in the UPC (CCABA analysis point).

The first TCS we used was the HP75000 Broadband Series Traffic Capture System (BSTS) [10]. This is a high cost ATM traffic analyser, which main purpose is to perform accurate ATM traffic analysis. Moreover, the BSTS can be configured to capture ATM cells at full link-speed. The capture is bounded by the size of the hardware buffers (131,072 ATM cells ≅7Mbytes). The ATM cells can be reassembled to obtain AAL5 frames and IP packets.

In 1998, a second capture platform was setup (MEHARI). It is a modification of the OC3MON [11] software for the PCA200 Fore ATM card adapter. The OC3MON traffic analysis platform relies on periodic IP flow records, while our modified software relies on periodic full IP packet samples. The TCS based on PC is 50 times cheaper compared to the BSTS. As shown in Figure 2, several analysis platforms are deployed in the NRN. The platform deployed in the MIRA project uses the same TCS and adds more complex AM.

[1] "Comunidad Autonoma" stands for state or political designed administrative country area.

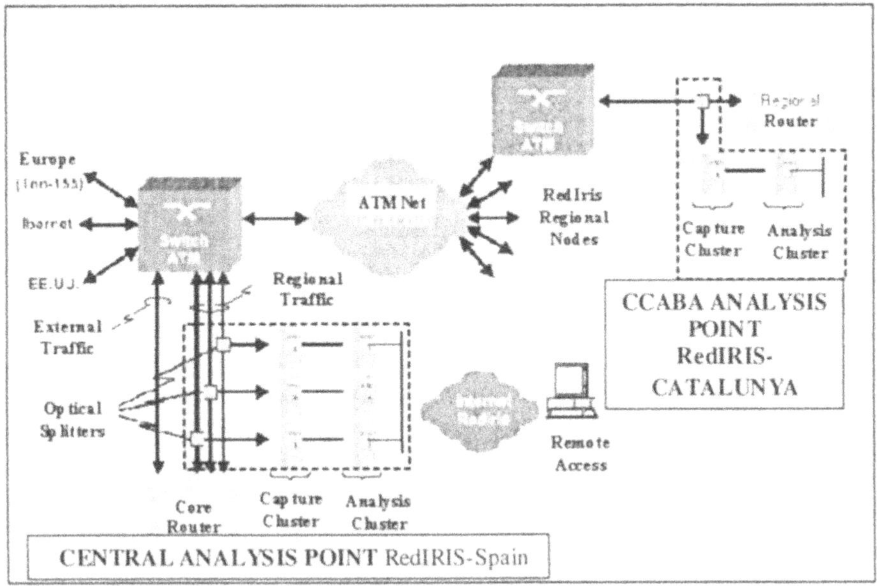

Figure 2. Traffic Capture And Analysis Points for CASTBA, MEHARI and MIRA projects

Now we are planing to use traffic capture specific cards like DAG cards [12]. While these cards are able to capture at full speed link at 155Mbps.

3. VALIDATION APPROACH FOR STATISTICAL TRAFFIC CAPTURE

The high cost of the BSTS equipment is justified, among other capabilities, for the ability to perform real-time traffic statistics at full link speed. The drawback is that the available real-time statistics are far from IP traffic parameters. But it is possible to account more IP parameters using pattern matching over ATM cells. A set of counters may be configured to perform bit pattern matching inside the ATM cells so that some IP and TCP/UDP header fields may be accounted during the capture.

There are some cases where a simple pattern matching over cells cannot find the desired data of the IP headers. When a packet contains options or an IP packet is fragmented, the transport protocol information (i.e. source and destination ports) are not detected. Nevertheless, the amount of those packets is small enough to be ignored in the study [3][5].

The validation approach takes as a reference a long period of capture using the BSTS and accounting several parameters. As this is a full traffic capture all comparisons are related to it. In order to validate different traffic capture and analysis platforms we model them and simulate their captures. It must be noticed that it is very difficult to obtain a full traffic capture and a statistical capture for a long period of time and have them synchronized in order to perform the same analysis. Moreover, the different capture platforms are not available at the same time. That is the main reason to use what we call the simulation approach.

Our Statistical Traffic Validation Platform (STVP) is based on real time traffic statistics measured with the BSTS and a sampler program that simulates the effect of other statistical TCS. This allows us to compare the differences of mean values of such parameters, comparing the full traffic mean to the simulated sampled mean of the same traffic. The BSTS average measurements are accounted every second, assuming no cell loss and a perfect clock (nanosecond precision).

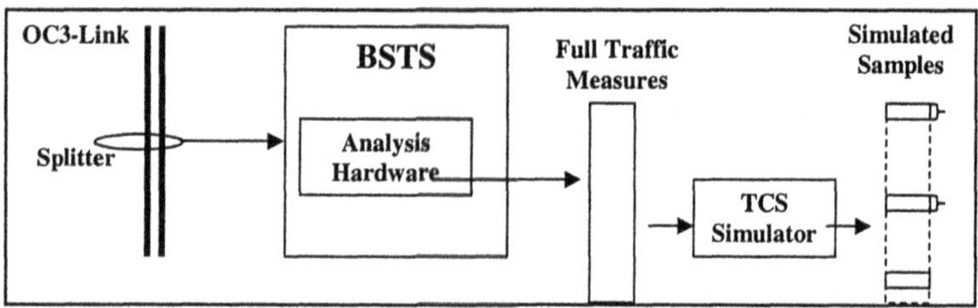

Figure3. Statistical traffic Validation Platform

The STVP simulator can be configured to produce samples of the whole traffic. The STVP can be configured to collect samples based on capture size of the capture buffers, and silence periods. The silence periods are related to the time required for dumping the buffers to the disk in the real TCS and for the preprocessing and analysis time between traffic captures. In particular, this is the model that fits our TCS. Other TCS where capture time does not depend on buffer size, but depends on time can be also simulated. In this case, the size of the capture is bounded by the capture time. This applies for all the systems that perform periodic sampling.

One important parameter is the integration period, that is the period of time that represents each sample. We defined an integration period higher than STVP Simulator sampling period for the mean calculation. Then, the mean of the full traffic measurements during such period, and the mean of the simulated samples during the same period, can be compared. We assume that the mean obtained with the BSTS is the real value of the traffic mean. Then, the statistical analysis via test for a zero mean for the difference of the means can be applied. Moreover, as we simulate the samples from a real trace, a Confidence Interval for the difference of paired observations can be used. A simple lineal regression (SLR), comparing both analysis methods, will give the measurement of the fairness of the statistic capture for any load of the link.

That is, while the confidence interval (C.I.) for the difference gives information about the statistic confidence about the sampling method, the SLR gives the same information but related to different loads of the link.

Figure 3 shows the architecture of the STVP. The BSTS collects real-time traffic parameters mean values. This is a continuous trace, one measurement per second. Then, a sampled trace based on configured TCS activity/silence periods and buffer size is given.

4. STATISTICAL TRAFFIC VALIDATION FOR MIRA PLATFORM

A long trace of real traffic has been obtained. The validation is performed considering two different cases. The first one takes into account the full traffic parameter estimation, and the second one is for classified traffic parameter estimation. The full traffic parameter validation includes the whole aggregated flows that compose the traffic. In our case of study they are the total number of bytes per second and packets per second. The classified traffic parameter validation stands for those parameters derived from some of the flows that compose the whole traffic. In our case, they are transport protocol packets per second (TCP and UDP), application protocol packets per second and network address packets per second. This latter validation is very important since it is very common to classify the traffic per flows, per protocol, per source or destination Autonomous System, per server, etc.

4.1 Description of the traffic traces

The full traffic trace[2] corresponds to the traffic in the CCABA (UPC) access point link during 37 days (from 20th July 2001 to 25th August 2001, 3196800 seconds) accounting cells per second, and AAL5 frames per second, in both directions (in/out). The number of cells multiplied by 53 (ATM bytes) is the value of IP bytes plus IP/ATM overhead. In [5][2] a study of the average IP/ATM overhead is about the 15%. However, all the ATM bytes can be considered for the study of an IP/ATM link. The average

[2] The traces from the real traffic which this paper is based, can be found at: http://www.ccaba.upc.es/projects/mira/E_mira_local.html

load of the link is 20,38Mbps/27,98Mbps (in/out). The number of AAL5 frames fits exactly the number of IP packets. This measurement is useful for the study of routing devices that are limited more by the number of packet routed than the size of those packets.

The second trace is also obtained from the same link, and at the same time that the first trace. The accounted parameters are based on bit pattern matching over ATM cells. Patterns that define some types of IP headers have been configured. This allows us to study the effect of traffic classification over sampled measurements. We would like to know the effect of sampling on the full traffic and on each class of traffic, in function of the percentage each class represents. The study of traffic classification is performed only for the number of packets, since real time statistics cannot provide byte counters per packet matched, only packet counters.

Tables 1,2 show the traces of real traffic used in the validation. Table 2 also shows the percentage of each class of traffic.

Table 1. Full traffic measurements

Full Traffic(3196800 s)	In	Out
GigaBytes	8147,23	11184,27
IP packets *10E6	14190,59	16767,21
Mean IP Packets per second	4439	5245
Mean bytes per second	2548558	3498583

Table 2. Classified Traffic measurements

Traffic class 362400s	InIP Packets	OutIP Packets
TCP	10926,66*10E6	14037,14*10E6
Mean	3418 pps	4391 pps
Percentage	76.99%	83.71%
UDP	364,43*10E6	620,17*10E6
Mean	114 pps	194 pps
Percentage	2.56%	3.69%
Big Network	786,41 *10E6	549,84*10E6
Mean	246 pps	172 pps
Percentage	5.54%	3.27%
Small Network	63,93*10E6	47,95*10E6
Mean	20 pps	15 pps
Percentage	0.45%	0.28%

The traffic classes shown in Table 2 are not intended to be exhaustive but an example of the validation. For each traffic class the total amount of packets, the mean number of packets per second and the percentage respect to the total traffic are given, both for input and output traffic. TCP and UDP classes deserve no more comments. The important fact to take into account is that as more detailed is the classification less traffic is captured and the measurements may not be significant enough. The row labeled "Big Network" corresponds to the input and output traffic for a medium-size University network provider identified by a range of IP addresses. This traffic class represents a classification per AS, per peer traffic, per entity, etc. Finally, the row labeled "Small Network" represents a small department inside one university.

4.2 TCS Simulation for MIRA

The TCS simulations are the result of different sampling schemes over the full traffic measurements. In fact, the different configurations of the STVP can produce the same results than other real TCS.

The BSTS reports real-time traffic statistics with a precision of one second. In the simulation, we model the real TCS considering that the traffic within a second is constant. Then, the proportional traffic to the capture time inside that second is calculated. The MIRA TCS reads 25 buffers of 1MB between preprocessing periods. This means an average capture time of 0.43 seconds at average link load. The traffic capture periods in MIRA simulation is configured based on buffer sizes. Then, the variable capture time is derived from the cell accounting in the BSTS trace, until the byte counter reaches 1MB. This short capture time means that most of the simulated samples are based on the proportional value of the average within a second. There is a silence time of about 1.25±0.25 seconds related to the dumping of each 1MB buffer to the disk. In addition, there is a preprocessing time of about 100±10 seconds between each batch of 25 files. A fixed time (90 seconds) is related to the sequential access to each packet of the file, and the variable time (20 seconds) is related to different analysis time depending on the complexity of the traffic captured. In summary, 25 buffers of 1 MB are captured every 2 minutes approximately.

5. RESULTS AND VALIDATION

This section shows the results of the comparison between the mean values obtained from BSTS trace (real traffic), and the mean values obtained from the simulated sampling process over the same trace. In order to have comparable mean values, both means are calculated over the same period. Then, we have paired observations obtained from two different sources, the real measurement and the sampled measurement. The difference of the mean is computed for each pair, then a 95% Confidence Interval is computed [13].

If the C.I. contains the zero value, there is no statistical difference for the mean value between the real measurement and the sampled measurement. We call it the test of zero.

Moreover, a Simple Lineal Regression (SLR) [13] study is applied in order to verify the confidence of the sampled model against the real samples for all traffic loads.

5.1 Full traffic parameter estimation

Table 3 shows the 95% C.I. for the test of zero under MIRA TCS conditions. The integration time for the mean calculation is 2 minutes, higher than MIRA TCS time between samples. The column labeled Sampled Mean gives the mean value to be compared with the error values. The C.I. does not contain the zero value for these conditions, but it is two orders of magnitude lower than the mean of packets and three orders of magnitude lower than the mean of bytes.

Table 3. 95% C.I. test of zero with 2 minutes integration period

Type	Sampled Mean	% Captured	C.I.
In IP packets/s	4476	14,59	36,041 ± 7,057
In Bytes/s	2561172	14,34	1910,173 ± 4238,463
Out IP packets/s	5298	8,17	0,387 ± 7,971
Out Bytes/s	3527468	8,15	2741,266 ± 4759,824

Table 4 shows the SLR analysis. The second column also shows the sampled measured mean value in order to have a reference for the errors. The third column shows the real percentage of traffic that has been captured in relation to the total traffic on the link. All straight lines are very close to the theoretic y=x (real average = sampled mean). In fact, there are small variations in the intercept and slope values compared to the mean values. Moreover, the intercept point represents a zero traffic load that almost never occurs. The slope is always below 1. This fact means that under these conditions the sampled measurement is always below the real value. The R^2 (Coefficient of determination) gives values above 90% in all cases. No differences are detected between in and out traffic, neither for packet average or bytes average comparison. Figure 4 shows an example for the UDP traffic, comparing the theoretic line x=y with the SLR analysis.

Table 4. SLR values for full traffic parameter estimation using with 2 minutes integration period

Type	Sampled Mean	% Captured	B0	B1	R^2
In IP packets/s	4476	14,59	288,902 ± 12,691	0,943 ± 0,002	94,25
In Bytes/s	2561172	14,34	73001,832 ± 5530,704	0,975 ± 0,001	97,61
Out IP packets/s	5298	8,17	447,699 ± 16,557	0,924 ± 0,002	92,35
Out Bytes/s	3527468	8,15	389608,597 ± 11263,180	0,896 ± 0,003	91,24

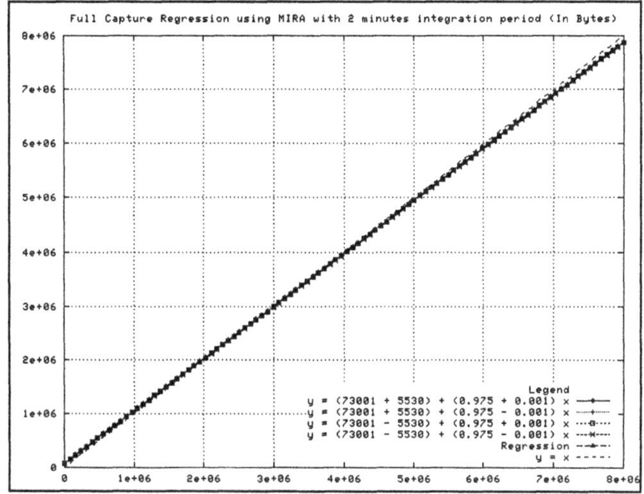

Figure 4. SLR Straight lines for Input traffic in bytes, with two minures integration period.

Table 5 shows the results of the C.I for the test of zero, with an integration period of one hour. In fact, this is the integration period used in the MIRA traffic estimation in the current version. Now, the order of magnitude of this parameter is always two orders of magnitude lower than the mean average for the packets and three orders of magnitude lower for the bytes.

Table 5. 95% C.I. test of zero with an hour integration period

Type	Sampled Mean	% Captured	C.I.
In IP packets/s	4361	14,59	-78,208 ± 13,536
In Bytes/s	2460101	14,34	-4145,024 ± 9192,585
Out IP packets/s	5182	8,17	0,01 ± 13,898
Out Bytes/s	3448180	8,15	3359,193 ± 6717,909

Table 6 shows the results of the SLR values for an integration period of one hour. It can be noticed that the increase of the integration period improves the validity of the b0, b1 and R2 values. Now, all R^2 values are better than 99. However, the slope values are still below one.

Table 6. SLR values for full traffic parameter estimation with an hour integration period

Type	Sampled Mean	% Captured	B0	B1	R^2
In IP packets/s	4361	14,59	-14,968 ± 25,655	0,985 ± 0,005	99,23
In Bytes/s	2460101	14,34	-53871,675 ± 12011,120	0,986 ± 0,003	99,62
Out IP packets/s	5182	8,17	19,850 ± 32,258	0,984 ± 0,005	99,06
Out Bytes/s	3448180	8,15	-27710,349 ± 17412,907	0,993 ± 0,004	99,38

Table 7 and 8 shows the test of zero and SLR values for full traffic parameter estimation with 15 minutes integration period. This table has been obtained in order to compare MIRA TCS with most SNMP systems, which usually report counters every 15 minutes.

The 15 minutes integration time gives C.I. with an error similar than one hour integration time, but containing zero in most cases (except for the In IP packets). For the SLR analysis, the R^2 values are always better than 98%. Moreover, the slope values contain the zero slope and the intercept point is clearly better than 2 minutes integration time case.

Table 7. 95% C.I. test of zero with 15 minutes integration period

Type	Sampled Mean	% Captured	C.I
In IP packets/s	4413	14,59	-26,29 ± 8,563
In Bytes/s	2509503	14,34	-1393,37 ± 5152,554
Out IP packets/s	5224	8,17	0,111 ± 7,742
Out Bytes/s	3477118	8,15	-1170,346 ± 3963,711

Table 8. SLR values for full traffic parameter estimation with 15 minutes integration period

Type	Sampled Mean	% Captured	B0	B1	R^2
In IP packets/s	4413	14,59	108,673 ± 15,463	0,9696 ± 0,003	98,86
In Bytes/s	2509603	14,34	-199,723 ± 6662,097	0,984 ± 0,002	99,53
Out IP packets/s	5224	8,17	110,319 ± 16,771	0,974 ± 0,002	98,98
Out Bytes/s	3477118	8,15	69972,113 ± 9692,829	0,973 ± 0,002	99,2

5.2 Traffic Classification

In this section, we want to analyze the effect of the sampling over meters that account more specific traffic characteristics.

For the classified traffic traces (Table 2), a 95% C.I. and a test of zero has been made, under the same conditions explained in section 5.1. The traffic classifications proposed in this section are only examples.

The SLR values have the same characteristics as the values for full traffic. We only present the C.I. for one hour (Table 9) and 15 minutes (Table 10) integration periods, in order to reduce the data.

Table 9 shows the mean comparison analysis over the real trace and the sampled trace for the MIRA TCS. All straight lines are also very near the theoretic y=x. Figure 5 shows the regression lines with confidence interval for the class with less traffic (Small Network). Also in this case, a value of R^2 about 99%, and the slope value contains the 1 value (Figure 5).

Once again, confidence interval for the mean is two orders of magnitude smaller compared to mean values.

Table 9. 95% C.I. test of zero with 1 hour integration period

Type	Sampled Average	C.I for the average of the errors
In TCP packets/s	3364	53,85 ± 8,708
In UDP packets/s	111	3,698 ± 5,372
In Big Network packets/s	242	4,81 ± 1,137
In Small Network packets/s	19	-0,382 ± 0,167
Out TCP packets/s	4350	-40,964 ± 9,971
Out UDP packets/s	186	-7,957 ± 4,646
Out Big Network packets/s	170	-2,39 ± 1,168
Out Small Network packets/s	15	0,01 ± 0,097

Table 10. 95% C.I. test of zero with 15 minutes integration period

Type	Sampled Average	C.I for the average of the errors
In TCP packets/s	3402	-17,038 ± 5,643
In UDP packets/s	112	-2,189 ± 3,065
In Big Network packets/s	246	-0,972 ± 0,967
In Small Network packets/s	20	-0,153 ± 0,134
Out TCP packets/s	4379	-12,452 ± 5,187
Out UDP packets/s	190	-4,033 ± 3,187
Out Big Network packets/s	171	-0,92 ± 0,982
Out Small Network packets/s	15	0,111 ± 0,088

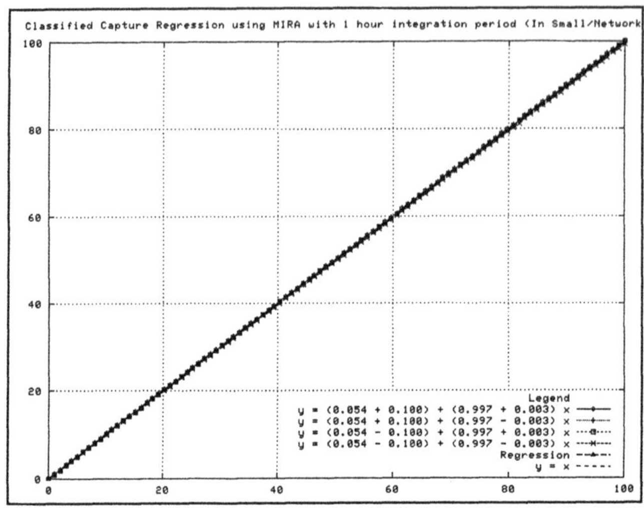

Figure 5. SLR Straight lines for MIRA UDP classified traffic, with two minutes integration period.

5.3 MIRA traffic classification validation

Some of the traffic classifications proposed in the MIRA project fit into the examples of traffic classification shown in this paper. Then, they may be useful for charging or cost sharing under great level of confidence. Some sampling-based analysis tools, that currently report trends about Internet traffic, could be used for charging and network provisioning if a confidence interval for the measurements is given. Also, some commercial charging methods like UUNet "Burstable and Metered"[14], can be improved with more detailed traffic classifications for charging. The MIRA project proposes several traffic classifications over sampled traffic.

1. Network Address: classifies the traffic based on source and destination address, accounting bytes and packets per AS, Network, and Host.
2. Application port: classifies the traffic based on source and destination port, extracting the information from the IP header and accounting bytes and packets per application (group of ports).
3. Application protocol: classifies the traffic based on application protocol analysis, extracting the information from the IP payload, and accounting bytes and packets per application.
4. Payload pattern matching: classifies the traffic based on application payload, and accounting bytes and packets.

The third and fourth classifications, cannot be verified with our method because it is not possible to perform such complex analysis with our real time traffic analyzer. However, we are working on some alternatives which allow real-time accounting via a smarter method than simple pattern matching over IP headers, using specialized hardware [12].

The Network Address classification seems to be unaltered by the sampling method, like we saw in the section 5.2, but a further study is needed for more complex and different size aggregations. In our example, also very small networks, with few packet per second means, can be estimated with good C.I. Other address aggregations like Autonomous Systems or singular networks are under study.

The Application Port classification is under study. Some preliminary results show that HTTP traffic sampled means seem to be unaltered by the sampling process. Since the HTTP traffic is usually 80% of the whole traffic, its behavior is usually the same as the whole traffic.

Most traffic classes in MIRA traffic classification are over 5% of the total traffic. Then, the traffic estimation from sampled averages seems correct, whenever low traffic classes compounds will be like full traffic.

6. CONCLUSIONS AND ONGOING WORK

Statistical capture subsystems are good for real traffic estimations under some conditions. In this paper we present an approach to validate the accuracy of the sampling methods, and to determine the significance of the results derived from the traffic analysis. The Statistical Traffic Validation Platform (STVP) is a simple method that allows the simulation of the behavior of some Traffic Capture Subsystems (TCS). It must be noted that it is required a traffic capture equipment able process or store all the traffic at line speed, since this is the reference trace for the validations. But, once the cheap TCS platform has been validated for the classes of traffic under study, the expensive equipment is not needed any more. Then, the deployment of many non-expensive TCS may provide a very good knowledge about the trends of the traffic in the network. Finally, these TCS may be used to collect significant information to be used for approximated billing or cost sharing.

The statistical analysis via confidence interval for the difference of the means, even though does not fulfil the zero test, gives an error values two orders of magnitude lower than mean values. This seems a good approximation, taking into account the simplicity of the hardware equipment and accounting process.

Our preliminary results show that very low capture ratios (lower than 1% for some traffic classifications like small networks) can produce approximations of average measurements with an error lower than two orders of magnitude compared to mean values.

The current work consist on a systematic verification of different traffic classifications, specially those based on address aggregations (Autonomous Systems, Networks and subnetworks), since the classification by application seems to be difficult for new peer-to-peer applications, web based services and encrypted services.

ACKNOWLEDGEMENTS

This work is funded by the CICYT (Spanish Education Ministry), under contract 2FD97-2234-C03-02. Some of the ideas of this work came from the participation on the MIRA project, together with UPM, UC3M, Telefónica I+D, and RedIRIS.

REFERENCES

[1] A.M. Odlyzko, "The history of communications and its implications for the Internet". http://www.research.att.com/~amo/doc/history.communications0.ps. June 2000
[2] J. Aspirdof et al., "OC3MON: Flexible, Affordable, High Performance Statistics Collection", INET'97, Malasya, June 1997.
[3] C. McCreary and KC Claffy, "Trends in Wide Area IP Traffic Patterns: A View from Ames Internet eXchange". In Proc. of 13th ITC Specialist Seminar: IP Traffic Measurement, Modeling and Management. Monterey, USA, September 18-20,2000.
[4] C. Fraleigh, S. Moon, C. Diot, B. Lyles, F. Tobagi. "Architecture of a Passive Monitoring System for Backbone IP Networks". Sprint technical report TR-00-ATL-101801. October.2000.
[5] M.Alvarez et al., "CASTBA: Internet Traffic Measurements over the Spanish R&D ATM Network", HP-OVUA Workshop, Rennes (France), April 1998.
[6] P. Lizcano et al., "MEHARI: A System for Analyzing the Use of the Internet Services", Computer Networks 31 (1999), pp. 2293-2307.
[7] C Veciana-Nogués, J. Domingo-Pascual and J. Solé-Pareta, "Server Location & Verification Tool for Backbone Access Points" In Proc. of 13th ITC Specialist Seminar: IP Traffic Measurement, Modeling and Management. Monterey, USA, September 18-20,2000.
[8] http://www.rediris.es
[9] Nevil Brownlee et al. "Traffic flow measurement: Architecture" RFC 2063, January 1997.
[10] HP75000 BSTS http://advanced.comms.agilent.com/bsts/datasheets/e4200b.htm
[11] http://www.c aida.org/tools/measurement/coralreef/
[12] http://dag.cs.waikato.ac.nz
[13] Raj Jain, "The art of computer systems performance analysis: techniques for experimental design, measurement, simulation, and modeling". Wiley professional Computing, 1991, ISBN 0-417-50336-3
[14] http://www.uunet.com/products/uudirect/uudirect

TESTING IP DIFFERENTIATED SERVICES IMPLEMENTATIONS

Carlos Parada, Jorge Carapinha, Francisco Fontes, Solange Lima and Paulo Carvalho

{carlos-f-parada, jorgec, fontes}@ptinovacao.pt, Portugal Telecom INovação, S.A., 3810-106 Aveiro, Portugal {solange, paulo}@uminho.pt, Departamento de Informática, Universidade do Minho, 4710-059 Braga, Portugal

Abstract Diffserv architecture is pointed out as a promising solution for the provision of QoS in the Internet in a scalable manner. The main objective of this work is to test, evaluate and discuss, from a practical point of view, two platforms for implementing Diffserv services: one developed at ICA/EPFL for the Linux OS and the other based on Cisco Systems routers. After comparing the configuration strategy in each platform, QoS related functionalities (e.g. classification, marking, policing, shaping) are tested and assessed. In particular, the implementation of EF and AF PHBs is analysed. The capacity of providing bandwidth guarantees and performing adequate traffic conditioning is evaluated as well as the impact background traffic has on delaying high priority traffic. Moreover, the computational effort Diffserv puts on routers is also measured in terms of CPU utilisation.

Keywords: QoS, Diffserv, PHB, Expedited Forwarding (EF), Assured Forwarding (AF), Best Effort (BE), Traffic Conditioning, Performance Testing.

1. INTRODUCTION

The Differentiated Services (Diffserv) architecture is considered a promising solution to implement Quality of Service (QoS) in the Internet in a scalable manner [1]. Bringing the network complexity to edge routers, it aims to keep the core network simple. In opposition to Integrated Services (*IntServ*) architecture [2], Diffserv does not require per-flow state and signalling at every hop [3]. Instead of dealing with individual flows, traffic is aggregated in a limited number of classes of service (CoS) according to its QoS requirements. Traffic belonging to each class is forwarded in each node according to a defined Per Hop Behaviour (PHB). The Internet Engineering Task Force has defined two PHB. The Expedited Forwarding (EF) PHB is intended to offer a low delay, low jitter, low loss and assured bandwidth service [4]. The Assured Forwarding (AF) PHB is intended to offer a group of four service classes with a certain assigned level of forwarding resources (buffers and bandwidth), and three drop precedence (DP) per class, assuring to each class a minimum bandwidth [5]. In a Diffserv network, services are provided using traffic classification and traffic conditioning (TC) at network edges coupled with the concatenation of PHBs along the transit path [1].

Diffserv routers are expected to perform different functions (not mutually exclusive) depending on their network or domain location herein called edge and core components. Edge components are located at DS domain boundaries and their main functions are classification and TC based on a set of pre-defined rules. The enforcement of TC is fundamental so that a Service Level Agreement may be established either between a customer and a DS domain or DS domains. Core components are located inside a DS domain and their main functions are classification of traffic aggregates and queuing.

The main objective of this work is to test, evaluate and discuss, from a practical point of view, two platforms for implementing Diffserv services: one developed at ICA/EPFL (*The Institute for Computer Communications and Applications / École Polytechnique Fédérale de Lausanne*) for the Linux OS [6] and the other based on Cisco Systems routers running IOS versions *12.1(1)T* and *12.1(3)T*. Although other Diffserv implementations exist [7, 8], the two chosen are widely used. While ICA/EPFL implementation is publicly available and open, Cisco equipment was already part of our network test infrastructure. The Linux testbed, involving edge and core routers, interconnects two networks geographically located at Portugal *Telecom Inovação* (PTIN) and *Instituto de Telecomunicações* (IT) in Aveiro city. The Cisco testbed is located at PTIN.

For a wide variety of test scenarios, this study analyses how differentiated services may be configured in both platforms, discussing their underlying functionalities. Edge and core components are assessed attending to their expected behaviour. The implementation of PHBs and DPs is appraised regarding bandwidth allocation and achieved throughput. On Cisco testbed, the impact of different background traffic on high priority classes is also measured in terms of delay. The impact on router performance is also measured in terms of CPU utilisation.

Recent studies [9,10] focused on particular aspects of this study. However, in our opinion, the wide variety of tests carried out identifying the main strengths, weaknesses and problems of the two platforms are an additional contribution to the field.

After a brief introduction, a summary of Diffserv functionalities under evaluation is presented in section 2. How these functions are supported in Linux and Cisco IOS is described in sections 3 and 4, respectively. The complete set of experiments and results are presented and discussed in section 5 and 6 for Linux and Cisco IOS testbeds, respectively. The main conclusions are reported in section 7.

2. EVALUATED DIFFSERV FUNCTIONALITIES

Diffserv functionalities can be divided in edge and core components. A brief description of their objectives is highlighted below before discussing their implementation on ICA/EPFL and Cisco IOS platforms.

2.1 Edge Component

An edge component may encompass the following functions: *Classification* selects packets based either on one or more header fields (Multi-Field/MF Classification) or on the DS CodePoint (DSCP) (Behaviour Aggregate/BA Classification). While the former is usually applied to individual flows, the latter is applied to traffic aggregates already marked. *Marking* sets the DS field to a particular DSCP [3] so that a particular PHB can be applied to them. *Metering* measures the temporal properties of traffic previously classified. This information, verified against the traffic profile specified in the Traffic Conditioning Agreement, is used by other TC functions to trigger according actions to packets in or out-of-profile. *Policing* enforces a specified traffic profile preventing non-conformant traffic from entering the network by dropping or remarking it with lower priority. *Shaping* regulates traffic submitted to the network by adjusting traffic characteristics to a defined profile. The Token Bucket (TB), Leaky Bucket (LB) or combinations thereof are common algorithms used for shaping.

2.2 Core Component

A core component may encompass the following functions: Classification selects traffic based on a single header field - the DSCP- (BA Classification). Queuing is essential to implement differentiation. Apart from FIFO, which per si is not oriented to packet differentiation, Priority Queuing (PQ) and Fair Queuing (FQ) are possible approaches to implement QoS-aware queuing. PQ implements a strict priority among existing queues. This means that while a high priority queue has traffic to be scheduled, low priority traffic will not be served. Although this mechanism may be particularly convenient to implement EF PHB, it may lead to traffic starvation. FQ aims to solve PQ limitations by controlling the bandwidth allocated to each class. Variants of this algorithm have been used to implement at the same time the EF and the AF PHBs. Congestion Avoidance prevents queue congestion by discarding packets according to a particular criterion. Initially proposed by Jacobson and Floyd [11], Random Early Detection (RED) algorithm is a reference in this context. RED parameters include a minimum and a maximum threshold (Min, Max), and a drop probability (DP) for Max (see Figure 3). RED variants have been developed such as WRED, GRED or RIO to deal with multiple AF DPs.

3. LINUX PLATFORM

The Linux implementation under study was developed at ICA/EPFL [6]. In order to establish a Diffserv network, the configuration strategy lays in the definition of a certain number of nested functions. This is achieved using mainly the *tc* tool. *ip*, *route* or *ipchains* can also be used. Three entities can be configured with *tc*: *nodes* (have a queuing discipline - *qdisc* - associated with them), *filters* (classifiers), and *classes*.

3.1 Edge Component

At the edge level, the main implemented functionalities are as follows: *Classification MF/BA* and *Marking* are achieved using *qdisc* DSMARK, being created as many classes as the number of existing CoS. *Policing* is also implemented using *qdisc* DSMARK. It is possible to define *Dropping* or *Remarking* of out-of-profile packets. *Shaping* is implemented using *qdisc* Token Bucket Filter (TBF), which follows a Token Bucket algorithm.

3.2 Core Component

At the core level, the main implemented functionalities are as follows: *Classification BA* is configured at the nodes level, using DSCP *filters*, based on the *tcindex* classifier. *Queuing* is configured mainly using *qdisc* Class-Based Queuing (CBQ). Although there are other *qdiscs* available (apart from FIFO), common policies may coexist in the same CBQ, for instance strict priority, proportional bandwidth sharing, guaranteed bandwidth, or traffic isolation. *Congestion Avoidance* is implemented resorting to *qdisc* RED and Generalised RED (GRED). The first one is an implementation of a RED-based algorithm, while the second one allows defining *n* simple REDs.

4. CISCO PLATFORM

The Cisco platform is configured through the usual Command Line Interface (CLI). Setting up DS services in this system is far simpler than in Linux, however, it is less flexible than the latter since nesting functionalities are not allowed. Individual mechanisms can be configured separately.

4.1 Edge Component

At the edge level, the main implemented functionalities are as follows: *Classification MF/BA* and *Marking*, such as in Linux, are not carried out separately. Cisco implementation uses Policy-Based Routing (PBR), which allows the classification of packets based on multiple fields. *Policing* is based on Committed Access Rate (CAR). Traffic exceeding CAR can be either dropped or remarked. *Shaping* is a functionality implemented through Generic Traffic Shaping (GTS). GTS follows the TB algorithm.

4.2 Core Component

At the core level, the main implemented functionalities are as follows: *Classification BA* is a function embedded in the queuing functions. *Queuing* includes three algorithms in addition to FIFO: PQ implementing a strict priority scheme; Custom Queuing (CQ) allowing a percentage bandwidth allocation scheme; Class-Based Weighted Fair Queuing (CB-WFQ) where a minimum guaranteed bandwidth can be defined for each class (useful to implement AF classes), being the remaining bandwidth divided proportionally to the reserved bandwidth. A high priority class can also be defined, having strict priority. *Congestion Avoidance* mechanisms are implemented through Weighted RED (WRED), which uses multiple drop probability profiles.

5. TESTING LINUX PLATFORM

In this section, the Linux differentiated services implementation is configured, tested and evaluated.

5.1 Traffic Related Tools and Equipment

Two traffic generation tools are used in the experiments: *mgen* for UDP traffic and *netperf* for TCP. While in *mgen* the volume of generated traffic needs to be specified, in *netperf* traffic is generated according to TCP ability to adapt to network load conditions. Traffic analysis is carried out resorting to the *tcpdump* tool and *PrismLite / RADCOM* equipment. While *tcpdump* is used for simple bandwidth measurements and debugging, and *PrismLite / RADCOM* allows more elaborated numerical and statistical analysis.

The main testbed equipment consists of routers and end systems running *Linux RedHat 6.X* and *Mandrake 7.X*. The *tc* version used in these tests is the one included in the *iproute2-000503* with the patch *ds-8* for *iproute2,* using the *kernel 2.3.40.*

5.2 Linux Testbed

The test platform running Diffserv over Linux is illustrated in Figure 1. The clouds represent the DS networks located at PTIN and at IT, respectively. The network layout consists of two Linux systems, a traffic sender and a receiver, and three Linux routers. These routers (two edge, one core) form a single DS domain.

All nodes are connected using Ethernet at 10Mbps, except the core router at PTIN and the edge router at IT, which use an ATM CBR connection, running classical IP over ATM. The ATM connection allows limiting the peak rate to a pre-defined value. This option is taken in most of the experiments in order to force a backbone bottleneck. In this way, a certain congestion level can be easily forced and managed. *PrismLite/RADCOM* measurements were carried out at core router outgoing ATM link.

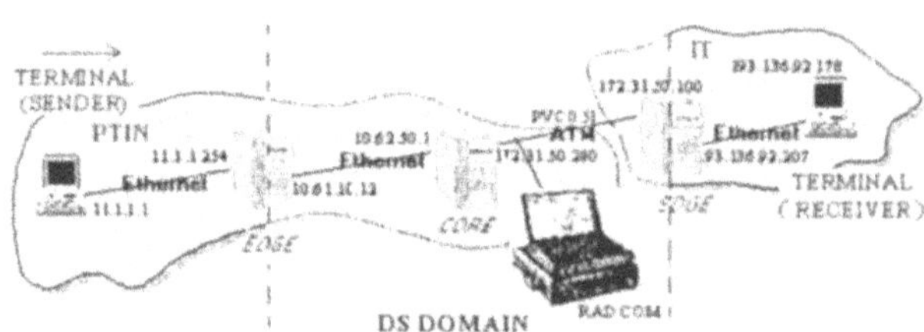

Figure 1. Testbed used in Linux tests.

5.2.1 Testing Edge Functionalities

The objective of this set of experiments is to assess the effectiveness of TC actions. *mgen* and *tcpdump* are used as traffic generator and traffic analyser respectively. Test scenarios for different traffic rates, packet sizes, source/destination address and ports are considered. Table 1 summarises the results obtained.

Table 1. Summary of the Linux test results (edge)

TEST	OBJECTIVE	RESULTS
Marking (DSMARK)	Check if all packets are correctly marked based on the traffic characteristics	The Marking is correct for all different traffic scenarios
Policing with Dropping (DSMARK drop)	Check if packets are policed and dropped (if needed) correctly	Inconclusive results (discussed below)
Policing with Remarking (DSMARK remark)	Check if packets are policed and remarked (if needed) correctly	Inconsistent behaviour (discussed below)
Shaping (TBF)	Check Traffic Shaping	Behaviour generally correct. The shaped rate was correct but the inter-packet time varied from about 1 to 15ms (discussed below)

In *Policing with Dropping*, after a large number of measurements, no packet drops were registered. The reason for this behaviour may be explained by the DS software version in use.

In *Policing with Remarking*, after exhaustive tests it was verified that *Policing* was accomplished correctly for rates up to 800Kbps. For upper rates, the behaviour is equal as if 800Kbps was defined. The reason for this is the low precision of the Linux system timer, which is unable to handle small time intervals. This also explains the large inter-packet time variation that occurs in *Shaping*. This behaviour has also been noticed and conveniently explained in [12].

5.2.2 Testing PHBs

This section covers an important set of experiments whose objective is to evaluate the traffic forwarding behaviour in the core router, assessing whether traffic is being differentiated as expected or not. The measurements focus on EF, AF and BE PHBs in terms of allocated and used bandwidth, in the presence of UDP and TCP traffic. CBQ is the Linux *qdisc* in use. Bandwidth in the ATM link was limited to 4Mbps and 6Mbps (approximately 3.7 and 5.5Mbps at IP level) depending of the test. Other test parameters are as follows: EF peak rate of 1Mbps; AF1x and AF4x minimum guaranteed rate of 1Mbps and 1.5Mbps, respectively.

PHBs testing results are similar for UDP (Figure 2-a) and 2-b)) and TCP traffic (2-c) and d)). Figure 2-a) and c) represent EF and BE achieved throughput, while b) and d) represent EF, AF11, AF41 and BE throughput, over a time period of one minute. The different traffic is launched along this period. In the TCP test, one connection is used for each PHB.

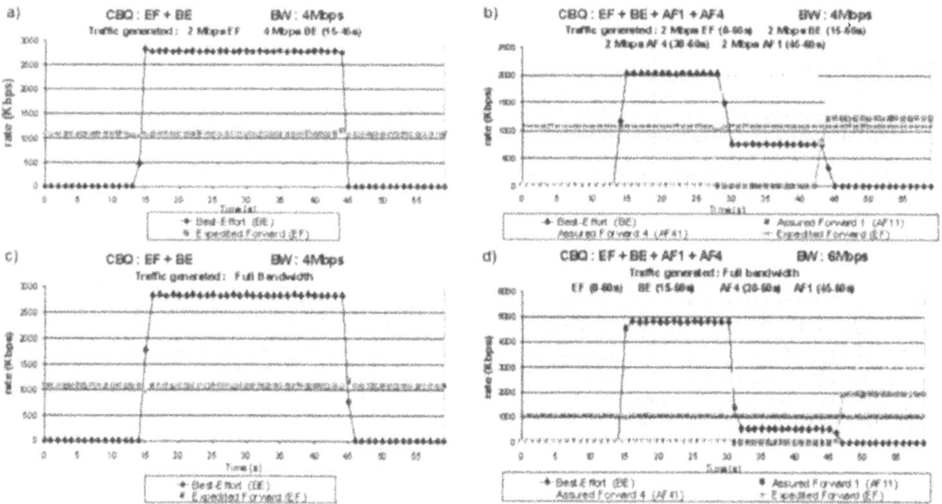

Figure 2. Throughput per PHB for UDP and TCP traffic (UDP – a) and b); TCP – c) and d)).

Figure 2 shows that EF traffic is clearly isolated from other traffic, i.e. both BE and AF packets do not interfere with EF (although a slight variation may occur when other traffic is injected in the network). Thus, EF throughput is independent of the remaining traffic and the allocated rate is guaranteed for traffic in-profile, i.e. above 1Mbps packets are dropped. For AF traffic, the minimum allocated bandwidth is also guaranteed. The remaining bandwidth (from 1Mbps to 1.5Mbps) is shared (not evenly) among the existing classes. As expected, BE traffic only gets through when high priority traffic does not take the maximum available bandwidth.

5.2.3 Testing Drop Precedence

This section focuses on how a class with different drop precedence is affected by congestion and by a particular congestion control mechanism – GRED. A single AF1x class with three DP is considered (both for UDP and TCP traffic). GRED parameters in use are illustrated in Figure 3.

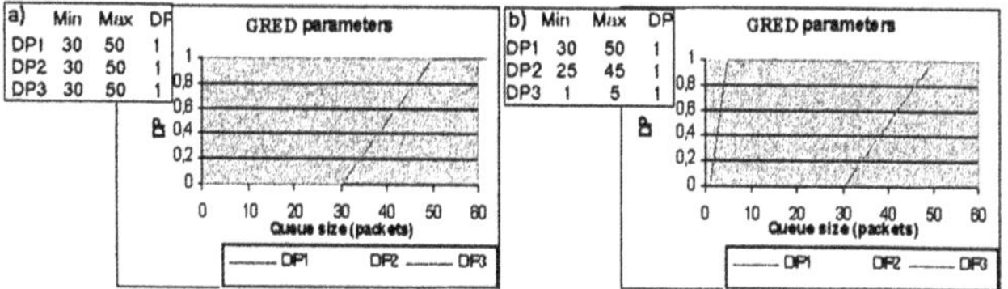

Figure 3. GRED parameters.

The ATM connection bandwidth was set to 2Mbps (about 1.8Mbps at IP level). The results for UDP and TCP traffic are shown below.

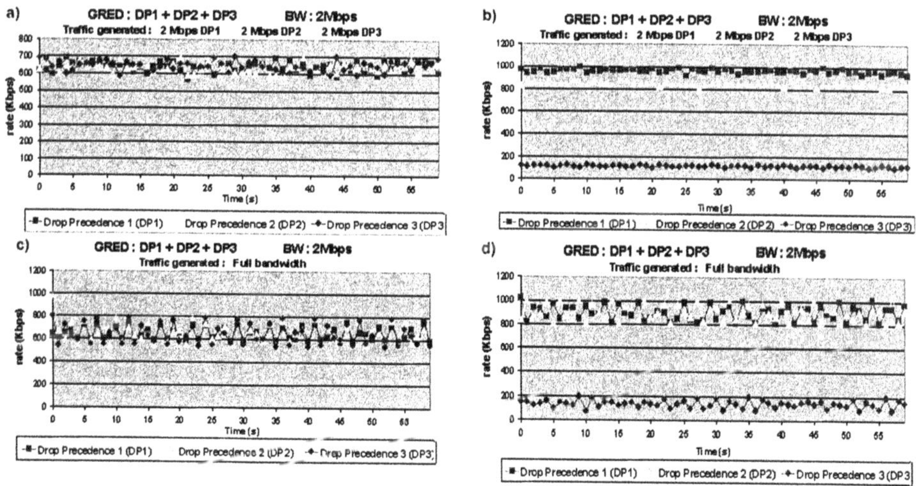

Figure 4. Throughput for the AF1x class (UDP – a) and b); TCP – c) and d)).

Figure 4 shows that, for equal GRED parameters, each AF1x receives identical treatment regarding throughput and packet loss. For different GRED parameters (*Min* and *Max*), AF1x behaviour evolves consistently, for instance, traffic with higher DP is drastically dropped and AF13 gets the smaller bandwidth share. Finally, AF1x throughput for TCP traffic shows more variability than the UDP traffic as consequence of TCP slow-start.

5.3 Linux Tests Summary

Positive aspects:

- great flexibility in the configuration of Diffserv mechanisms due to the capacity of nesting functionalities;
- number of Diffserv functionalities implemented;
- Marking and Shaping work correctly;
- easy to implement standard PHBs with the existing Queuing and Congestion Avoidance mechanisms;
- good performance both for UDP and TCP traffic.

Negative aspects:

- complexity and size of the configuration scripts;
- lack of documentation;
- problems with Policing (Dropping/Remarking) and Shaping (jitter).

6. TESTING CISCO IOS PLATFORM

In this section, the Cisco IOS differentiated services implementation is configured, tested and evaluated.

6.1 Traffic Related Tools and Equipment

The traffic generation tools used in the experiments are *mgen* for UDP traffic and *netperf* for TCP. Traffic analysis is carried out using *tcpdump* and *PrismLite / RADCOM. SmartBits* equipment is used for delay analysis (it solves clock synchronisation problem). The main testbed equipment consists of one *Cisco 7200* with *IOS 12.1(3)T*, one *Cisco 7500* with *IOS 12.1(1)T*, routers and end-systems running *Linux RedHat 6.X* and *Mandrake 7.X.*

6.2 Cisco Testbed

The test platform using Cisco routers is illustrated in Figure 5.

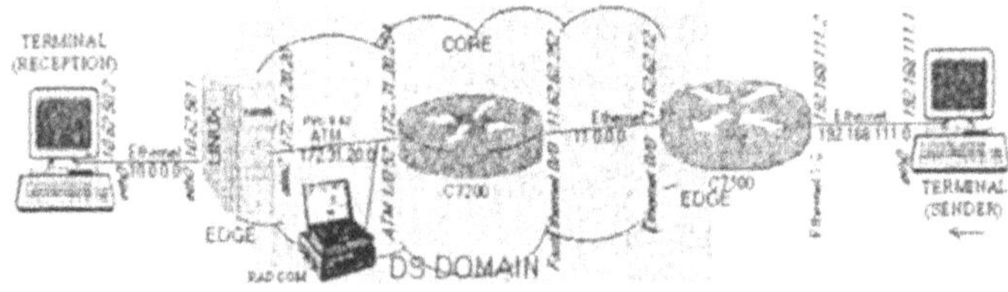

Figure 5. Testbed used in Cisco tests.

All nodes (located at PTIN headquarters) are connected using Ethernet at 10Mbps, except the core and Linux router, which use an ATM nrt-VBR connection with classical IP over ATM. Such as in Linux, this connection allows forcing a bandwidth bottleneck in the routers. *PrismLite / RADCOM* measurements were carried out at core router ATM outgoing link. Due to the lack of support for the DSCP field in the used IOS versions we have used the *precedence* field (this problem was solved in IOS 12.1(5)T).

6.2.1 Testing Edge Functionalities

Following the sort of experiments reported for Linux, this set of tests assesses the effectiveness of TC actions such as Marking, Policing and Shaping. As in Linux, *mgen* and *tcpdump* are used as traffic generator and traffic analyser, respectively. Table 2 summarises the results obtained.

Table 2. Summary of the Cisco test results (edge)

TEST	OBJECTIVE	RESULTS
Marking (PBR)	Check if all packets are correctly marked based on the traffic characteristics	Marking correct for different source rates, traffic types and packet lengths
Policing with Dropping (CAR drop)	Check if packets are policed and dropped (if needed) correctly	Policing / Dropping correct for different source rates, traffic types and packet lengths
Policing with remarking (CAR remark)	Check if packets are policed and remarked (if needed) correctly	Policing / Remarking correct for different source rates, traffic types and packet lengths
Shaping (GTS)	Check Traffic Shaping	Shaping correct for different traffic types and bucket sizes. Both rate and inter-packet time are shaped correctly

6.2.2 Testing PHBs

Our objective is to assess how EF, AF and BE PHBs perform on Cisco equipment regarding the allocated and used bandwidth, with either UDP or TCP traffic. The ATM connection bandwidth was set to 5Mbps, EF peak rate to 1Mbps, AF1 and AF4 minimum guaranteed rates to 1Mbps and 1.5Mbps, respectively, and CB-WFQ (see results in Figure 6). Traffic corresponding to a given class is transmitted along pre-defined time periods.

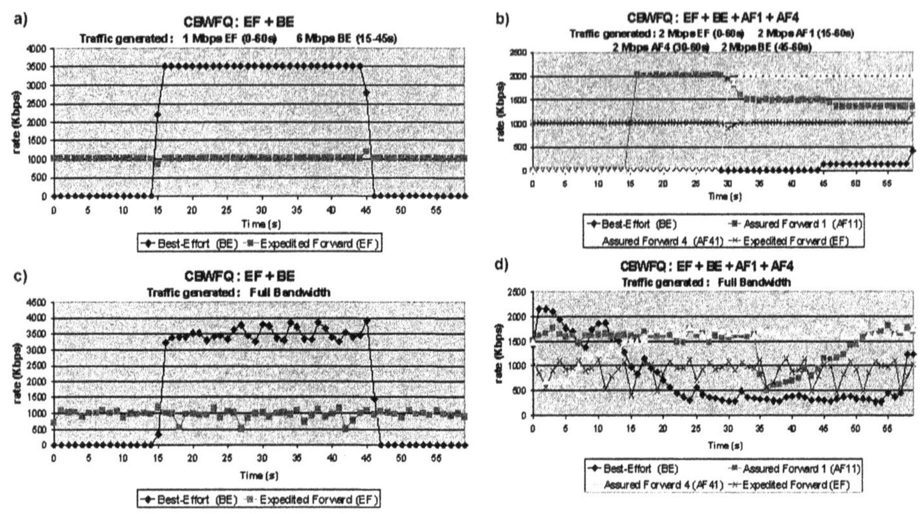

Figure 6. Throughput per PHB for UDP and TCP traffic (UDP - a) and b); TCP c) and d)).

The results obtained for UDP and TCP traffic differ considerably. In fact, throughput measurements for UDP traffic follow our expectations. The rate achieved by EF is constant and limited by its peak rate. AF classes receive their minimum allocated rate, being the remaining bandwidth divided by them proportionally to the reserved bandwidth. As [1, 3] do not state how the remaining bandwidth is distributed, BE traffic also shares (by option) this bandwidth in the same way as other classes (see Figure 6-b)). For TCP traffic the instability around reserved bandwidth value is notorious. Figure 6-d) shows that AF11 throughput is kept below the minimum rate during more than 10s. In our opinion, this behaviour is a result of heavy packet dropping at the router and consequent TCP slow-start adaptation.

6.2.3 Testing Drop Precedence

In the following experiment AF1x behaviour is tested for WRED. Traffic is generated as AF11, AF12 and AF13 over an ATM connection limited to 2Mbps. The tests were carried out for UDP and TCP traffic and the results are shown in Figures 7-a) and 7-b), respectively.

Unexpectedly, throughput measurements showed invariance for the set of WRED parameters shown in Figure 3. AF1x throughput results were expected to be close to the ones presented in Figure 4. However, for UDP traffic, either AF11 or AF12 or AF13 can take over (almost) the maximum allocated bandwidth randomly (Figure 7-a). For TCP traffic, the available link capacity is always used in a balanced way among the existing AF1x traffic (Figure 7-b). Once again, the variability of TCP rates is clear.

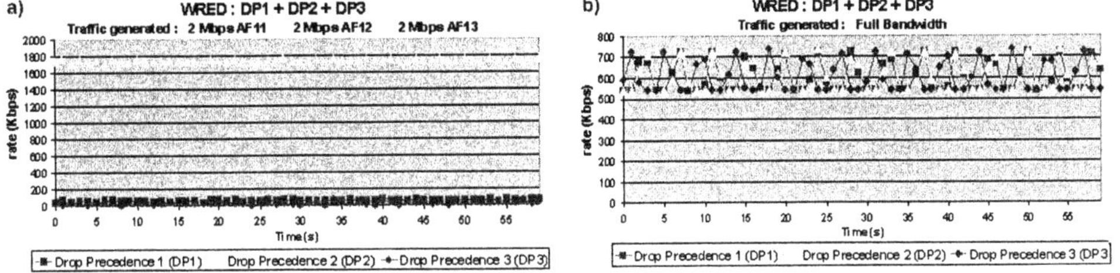

Figure 7. Throughput for the AF1x class (UDP – a); TCP – b)).

This unexpected and incorrect behaviour may be due to the use of ATM PVC interfaces where WRED cannot be configured at the interface level. In order to solve this, CB-WFQ was defined at ATM sub-interface level, where WRED was configured. Although this allowed proceeding with the tests, the WRED parameterisation appeared not to be effective.

6.2.4 CPU Utilisation

In this section, the impact of supporting Diffserv functionalities is evaluated in terms of additional CPU utilisation. An UDP traffic load of 8Mbps is equally distributed among EF, AF1, AF4 and BE (2Mbps each). Policing and Shaping is done at 1Mbps for each traffic class.

Graphs a) and b) in Figure 8 illustrates the CPU utilisation at the ingress router for packet sizes of 500 and 50 bytes, respectively. Graphs c) and d) correspond to equivalent measurements carried out at the core router.

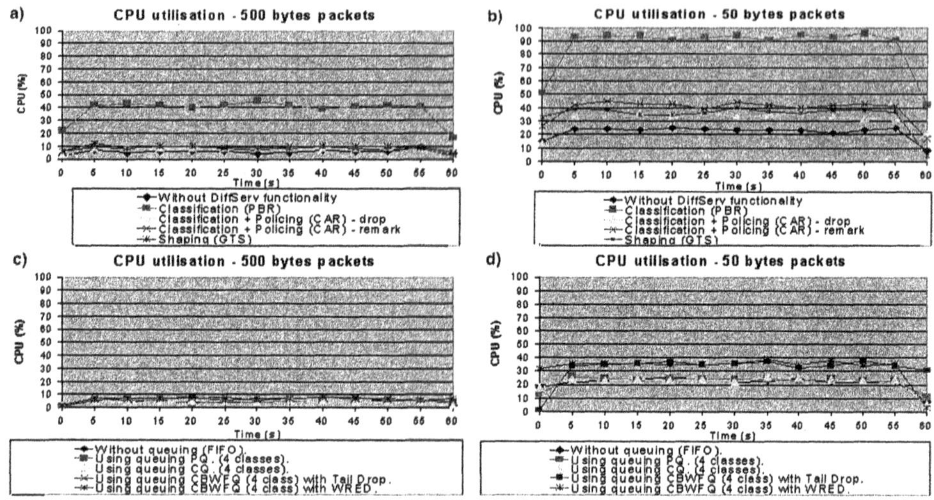

Figure 8. CPU utilisation.

The results presented show that edge functionalities require higher computational effort when comparing with the *without Diffserv* case, especially, for small packet sizes. Supporting *MF Classification* (PBR) is a CPU-consuming task. This behaviour is unexpected as *Classification and Policing* using CAR adds *Policing* to *Classification* and remains a lighter task. These results illustrate that PBR is significantly more inefficient than CAR. Figure 8-a) shows an increase from below 10% to over 40% in CPU utilisation, while for small packets (50 bytes) this value goes above 90%. CPU utilisation almost doubles when running *Classification and Policing (CAR) with remarking;* this increase is smaller when *dropping* is carried out instead of *remarking*.

Most of the tested core functionalities require a negligible increase on CPU utilisation, either for packets of 50 or 500 bytes. Only CB-WFQ implementation causes an additional utilisation of around 10%, for the smaller packet sizes. Generically, the results show that reducing packet size (the total number of packets increases as the rate is kept constant) requires additional processing from DS routers, especially at the network edge. For higher traffic rates the CPU requirements may increase substantially.

6.2.5 Delay Measurements

The main objective of delay measurements was to assess the ability to offer low delays to high priority traffic. The initial network layout presented in Figure 5 was slightly modified so that traffic is sent and received at the same equipment (*SmartBits*) (Figure 9). This solves clock synchronisation problem when measuring absolute delays. To increase accuracy, the delay results presented below are taken from the average of 100 measurements.

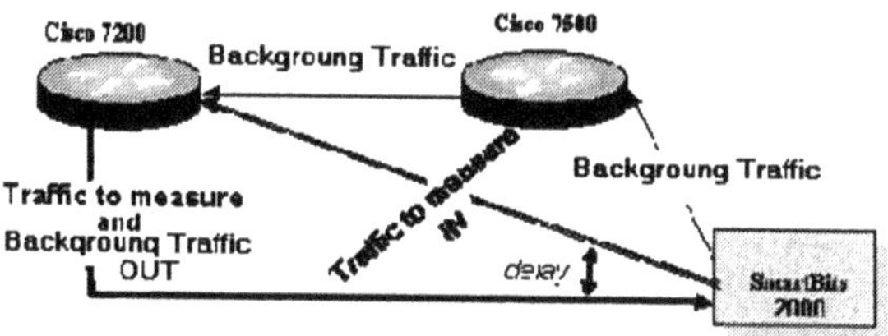

Figure 9. Testbed used for delay measurements.

These tests focused on EF PHB in order to assess if a low delay can be guaranteed in the presence of low priority background traffic. The ATM connection was set to 5Mbps. The traffic is generated so that the network operates without packet loss. The test scenario includes different types of background traffic competing with a single EF traffic flow. Background traffic can be either BE (CBR or on-off (bursty)) or AF (CBR), for different packet size and for two link loads (see results in Figure 10).

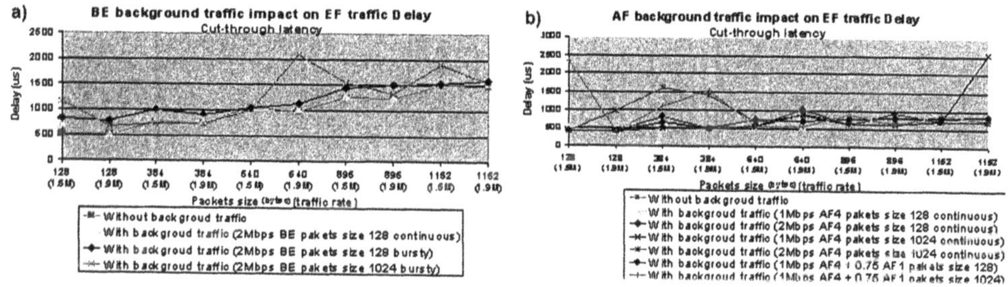

Figure 10. Impact of background traffic on EF PHB.

Note that, EF traffic is slightly delayed by BE background traffic essentially in the presence of bursty (ON-OFF) traffic. EF delay is also influenced by BE packet sizes, as serialisation delay increases (as peaks in Figure 10-a demonstrate). When a background packet is being transmitted, even if an EF packet arrives it has to wait until the BE packet transmission is completed (recall that the implemented CB-WFQ defines a low-latency queue for EF traffic). Thus, the higher BE packet size is, the longer EF traffic waits for being scheduled. In the presence of bursty BE traffic this effect is stressed as the BE queue has periods of high activity. The difference of having AF or BE as background traffic is not significant.

6.3 Cisco Tests Summary

Positive aspects:

- configuration of services using simple and few commands;
- number of Diffserv functionalities;
- TC mechanisms and Queuing generally work as expected;
- amount and quality of available documentation;
- platform used worldwide.

Negative aspects:

- lack of DSCP support (included from Cisco IOS version 12.1(5)T on);
- mapping to layer two with some limitations (e.g. ATM);
- problems in running WRED in ATM interfaces;
- CB-WFQ queuing discipline for TCP traffic showed problems;
- less flexible than the Linux implementation, but much simpler.

7. CONCLUSIONS

The implementation of IP differentiated services on two platforms – a Linux and a Cisco IOS based testbed – has been established, configured, tested and evaluated regarding both Diffserv functionalities and algorithms supported. This work also assessed the impact edge and core functionalities have on Cisco routers and the impact background traffic has on EF traffic.

The Diffserv implementation developed at ICA/EPFL for Linux allows a flexible set up of services through a configuration strategy based on nested functionalities. This flexibility may however lead to intricate and long configurations. The Cisco testbed, including a smaller number of functionalities oriented to traffic differentiation, is able to provide Diffserv services while keeping the overall configuration simple. Concerning Diffserv functionalities, ICA/EPFL implementation allows the correct definition of rules and mechanisms to provide efficient traffic differentiation. EF traffic rate is not impaired by other competing traffic and AF traffic can achieve minimum bandwidth guarantees. The drop precedence for AF PHB group worked as expected for UDP and TCP traffic, under GRED. Policing showed problems in remarking, for rates above a certain (machine-dependent) value.

Cisco platform was very effective on edge component implementation, where traffic policing and shaping were strictly enforced. In our testbed, the core component showed poor performance and unexpected behaviour on TCP traffic differentiation. Drop precedence tests did not lead to meaningful results due to limitations in configuring WRED effectively at the ATM level.

Measuring CPU utilisation, it was found that while the increase of CPU demand at core routers is negligible, at edge routers it may be significant depending on how classification and policing/remarking are accomplished. The increase on CPU utilisation in edge and core routers may be notorious as packet size decreases. Regarding the impact background traffic has on EF traffic, the measurements showed a slight increase on delay essentially in the presence of bursty traffic and for large packets.

Future work will include test tuning in both platforms using upgraded software versions. PHB concatenation and PDB testing will also be covered.

ACKNOWLEDGMENTS

This work is part of EURESCOM P1006/DISCMAN Project framework.

REFERENCES

[1] S. Blake et al., RFC 2475 - An Architecture for Differentiated Services, 1998.
[2] R. Braden et al., RFC 1633 – Integrated Services in the Internet Architecture: an Overview, June 1994.
[3] K. Nichols et al., RFC 2474 - Definition of the Differentiated Services Field (DS Field) in the IPv4 and IPv6 Headers, December 1998.
[4] V. Jacobson et al., RFC 2598 - An Expedited Forwarding PHB, June 1999.
[5] J. Heinanen et al., RFC 2597 - Assured Forwarding PHB Group, June 1999.
[6] W. Almesberger, http://icawww.epfl.ch/linux-Diffserv/, November 1999.
[7] NEC, http://www.nec-cx.com/products/, September 2001.
[8] IBM, http://www.networking.ibm.com/netprod.html, September 2001.
[9] T. Ferrari, P. Chimento, A Measurement-based Analysis of EF PHB Mechanisms, 2000.
[10] S. Radhakrishan, Internet Protocol QoS Page, http://qos.ittc.ukans.edu.
[11] S. Floyd, V. Jacobson, Random Early Detection gateways for Congestion Avoidance, IEEE/ACM Transactions on Networking, V.1 N.4, August 1993, pp 397-413.
[12] K.Wehrle, H. Ritter, Problems of Traffic Shaping in ATM and IP Networks Using Standard End Systems, ATM2000 Conference, http://atm2000.ccrle.nec.de/.

INVITED TALK I – ABSTRACT

ACHIEVING HIGH RELIABILITY FOR UBIQUITOUS INFORMATION TECHNOLOGY

Robert V. Binder
RBSC Corporation, Chicago, USA
rbinder@rbsc.com

Abstract Emerging information technology promises to take us from the wired web to a wireless "hive mind". This talk considers how can we achieve the necessary reliability. Some lessons from testing object-oriented systems and my work in advanced automated testing are presented. A strategy to apply these lessons to new technical challenges concludes the talk.

Outline:

What is ubiquitous information technology?
- New applications, new technology
- "Five nines": why should you care?

What have we learned about achieving high reliability?
- Object-oriented systems
- Distributed systems
- Usage versus bugs
- Testing and verification strategies

New challenges for 21st Century systems
- Scope and complexity
- Components -- the good, the bad, and the ugly
- Risks to the public

Strategies for high reliability
- The elusive optimal development cycle
- Testing as a requirements process
- User simulation and system behavior models
- Automated testing

SESSION II

TESTING INTERNET SYSTEMS

AN AUTOMATED, FLEXIBLE TESTING ENVIRONMENT FOR UMTS

Jan Bredereke, Bernd-Holger Schlingloff
Universität Bremen, TZi · P.O. box 330 440 · D-28334 Bremen · Germany
{brederek,hs}@tzi.de · www.tzi.de/{~brederek,~hs}

Abstract We describe an automated, flexible testing environment for UMTS systems which are specified and developed with SDL. For testing these systems, we use a testing tool which generates black box tests from a formal specification of the desired properties. Since the requirements are subject to considerable change at any time, it is important to guarantee consistency between the interfaces of the test specification and the system under test. Therefore, we defined rules for the modularization of the requirements according to functional properties. Furthermore, we devised and implemented a generator tool which automatically produces all necessary interface code. This is a first step towards a general configuration utility for the automatic creation of runtime interfaces and adapters. We report on testing results and experiences with our setup.

Keywords: test tools; test interface generation; industrial testing experience; test selection and management; UMTS; SDL; conformance testing.

1. INTRODUCTION

UMTS (Universal Mobile Telecommunication System) is an evolving standard for a new generation of high-speed, multi-media mobile phone systems. It is being defined by the 3GPP consortium (the 3rd Generation Partnership Project [1]), and currently the equipment is being developed at different sites. Even though the standard has been released already in 1999, there have been a number of significant changes and additions, and further have to be expected. In a black box testing approach, all interfaces and parameters have to be provided to the testing environment in detail. Therefore, it is important that a testing environment for UMTS software is flexible and easily adaptable. If the interfaces and requirements are modified, the necessary changes in the testing specification and environment should be as small as possible.

In this paper, we describe an automated, flexible testing environment for UMTS systems which are specified and developed with SDL (Specification and Description Language, see [2]). For testing the SDL system, we use a tool in which test suites can be described in the formal specification language CSP (Communicating Sequential Processes, see [3]). We developed a generator tool which automatically produces all necessary interface code to connect the SDL development suite and the CSP testing tool. Since the generation is completely automated, consistency between the interfaces is guaranteed.

This work evolved from testing needs in the development of the Radio Link Control (RLC) protocol layer of UMTS. It was done in cooperation with Siemens AG, Salzgitter. For this system, it was decided to apply specification based testing (black-box-testing) rather than structural testing, for the following reasons. In the case of UMTS, user equipment and base stations are developed by different companies. Moreover, even the development of the software for different layers of the protocol is distributed between different sites within Siemens AG. For the correct functioning of the whole system, it is extremely important that the standard is implemented by all participating developers in a consistent way. Therefore, in order to ensure inter-operability between devices from different providers, it is mandatory to base test suites solely on the 3GPP standards (plus additional site-specific requirements) rather than on individual program code from specific developers.

In specification-based testing, the requirements are described separately from the implementation in a formal language. Thus, a need to interface the testing specification and the implementation arises. As mentioned above, in the case of UMTS the interfaces of specification and implementation are subject to change; all changes must be carried out consistently. For example, in release 4 of the RLC layer standard, for the primitive `CRLC_CONFIG_Req` additional parameters `Stop` and `Continue` have been added. They indicate that the RLC entity shall not transmit or receive RLC PDUs or shall continue transmission and reception, respectively. If these additional parameters are taken into account either in the implementation or in the test case specification, it must be ensured that these still fit together. Additionally, the interface code between the implementation and the testing environment must be re-generated. The `CRLC_CONFIG_Req` primitive has hundreds of parameters, with more than one kilobyte of heavily structured data. Thus, without automated support, these tasks are tedious and error-prone. Especially, if the test specification and the implementation are developed by separate teams, automated consistency checks and code generation are extremely useful. We therefore devised a tool which allows to perform these tasks with minimal manual efforts. Subsequently, we describe its design and underlying principles. Details of the interface generation part of our tool can be found in a companion paper ([4]).

This paper is organized as follows: in Section 2, we briefly introduce our specification language and testing tool. Section 3 is the main part, it presents the principles of the automated, flexible testing environment. This environment generates the interface to the implementation automatically while also automatically checking the consistency of the implementation's and the specification's interface. We present rules for the modularization of the requirements which prepare for a flexible maintenance of the initial test specification and which reduce the work necessary for modifications. In Section 4, we report on the application of the environment to a part of the UMTS protocol stack; and we describe and interpret the testing results. Section 5 summarizes our work.

2. FORMAL CSP SPECIFICATIONS AND RT-TESTER

CSP (Communicating Sequential Processes, see [3]) is a specification language which allows to give a description of a system on a high level of abstraction. The structure of the requirements is reflected by particular operators such as sequential or parallel composition, choice, iteration and hiding. Communication between the processes and with the outside is by the exchange of events. In contrast to SDL, however, this communication is synchronous (handshake); buffered communication has to be modelled explicitly. We use a timed version of CSP, where it is possible to set timers which generate events upon elapse. This way, it is possible to test real-time behaviour of applications, which is especially important for embedded systems.

Since CSP arose from theoretical considerations, it has a well-defined formal semantics and a rich theory. Several elaborate verification tools have been developed for CSP, most notably the FDR system (**F**ailure **D**ivergence **R**efinement) by Formal Systems, Ltd. At present, FDR forms a basis for our testing system RT-TESTER.

Compared to other specification languages such as TTCN-3 [5], the parallel composition is treated differently in the test case generation from CSP specifications. The testing system first constructs a *transition graph* which is a representation of all possible interleavings of the parallel tasks. The test driver then enumerates all paths through this graph and uses them as test sequences for the SUT. This way it is possible to specify separate requirements on the same interfaces as independent parallel testing tasks, which allows a modular description of testing objectives.

Example 1 A vending machine specification featuring a few basic CSP operators.

```
include "timers.csp"
pragma AM_INPUT
channel coin, buttonCoffee, buttonTea
nametype MonEv = { coin, buttonCoffee, buttonTea }
pragma AM_OUTPUT
channel coffee, tea
nametype CtrlEv = { coffee, tea }

OBSERVER = (  (coin -> HAVE_COIN)
           [] (buttonCoffee -> OBSERVER)
           [] (buttonTea -> OBSERVER))
HAVE_COIN = (  (coin -> HAVE_COIN))
            [] (buttonTea -> AWAIT({tea}) ; OBSERVER)
            [] (buttonCoffee -> AWAIT({coffee}); OBSERVER)

RANDOM_STIMULI = (|~| x: MonEv @ x -> PAUSE; RANDOM_STIMULI)

TEST_SPEC = RANDOM_STIMULI [| MonEv |] OBSERVER
```

A system described by the process `OBSERVER` accepts either of the three inputs listed (external choice "`[]`"). If the input is a `coin`, then the system behaves like the process `HAVE_COIN` (event prefix "`->`"). A system described by the process `HAVE_COIN` outputs the desired drink after the corresponding button press. In this, the subprocess `AWAIT` waits for any of the outputs specified (sequential process composition "`;`"). The definition of this process is listed in Example 2 on page 88 below. The process `RANDOM_STIMULI` non-deterministically selects one event from the set `MonEv` (replicated internal choice "`|~| x : S @ P(x)`"), waits a short time, and starts all over (recursion). The process `TEST_SPEC` describes the complete test suite: the process `RANDOM_STIMULI` provides all the test inputs, which are also tracked by the process `OBSERVER`. The latter additionally tracks the test outputs. They are combined by sharing ("`P [| S |] Q`") the input events in the set `MonEv`.

Example 1 introduces a few basic operators of CSP, in particular the event prefix, the external choice, and one of the parallel composition operators.

From formal CSP test specifications, test cases can be generated and executed on-the-fly. Our tool RT-TESTER [6] reads the CSP input and uses FDR to generate the transition graph from it. In a separate stage, this transition graph is used by RT-TESTER to generate test scripts, which are executed on a separate testing machine automatically and in real time. They may run over long periods of time: hours, days, weeks and more – without the necessity of manually writing test scripts of an according length. The testing machine and the SUT (system under test) communicate via TCP/IP sockets, and test results are evaluated on the fly in real time during the run of the SUT, by using the compiled CSP description as a test oracle. To ensure that the tests cover the whole bandwidth of all possible system situations, a mathematically proven testing strategy is used [7].

3. AN AUTOMATED, FLEXIBLE TESTING ENVIRONMENT FOR SDL WITH CSP

The 3GPP standard is written in a mixture of formalisms. The main part is plain English and annotated figures. These are accompanied by tables describing bit-level data formats, small state transition diagrams for the different modes and control commands, plus message sequence charts for the procedural communication between sending and receiving protocol instances. Earlier versions of the standard were accompanied by a detailed implementation suggestion described in the specification and description language SDL [2].

The implementation is developed at various sites from these and similar sources with the help of suitable tools. In particular, there are commercial tools which can execute an SDL system in an emulated runtime environment, and which can compile a set of SDL diagrams plus a set of data type descriptions written in ASN.1 or as C headers into executable machine code for embedded targets.

A particular problem for the development of test suites for UMTS is that the standard describing the requirements still is subject to considerable change. Even after the "December 1999" release, which was supposed to be stable, a large number of changes were made, and more have to be expected. This concerns, for example, the parameters of the service primitives and the details of the data at the interfaces, such as the structure of the protocol data units. Even the behaviour of the protocol machines is still expected to change, in particular for error handling. Similarly, not all implementation decisions have been finalized, some details of the machine representation of data at the interfaces are not yet fixed. We therefore designed the testing environment to be highly flexible by

- defining the interface in terms of SDL signals and data structures instead of low level descriptions,
- performing an automated consistency check between the SDL description of the interface and the formal CSP specification of the interface, and
- defining rules for modularizing the formal behaviour specifications into largely independent functional requirements.

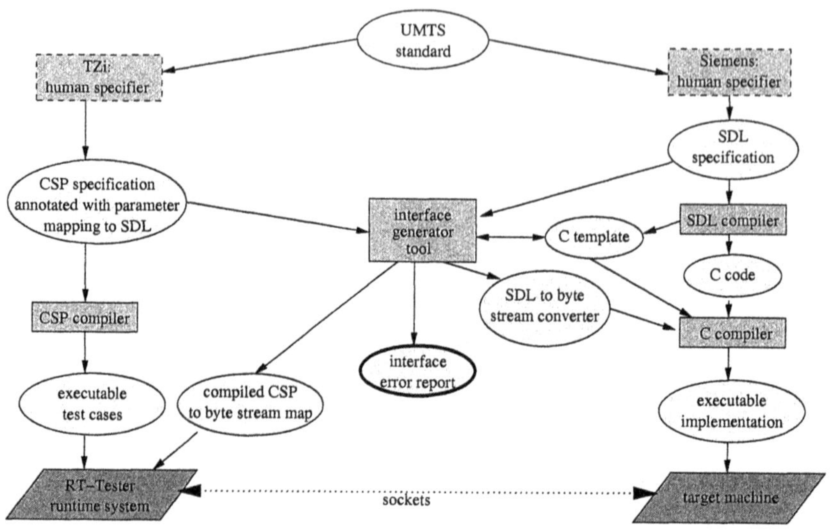

Figure 1. Automatic interface generation

3.1 Interfacing SDL and CSP

The interfaces of the UMTS protocol layers relevant for testing are specified in SDL. Our automated approach makes them the only relevant interfaces. The goal of the tests is to ensure that we can combine the tested SDL processes into a larger SDL system and achieve the desired behaviour. The actual representation of the internal interfaces between the components is not part of the visible behaviour of the combined system.

Only these internal interfaces have to be consistent. On one hand, the SDL and C compilers do this type check. On the other hand, RT-TESTER can check whether the intended inter-process cooperation indeed occurs by performing (black box) integration tests of several components.

An interface in terms of SDL signals must be mapped to an interface in terms of RT-TESTER's native CSP channels. Therefore, a translation between the two forms of syntax is needed. Due to its changing nature, we decided to automate the mapping by a generator tool. This generator tool also flags any inconsistencies between the interfaces of the two specifications. If the SDL specification is changed, the generator tool simply needs to be re-run. If it does not flag any error, the interface descriptions of the SDL specification and the CSP specification are guaranteed to be consistent. Consistency of the behaviour can then be checked in a subsequent test run. If the SDL interface has been changed in a part that is relevant to the CSP tests, all items which do not match are logged and the problem can directly be investigated. In the case of the the RLC layer of the UMTS protocol stack, this feature is especially important. This module uses large and complex signal parameters, which are difficult to keep in sync manually. There are signals with more than one kilobyte of heavily structured parameter data; comparing their definitions manually would be extremely tedious and error-prone.

Figure 1 on the facing page presents the concept of the automated interfacing. Detailled information on the automatic generation of the interfacing software can be found in a companion paper; see [4].

Our automated approach for mapping signals obsoletes the need for a manual description of the machine representations, and it does not demand any user interaction after a change. Since we confine the machine representation of the data in the target entirely to that machine, it is sufficient to rebuild the generated files and recompile them. The socket communication with RT-TESTER uses our own byte string format which is independent of any machine representation.

3.2 Flexible Maintenance of CSP Specification

Usually, all test cases have to be revised and reorganized a number of times in the software development process. It is advisable to consider the maintenance tasks associated with a test suite already during its design. With a suitable structuring, the efforts for rewriting and recombination of test cases can be significantly reduced.

In our application, we identified two such maintenance tasks: we had to expect considerable *changes to the requirements* of UMTS, as discussed in the introduction of this paper. And we had to support *variants of our test suites* using as little duplication of description as possible. Test suite variants result from three orthogonal sources of variation: adjustments of the test coverage, stepping from component tests to integration tests, and stepping from active testing to passive testing.

The need to *adjust the test coverage* in different test suites derived from the same requirements arises for the following reasons: we have to test the SUT with *selected*, interesting sets of *signal parameters*, while using the same behaviour description. Furthermore, we want to test the SUT with different choices of its possible *behaviour*, which are either completely *random*, or which have a selectively *increased probability* for certain choices, or which are manually selected, fixed and *deterministic* test traces. All these test cases use the same description of admissible behaviour.

While starting to design *component tests* for an individual layer of the UMTS protocol stack, we already had to *prepare for integration tests* of several layers tested together, using the same description of admissible behaviour of the individual layers. Furthermore, already the RLC layer allows for multiple parallel instances of the same protocol machine. These run independently, at least at the black box behaviour level, but the implementation in SDL has a different, less decoupled structure. Therefore, integration tests for the protocol machine instances of this protocol layer were necessary.

All these tests had to be *active tests* where the test specification generates the test stimuli. It was nevertheless envisioned already at this stage to use the same behaviour descriptions in *passive tests*, where real UMTS air interfaces and upper protocol layers provide the stimuli to the SUT, and where the testing system can not monitor internal signals, but only external stimuli and reactions.

Integration of test suites and replacement of simulated by real environment are common maintenance tasks in test development. We designed the testing requirements as a *family of test suites*, with a modular structure. During this task, we identified the following *rules for modularizing requirements.*

There are two basic rules which lead to further, more specific rules:

- separate the description of the signature of a module from the description of the properties of its behaviour, and

- identify which requirements will likely change together, and to put them into one requirements module.

For the first of these rules, we discuss the case of CSP. A CSP signature consists of a set of channels with their parameters, and the behaviour is described by a composition of CSP processes over these channels. This separation allows to change the description of the behaviour of a module without changing the description of other modules that communicate with this module. The properties of the behaviour are hidden within the behaviour module. For example, with this strategy we can change the level of test coverage without changing the interfaces. Similarly, this separation enables to step from active to passive testing and from integration tests to component tests, as discussed below.

For the second rule, we note that it implies that all changes are within a particular module and do not affect the rest of the specification. Thus, the effects of a change remain local and manageable. The rule can be instantiated into several more specific rules, using the analysis of the expected changes:

- separate test stimulus generation from test observation;
- separate application specific and tester specific issues;
- for real-time testing, separate timer handling from application description; and
- for protocol testing, separate protocol layer specifications.

The modularization of requirements can be applied recursively. One example is the sub-structuring of a module into its signature and its behaviour.

In the remainder of this subsection, we discuss these specific rules. The *separation of test stimulus generation from test observation* was demonstrated in the vending machine example in Example 1 on page 82, where `RANDOM_STIMULI` and `OBSERVER` are separate CSP processes. We used the same structure for the UMTS protocol layers (see Figure 2):

In this modelling, a test stimulus generator, written in CSP, generates an input to the implementation under test and waits some defined amount of time, then it loops and generates the next input. Concurrently, a test observer process, also written in CSP, observes both the input stimuli and the output reactions of the system under test. If the behaviour of the system under test is incorrect, an error is flagged.

The choice of test coverage is private to the test stimulus generator, and the definition of the correct behaviour is private to the test observer. Therefore, this separation allows for several test suites which concentrate their coverage on a specific issue each but which use the same behaviour description, and it also allows for additional passive test suites which use only the behaviour description, but not the test stimulus generator at all.

The *separation of application specific and of tester specific issues* is a consequence of the fact that the testing tool usually is much more stable than the application requirements. Therefore, these should be put into a separate module. For our testing tool, tester specific events include `wrong_reaction` and `no_reaction`, which go into the test log, and the timer events.

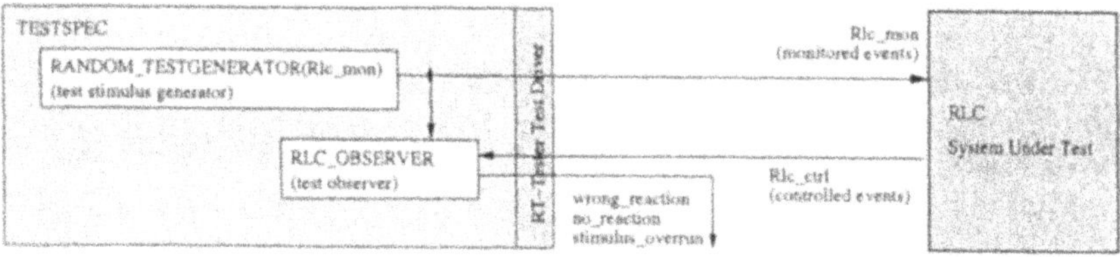

Figure 2. Separation of test stimulus generator and test observer.

Example 2 The timer-related CSP processes for Example 1 on page 82.

```
pragma AM_SET_TIMER
channel setTimer : { 0, 1 }
pragma AM_ELAPSED_TIMER
channel elapsedTimer : { 0, 1 }
pragma AM_ERROR
channel wrong_reaction, stimulus_overrun
pragma AM_WARNING
channel no_reaction

PAUSE = setTimer!0 -> elapsedTimer.0 -> SKIP

AWAIT(ExpectedEvSet) =
(   -- start timer and wait for things to come:
    setTimer!1 ->
    (   -- Accept correct reaction:
        ([] x: ExpectedEvSet @ x -> SKIP)
     [] -- Flag wrong reaction:
        ([] x: diff(CtrlEv + MonEv, ExpectedEvSet) @
            x -> wrong_reaction -> SKIP)
     [] -- Flag no reaction (timeout):
        elapsedTimer.1 -> no_reaction -> SKIP))
```

The process `PAUSE` sets a timer and waits until it elapses. Then it terminates and thereby returns to its calling process.

The process `AWAIT` assures that one of the specified set of legal outputs occurs in due time. If not, it performs one of the events `wrong_reaction` `no_reaction`, ... which go into the test log. This process also terminates and thereby returns to its calling process.

The *separation of timer handling from application description*, which should be done for real-time testing, is a particular instance of the previous rule. The realization of high-level timing processes by primitive set/elapse events of timers is completely internal to the timer handling module. Example 2 shows the definition of the CSP process `AWAIT` from Example 1 on page 82 which assures that one of the specified set of legal outputs occurs in due time.

Finally, the *separation of protocol layer specifications*, when testing protocols, encapsulates the behaviour of each layer into a separate module. Together with the separation of signatures and behaviours, this facilitates the generation of integration test suites from test suites for the components. If the rule is being followed, then specifications of admissible behaviour for the components can be re-used to get a description of the admissible system behaviour.

All these modularization rules must be implemented by mapping them to existing expressive means of the specification language. The dialect of CSP which we used allows to partition specifications into several files, to organize these in a directory structure, and to compose the parts by an `include` statement. Example 1 on page 82 uses such an `include` statement in its first line to compose Example 2 into the specification.

In a large application, sub-directories can be used to express the hierarchical module structure, and individual files to express leaf-node modules. For example, in our UMTS application there is a sub-directory for each protocol layer. The sub-directory for the tester specific issues contains a further sub-directory for timer specific issues. All of these directories typically contain several variants of a specification part.

We have a separate directory tree which contains the actual test suites. Each sub-directory contains a file which composes the particular test specification from the requirements modules, and which contains further test-related data such as test result reports.

During integration testing, several protocol layer instances must be executed at the same time. This can be implemented by the parallel composition operator of CSP. In this composition, CSP process instances are parameterized with an instance number. These processes then run concurrently in parallel. Each process generates test stimuli for one of the protocol instances, and checks the corresponding reactions separately. The RT-TESTER tool allows to run several CSP specifications in parallel, with different interleaving strategies for the processes.

4. APPLICATION OF THE TESTING ENVIRONMENT

Subsequently, we describe a first experimental application of our testing environment in an industrial context. We provided testing support for a specific protocol stack layer in the user equipment of a mobile phone system.

4.1 The RLC Layer of the UMTS Protocol Stack

UMTS is a new international wireless telecommunication standard developed by the 3GPP consortium [1]. The standard comprises a layered architecture, where each layer relies on primitive services from the layer below and provides complex services to the layer above. Conceptually, each layer in the user equipment communicates with the same layer in the UMTS terrestrial radio access network.

Layer 1 is the physical layer of hardware services provided by the chip-set. Layer 2 is the data link layer. It provides the concept of a point-to-point connection to the network layer above. Layer 3, the network layer, provides network services such as establishment / release of a connection, hand-over, broadcast of messages to all users in a certain geographical area, and notification of information to specific users. It includes the Radio Resource Control (RRC), which assigns, configures and releases wireless bandwidth (codes, frequencies etc.). Above layer 3 there are application layers containing functionality such as Call Control (CC) and Mobility Management (MM).

Layer 2 consists of several sub-layers: Medium Access Control (MAC), Radio Link Control (RLC), Packet Data Convergence Protocol (PDCP), and Broadcast and Multicast Control (BMC). The MAC provides unacknowledged transfer of service data units, reallocation of parameters such as user identity number and transport format. It furthermore reports local measurements such as traffic volume and quality of service indication to the RRC. The main task of the RLC is segmentation and reassembly of long data packets from higher layers into fixed width protocol data units, respectively. This includes flow control, error detection, retransmission, duplicate removal, and similar tasks.

The RLC layer of the UMTS protocol stack [8] provides three modes of data transfer: acknowledged (error-free), unacknowledged (immediate), and transparent (unchanged) mode. In acknowledged mode, the correct transmission of data is guaranteed to the upper layer; if unrecoverable errors occur, a notification is sent. In unacknowledged mode, erroneous and duplicate packets are deleted, but there is no retransmission or error correction: messages are delivered as soon as a complete set of packets is received. In transparent mode, higher layer data is forwarded without adding any protocol information; thus no error correction or duplicate removal can be done.

In all of these modes, the variable-length data packets received from the upper layer must be segmented into fixed-length RLC protocol data units (PDUs). Vice versa, for delivery to the higher layer, received PDUs have to be reassembled according to the attached sequence numbers. As additional services, the RLC offers a cipher mechanism preventing unauthorized access to message data. Thus, to transmit data, the RLC reads messages from the upper layer service access points (SAPs), performs segmentation and concatenation with other packets as needed, optionally encrypts the data, adds header information such as sequence numbers, and puts the packets into the transmission buffer. From there, the MAC assigns a channel for the packet and transmits it via layer 1 and radio waves. On the opposite side, packets arriving from the MAC in the receiver buffer are investigated for retransmissions, stripped from the RLC header information, decrypted if necessary and then reassembled according to the sequence numbering, before they are made accessible to the upper layers via the corresponding SAP.

Example 3 CSP specification of the initialization of an RLC connection in acknowledged mode.

```
-- The null state of the RLC abstract machine:
RLC_AM_NULL(instance_id) = instate_rlc_am_null.instance_id ->
(   -- Wait for crlc_config_req setup request and honour it:
    crlc_config_req.rbSetup.1.instance_id?dummy ->
        RLC_CONFIG_AM(instance_id,rlc_to_rrc)
 []
    -- No data transfer is yet possible, since the instance does not
    -- yet exist, thus no reaction is expected otherwise:
    -- (A release request is discarded in this state, too.)
    ([] x : diff(Rlc_mon,
            {| crlc_config_req.rbSetup.1.instance_id |}) @
        x -> RLC_AM_NULL(instance_id))
 []
    -- any spontaneous reaction produces a warning:
    ([] x : Rlc_ctrl @ x -> warn_spontaneous_event -> RLC_AM_NULL(instance_id))
)

-- The other states are omitted here:
RLC_CONFIG_AM(instance_id,rlc_dest) = ...

-- The main process:
RLC_AM_OBSERVER(instance_id) = RLC_AM_NULL(instance_id)
```

The observer for the RLC instance with the number `instance_id` starts in the state `RLC_AM_NULL` and waits for a configuration request event. If the event occurs, the instance goes to the next state. All other events to the SUT are ignored. Any spontaneous output from the SUT would be an error and is flagged.

A particular feature of the RLC is that there may be several instances coexisting at the same time. This is necessary since the services to the upper layers provide a variable number of connections, whereas the service of the lower layer provides a fixed number of logical channels. For efficiency reasons, however, the maximum number of parallel instances is statically fixed in the system.

Example 3 presents a CSP text fragment from our RLC layer specification. It describes part of the initialization of a connection in acknowledged mode.

4.2 Ambiguities in the Standards Document

Our tests yielded two kinds of results: the first kind are ambiguities and misinterpretations in the UMTS standards document. The second kind, discussed in Section 4.3 below, are deviations of the actual from the expected behaviour of the SUT.

One of the advantages of specification based testing is that it requires a formalization of the specification whose interfaces must be compared to the implementation's interface. Writing this formalization, we found several ambiguities in the standard which can be subject to different, equally legal, incompatible interpretations.

For example, the RLC layer must accept several kinds of data as PDUs from the underlying MAC layer and forward it through the appropriate service access points (SAPs) of itself to its upper layers. Similarly, the RLC layer must forward data arriving through its SAPs as service primitives down to the appropriate "logical channels" of the underlying MAC layer. In both cases, the appropriate destination cannot be determined from a service primitive or PDU and their parameters alone, as given in the standard. Therefore the RLC SAP was split into two SAPs, distinguishing whether an upward bound signal should go to the RRC layer or to a different upper layer, and another parameter was added to most service primitives and PDUs which identifies the destination inside one layer. These necessary extensions have the consequence that the RLC layer can be used only with MAC and upper layers which add the same parameter and which use the same SAP split.

Another much less obvious, but potentially even more serious example is that we did not find any precise definition of the properties of a service access point (SAP), or of the MAC layer's logical channel. In particular, there is no definition of

- whether signals are forwarded instantaneously or whether they are buffered,
- a queueing discipline (FIFO, ...) in the case of buffering,
- queue delivery dependences between different SAPs (single queue/multiple queues),
- possible minimum/maximum delays between delivery and availability,
- the handling of signals that cannot be received.

The implementors had to make decisions on the above issues. Several of them were made more or less implicitly by choosing SDL as the implementation language, since the endpoint of an SDL signal route or channel has a precise, specific semantics. Further decisions were made by choosing a particular structure of SDL processes inside a layer (e.g., the number of independent queues per layer).

4.3 Testing of the SUT's Behaviour

There were several situations in which the SUT did not behave as expected. For example, in a certain state the SUT reacts to a certain signal where no reaction was intended: an RLC protocol machine is created by the event `crlc_config_req.rbSetup` from the upper layers, and it becomes operational after receiving the event `mac_status_ind` from the underlying MAC layer. Immediately after that, the random test stimulus generator sometimes generated another (nonsensical) `mac_status_ind` event, to which the RLC layer sometimes, but not always, reacted by generating a data packet, i.e., with a `mac_data_req` event. Since no data transmission requests had been issued yet, and thus no buffered data could possibly be pending, this is unexpected. Probably no explicit test script would have been written that checks for a non-reaction in this state. The systematic random exploration of the state space in our approach found this problem automatically.

Furthermore, the tests revealed interactions between multiple instances of the RLC protocol machines. The requirements allow several instances of these machines which behave completely independent. Each instance could be tested separately. But we also performed a test where several protocol machines were tested at the same time, each one against its own copy of the requirements specification. It turned out that in such a setup there was the possibility that the entire SUT could deadlock. The reason for this effect was that the various instances of the RLC protocol machines are not implemented as entirely separate copies. Rather, there is a centralized routing SDL process which forwards data transmission requests to a set of SDL processes which implement one RLC instance each. This routing process did not handle the following case properly: if a signal arrived addressed to an RLC instance which does not currently exist, the process could loop infinitely during the instance look-up. It then ceased to perform its routing job. Even though the implementation was built with sophisticated error recovery mechanisms, this situation could not possibly have been foreseen in the development.

5. SUMMARY

In this paper, we described a testing setup for the UMTS protocol stack. A specific feature of this setup is that the interface between the system under test and the requirements specification is generated by an automated tool, which also performs consistency checks. This allows last-minute changes in the data formats.

The tool is complemented by a set of rules for designing the testing requirements as a family of test suites, with a modular structure. This prepares for a flexible maintenance of the initial test specification and reduces the work necessary for modifications.

Whereas our particular tool is tailored towards the development of UMTS software with SDL, the underlying ideas are applicable for other developments as well. Automating the interface generation between the testing tool and the system under test, and modularizing the requirements specification, is profitable under the following circumstances:

- a requirements document with complex interface definitions, which is authoritative for the final product, is being developed by an independent party;
- for the most part of the development time, the interface definition is in a draft state, with substantial changes to be expected and templates still to be filled in;
- after completion of the requirements document, an extremely short time to market is crucial for the success of the project.

Whenever these conditions are met, it is of advantage to shift verification and validation efforts into earlier design phases. By implementing automated interface generation tools already in the project preparation phase, and by additional up-front efforts for analyzing potential changes and for modularizing the requirements, the duration of the system integration and testing phase can be significantly reduced.

References

[1] 3rd Generation Partnership Project. http://www.3gpp.org.

[2] J. Ellsberger, D. Hogrefe, and A. Sarma: *SDL – Formal Object-oriented Language for Communicating Systems.* Prentice-Hall 1997.

[3] A. W. Roscoe: *The Theory and Practice of Concurrency.* Prentice-Hall 1997.

[4] J. Bredereke and B.-H. Schlingloff: Specification Based Testing of the UMTS Protocol Stack; in: *Proc. 14th Int. Software & Internet Quality Week (QW2001)*, San Francisco (May 2001).

[5] J. Grabowski, A. Wiles, C. Willcock, and D. Hogrefe: On the design of the new testing language TTCN-3. In: H. Ural, R. L. Probert, and G. v. Bochmann, *Testing of Communicating Systems - Tools and Techniques*, vol. 176 of IFIP Conf. Kluwer Academic Publishers (Aug. 2000).

[6] Verified Systems International GmbH. `http://www.verified.de`

[7] Jan Peleska: *Formal Methods and the Development of Dependable Systems.* Habilitation thesis, Report No. 9612, Christian-Albrechts-Universität Kiel, and UniForM project, Technical Report 9601, Universität Bremen, Germany Dec. 1996.

[8] 3rd Generation Partnership Project, 3GPP TS 25.322 V4.0.0. RLC protocol specification (Mar. 2001).

TESTING MOBILE AGENTS

SAM: a tool based on a simulation approach

Mikael Marche, Yves-Marie Quemener, Roland Groz
France Télécom R&D/DTL/MSV,
2 Avenue Pierre Marzin, F-22307 Lannion CEDEX, France,
Tel +33 2 96 05 20 12
mikael.marche, yvesmarie.quemener, roland.groz @rd.francetelecom.com

Abstract For years to come, we can predict an important increase in the use of software systems using mobile code. Those systems give birth to new development problems compared to current distributed systems. In particular, testing for such systems must take into account the mobility of tested processes, which makes it difficult to maintain contact points between testing and tested processes. We propose a solution based on the simulation of the environment of mobile processes. For developing such a simulator, we need to abstract the notions found in different platforms enabling the execution of mobile processes, by giving a common API between those platforms and our simulator.

Keywords: Mobile code, mobile agents, testing, simulation, MASIF

1. INTRODUCTION

The changing nature of distributed computing, the availability of common middleware, the adaptability of software code to various environments due to the variety of terminals and the interlinking of servers on the Internet have raised the interest in the mobility of code over networks.

Just as the need for interoperability in distributed networks raised interest for testing protocols in the 1980's, the need for solutions in testing new types of distributed communicating software based on mobile code should come up rapidly. We found that software developers in our environment using e.g. agent technology were lacking test methods and tools, because very little research has been done on the specific problems implied by code mobility.

Various types of mobility [9] may be considered, from applets and code downloading, to full mobility of the code along with its execution context such as in the agent paradigm and script languages in the sense initiated by Telescript [18]. All notions of mobility rely on the fact that a given software code may be executed on different hardware execution environments over time. In the most static form, the code may simply be moved along with the support on which it is stored, such as a smart card, for instance the SIM card of a GSM telephone handset. It can also be stored on a laptop or a handheld which may move to different locations on a network and interact with other software processes depending on the location from where it accesses the network. In a more dynamic form, no physical support moves, but the code is transfered over a network from one location to another. Of course, both types of mobility can be combined. And then, we have to take into account the nature of the code we are talking about: is it source code, bytecode to be interpreted or a compiled binary? Does it include the execution contexts, or at least dynamic bindings? Depending on which type of mobility we are considering, the test of software applications based on mobile code may entail different problems.

In this paper, we address the problem of testing an application based on a rich notion of mobility, where

- the execution context is moved along with the code;
- moves can be triggered by the code itself.

The first clause specifies that we are moving not just code, but processes, and the second clause further specifies that we are in fact dealing with autonomous processes. These characteristics correspond to what can be found in the mobile agent paradigm [5, 9]. Typically, an agent A would transfer its own execution from a given location S_1 to move to location S_2 where it would resume processing. Moving to S_2 might typically be decided by agent A to access specific resources available on S_2. In order to work on a relevant set of concepts with some potential impact on the development of telecommunication services, we decided to start from existing standards defining an infrastructure for mobile agents. Although FIPA [8] proposes a standard interface for interactions with agents, it does not really address mobility issues. Therefore we started mainly from the OMG MASIF specifications [15], although we consider also the primitives offered by various platforms offering an agent-based infrastructure which may be more or less compliant to MASIF.

Of course, applications based on mobile code are distributed software applications, and much of the theory and practice on software testing, as well as the theory of testing in distributed contexts (such as embodied in the ITU Z.500 standard for instance) is relevant. But there are specific problems in testing mobile applications, and we are interested in addressing those problems.

Although the previous research orientation in our group was mainly towards test generation [11], in the case of mobile code we consider that the problems related to test execution should be solved first, before we move to higher degrees of test design. It is as yet unclear in our context of telecommunication services whether there would be a strong case for testing conformity of mobile agents to a given specification, or whether testing is well suited to address security issues such as the use of local resources by an incoming agent, or the protection of the integrity agents from their execution environment.

We identified three main problems raising specific issues in test execution when the Implementation Under Test (IUT) is a mobile process.

First, it is clear that what can be tested, in any setting, depends on what can be observed. In a mobile setting, the IUT interacts with an execution platform which provides mobility and other services. Those actions are the ones which have to be tested, but they are typically not observable in common platforms such as Grasshopper [1] and Jade [2]. *Our first problem will be to make the interactions of the IUT with its execution platform observable.*

Second, the interaction between a tester or test system and the IUT goes through so-called Points of Control and Observation (PCOs). When the IUT is a mobile process, PCOs are attached to a mobile entity, i.e. they have to be dynamically modified after each migration of the IUT. It should be noted that PCOs are defined through primitives offered by execution platforms, which implies that the first problem of non-observability of those platforms have also to be taken into account here. *So the first problem, observability, has to be solved by adding PCOs to the system, and the second problem is that those PCOs are dynamic.*

Last, it is clear that a mobile process will be executed in several locations, existing in various configurations. Hence, the test environment should offer a way to define easily various configurations, in a tightly controlled way. In that way, tests would be able to validate an IUT sufficiently enough by defining the different configurations with which the IUT is bound to interact. Contrary to traditional network testing, where the number of configurations to address in a test is limited and static, so that it can be described enumeratively, *mobile code should be tested against a rich set of dynamic configurations.*

To solve those problems, we decided to go for an approach based on simulation of the environment representing the locations and services typically offered by a mobile agent platform. This is a natural choice as it provides the needed level of observability, control of the configurations and some control over the execution. We have implemented those ideas in a tool called SAM.

The rest of the paper is organized as follows. In section 2, we present the notion of code mobility we retain, and the MASIF framework. In section 3, we describe with more details the problems raised by testing mobile code and the specific issues we address. Section 4 describes our simulation tool, and how it helps in solving the problems of testing mobile processes. We conclude with a few results about our implementation.

2. CODE MOBILITY FRAMEWORK CONSIDERED

Simple mobile code techniques are based on code on demand and remote evaluation (e.g. applets, RMI). This results in moving static code and/or data. As mentioned in the introduction, we consider in this paper a richer form of mobility corresponding to mobile agent techniques which bring everything together and enable the autonomous migration of active processes under execution. This concept has been introduced by Telescript [18] to reduce network load and latency and to suit temporary network connectivity.

The technology supporting mobile agent takes a perspective which differs from classical distributed systems. In a mobile paradigm, as shown in Figure 1, the structure of the underlying computer network consists of execution sites layered upon the operating system. The purpose of these execution sites is to provide an execution context to agent applications which are able to dynamically relocate their execution. The concept of mobile agent raises two significant problems, related for the first one to the heterogeneity of the host systems (operating system and hardware) and for the second one to the management of the execution environment. More precisely, an environment for mobile agents must bring a solution to the following points: portability and code migration; mobility management; communication management; resources management; security management.

Portability and code migration problems are solved by the use of *MCLs(mobile code languages)* [6, 16], particularly adapted to the mechanisms of mobility. Indeed, these languages such as Java, Obliq, Objective Caml, Tcl, etc, are interpreted and offer a *runtime* allowing code insulation and migration, although some languages, for example Java, propose only a serialization mechanism of the code. In this case, the agent's state is not completely restored after its migration.

The other problems which are linked to the agent's execution management (migration, communication, authorization, ...) are solved in an

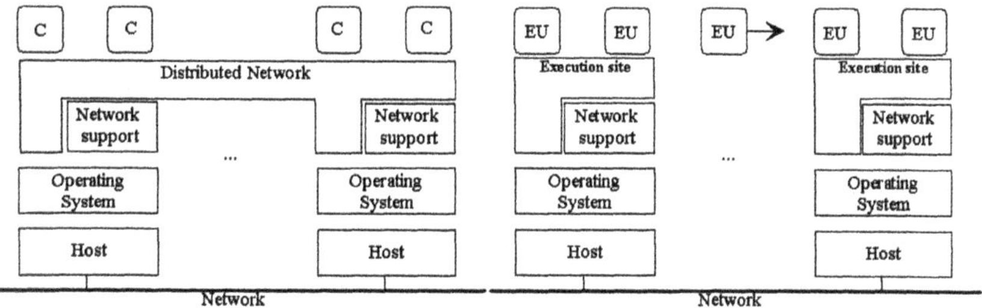

Figure 1. Classical distributed structures vs Mobile distributed structures

applicative way. A uniform solution is to consider the execution sites as a service-providing environment. The agent in this environment reaches the various services it needs by calling methods of an application which plays the role of the execution site.

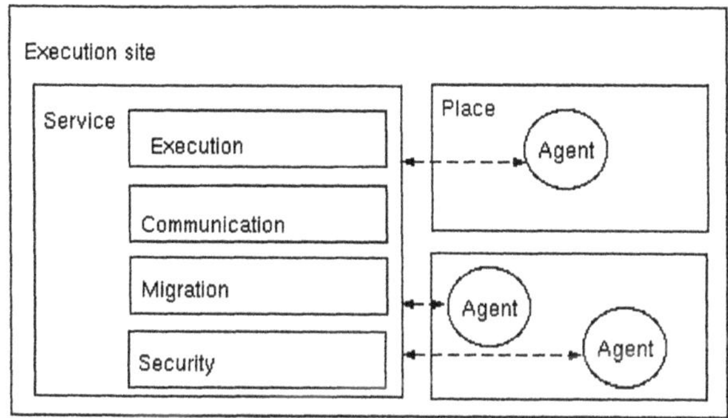

Figure 2. Hierarchical structure of the components (MASIF)

MASIF [15] clearly defines this hierarchy between agent and execution sites, as shown in Figure 2. However, MASIF is limited to interoperability between execution sites. Hence, it addresses the site interface and concepts, but not the problems of language interoperability and the standardization of agents' actions, such as migration and communication. So, it can be said that MASIF defines the interfaces at the execution site level rather than at agent level. MASIF standardizes agent management primitives (creation, execution, suspension, termination..), agent transfert primitives (sending and reception) and syntaxes and terms defining for example agent and execution site names, their characteristics and their properties.

In the rest of this paper, our study of test for mobile process is based on the MASIF framework. In this framework, agents encapsulated by an execution unit act on behalf of a person and are executed in logical places hosted by an execution site. Agents have the ability to move from place to place and to communicate with other agents to perform their computation task.

3. TESTING ISSUES ADDRESSED

3.1 Testing problems addressed

Testing is an operational way to check the correctness of a system implementation by means of experimenting with it. Testing a software system built on agents can be addressed from different points of views. Our choices were motivated by the current concerns of developers of telecommunication services based on this technology. They can be summed up as follows.

We address black-box testing of agents The test system interacts with agents only through their interfaces, either with the "upper" environment (consisting of other agents, user requests...) or with the underlying platform.

We are dealing with systems of multiple interacting agents In a sense, at that level, we are doing grey-box testing as we have access to interactions between agents and platforms. We are not testing agent platforms.

We concentrate on *functional* testing of those systems. We are not addressing the specific problems of other types of tests, such as load and stress tests. Also, our framework is not that of conformance testing as we are in a situation where there would be well defined reference specifications to which we would have to compare several implementations.

We address functional *interoperability* testing beetwen agents. One key point is that we consider software built on multiple agents running on different types of platforms, languages and paradigms. Therefore we tackle specifically the problems raised by *interoperability* (functional) testing of multiple platforms, interconnected through a MASIF framework.

We do not address the problem of test design, test selection. On the other hand, we provide a basis for expressing tests to be run on our testing environment. We provide a test language, which is abstract in the sense that it provides means of expressing tests which are independent from the platforms, and can adapt to various types of platforms.

Finally, in our research, we concentrate on features specific to mobile code. Although multi-agent systems are distributed systems, we do not deal with problems already studied in the considerable amount of research done for distributed systems, such as synchronization of testers, timing of events.

Capitalizing on the advances done in the theory of network testing e.g. [17], we first tried [13] to give a semantic basis to the test of mobile processes by extending IOLTS with a notion of location and atomic mobility actions. This amounted to suppose that the mobility of processes is part of their observable behaviour. We then showed it was possible to automatically generate sound tests which take into account mobility. However we did not continue this line of work, because this preliminary study showed that migration actions must be observable if we want testing of mobile processes to be significant. Unfortunately, this is not true for common execution platforms. This is what sparked our interest in the problems of test execution for mobile processes.

3.2 Test environment: our choice of simulation

Mobile agents depend upon their execution platforms for their execution, and specially for executing migration and communication actions. Those execution platforms are typically neither controllable nor observable: for example, migration is defined as a primitive service of the platforms, and are executed through system calls to the platform. So, the question for testing mobile agents is how to establish so-called Points of Control and Observation (PCOs)?

Testing mobile agents makes it necessary to define a testing context which will be able to fulfill two different goals. First, it will be used for the execution of mobile agents; second, it will enable the observation of those agents and their controllability.

A first solution could be to *instrument* existing execution platforms. Execution of mobile agents implies calls to platform primitives, which could be made observable and controllable by modifying the platform itself. This raises a few problems. First, such an instrumentation would probably require to have access to the source code of the execution platform, which is generally not available. Second, a different instrumentation work should be made for each different platform. And last, tests written for one mobile agent executing on a given platform could not be directly reused if this agent was rewritten for executing on another platform, because the tests would be written for observing (and controlling) actions which are executed as primitives specific to each platform.

Similar problems of control and observation exist in the field of embedded software. Indeed, as soon as software is placed inside an embedded environment, it is very difficult to observe it thoroughly. Hence, prior testing is made using a simulator which will emulate the embedding context of such software. A simulator makes it easy to test the software in various different contexts which correspond to the different possible embedding contexts. Likewise, in the context of testing mobile agents, we also propose to use a simulation tool.

This tool should incorporate what are the common points between different execution platforms, in that way offering a generic context for testing mobile agents. A standard such as MASIF [15] can be used as a starting point to identify common concepts between different platforms. Mappings between specific execution platforms and this generic simulation tool will have to be implemented. In that way, mobile agents designed for a specific platform could be executed without modification. Their calls to primitives of the platform would in fact be directed to the simulation tool through the mappings defined for each platform. Such calls would of course be made controllable and observable, enabling the execution of tests on the mobile agent coupled with the simulator. This also would enable to reuse tests when rewriting mobile agents for different platforms, since tests will not be attached to a given platform but could be defined directly in terms of the simulator's primitives.

We implemented those principles in a tool called SAM (*Simulation d'Agents Mobiles*), presented in detail in the following section.

4. A TOOL FOR TESTING MOBILE AGENT SYSTEMS

4.1 Goals and overview

Our goal is to offer an observable and controllable environment for executing systems made of mobile agents. Those multi-agent systems could then be tested, once they are made observable and controllable.

We want to be able to test systems targetting various execution platforms. We use MASIF and FIPA standards for defining a common model, generic enough for encompassing the maximum number of existing execution platforms. We describe in 4.2 the general architecture of our execution platform, and how it enables to execute agents defined for other platforms, and we see in 4.3 the different services offered to mobile agent systems by SAM.

Tests will have to be executed in this multi-agent setting, and for preserving the unity of this framework, we decide to consider test programs themselves as multi-agent systems. We defined our own test language, based on ideas originating in the notion of observers [10], using as starting point the reactive script language [4]. We call such test programs observation agents. We describe these notions with more detail in 4.4.

4.2 General architecture

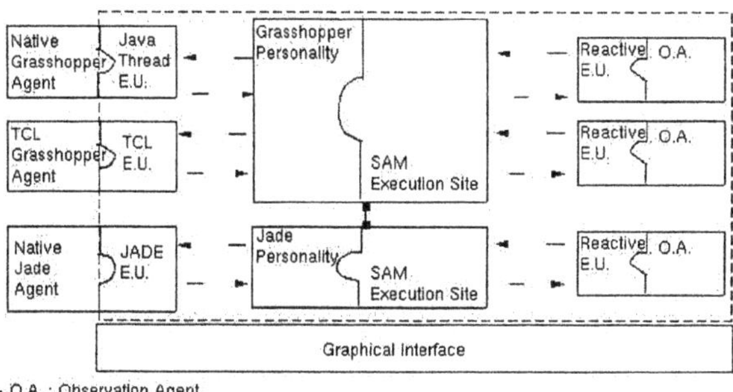

Figure 3. Tool architecture

The general architecture of our tool is described on Figure 3. This shows an example of what kind of system could be executed and tested using SAM. On the one hand, the Implementation Under Test is made of three agents executing and possibly migrating between two execution sites. One of the site is a simulated Grasshopper platform, with one native Grasshopper agent and a TCL one. The other site is a simulated Jade platform. On the other hand, the test program is made of three observation agents, written in our own test language. All those agents can migrate, and communicate with each other, and the observation agents can moreover react to specific actions of the IUT such as specific migrations or communications. For such an interaction to take place, without ever modifying the initial agents comprising the IUT, it is necessary to devise an architecture where different adapters can fit.

4.2.1 Generic execution sites. The main module defined by SAM are the execution sites. They are named environments that can create, interpret, execute, transfer and terminate agents. More generally, they offer all services (or primitives) defined by the MASIF and FIPA standards to all agents requesting them. As a starting point for our implementation, we used an user-custimizable MASIF implementation designed at France Telecom R&D, called MobiliTools [7].

SAM is designed to make the calls to those primitives observable by the observation agents. For this, SAM generates for each call an event in the execution runtimes of observation events. Those runtimes are synchronized virtual machines which enable to have events known simultaneously to all observation agents. See 4.4 for more details on this mechanism. Execution sites also have to manage the presence of agents, and for example they give access to management data such as the number of agents executing at a given moment.

Those generic sites can be customized by what we call personalities. Personalities propose a set of entry points making it possible to define specific execution environments. In this way, generic sites can offer interfaces similar to those provided by existing platforms.

4.2.2 Personalities. Personalities are adapters which enable generic sites to be seen as already existing platforms such as Grasshopper. They realize a mapping between the primitives specific to a given platform and those offered by the generic sites. For developing those personalities, we are helped by the emergence of standards such as MASIF. The concepts behind different platforms are very close to those defined for our generic sites, and the mappings are often only syntactic.

More than a simple adapter, a personality can encode the specificities of the simulated platform by a call-back mechanism. A call-back defines which procedures are invoked on the personality when one of the primitives of the generic execution site is performed. This call-back can modify the generic execution.

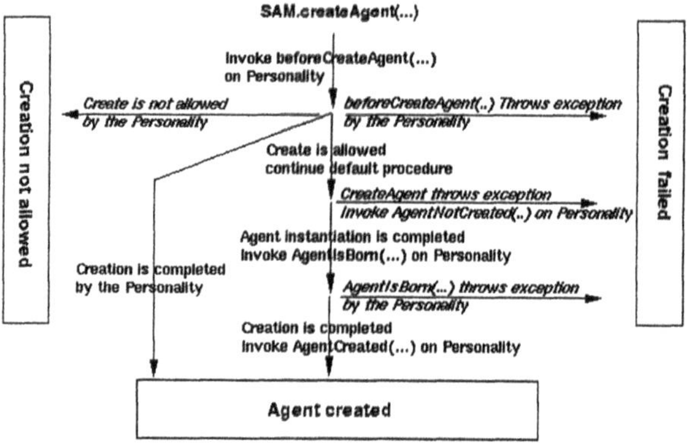

Figure 4. Call-back mechanism on personality: agent creation procedure

For example, when creating an agent (see Figure 4), the personality is notified by an agent creation request. The personality can then execute the request and return the reference of the created agent; refuse the action; or accept the default creation procedure initiated by SAM. In the last case, SAM carries out the creation action and notifies again the personality through the call-back *agentIsBorn*. The personality can then modify the reference of the created agent and realize some initializations on the agent or throw an exception to stop the initiated creation procedure.

4.2.3 Abstract execution unit. SAM does not handle directly the executed agents but abstracts them to an entity which we name execution unit. Indeed, since an agent represents the sequential flow of computation of a process, according to its type the execution and the control of the process can be basically different. For example, agent run-time can be a Java or C++ thread, and the agent activity can be controlled by the agent (reactive control) or by the execution site (proactive control). Thus, to integrate those different models, SAM does not enforce any execution and activity model on the level of execution sites, and only gives entry points for implementing them. Section 4.3.1 gives an example of interaction between SAM and execution units.

Just as personalities, an execution unit is an adapter which enable generic sites to manage an agent. This adapter mainly consists of callbacks related to the management of agents. For example, when an agent should be suspended, the generic execution site calls the execution unit to suspend it, then the execution unit computes or not the action and returns the result. Thus, the interface representing the abstraction of the execution unit defines the runtime of the agent implementation.

We choose to move the execution environment of the agent on agent level, because it makes it possible to dissociate the agent behaviour linked to the functionalities of the simulated system of the mechanism which execute and manage it. For example, as Figure 3 shows, agents implemented in different languages can be executed on a same site because they offer the same interface through the execution unit.

4.2.4 Graphical interface. We developed a simple interface for accessing SAM. It enables to visualize the existing execution sites, and which agents execute on them. It also provides a little shell language for enabling a human tester to manage the system under test (e.g. launching and destroying agents as required by the tests).

4.3 Services

4.3.1 Activity management. Activity management in SAM is related to the agent life-cycle defined in MASIF. An agent can be activated, suspended, resumed and finished. As we saw before, activity management and run-time of the agents are moved on execution unit level. This one being informed by the execution site of a change of activity can compute it. Let us note that the personality can also refuse the change of activity (see Figure 5).

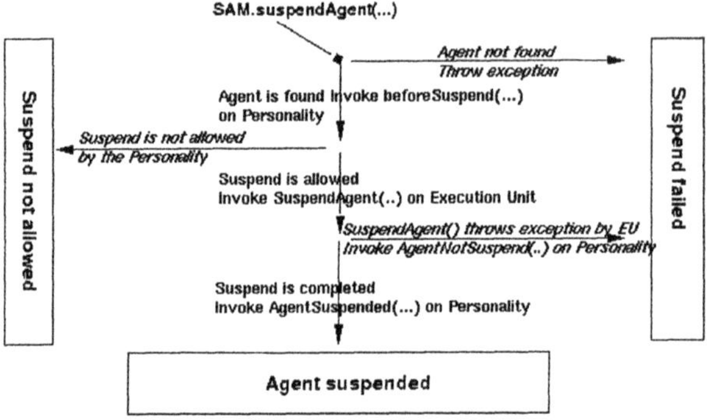

Figure 5. Call-back mechanism: suspend activity procedure

4.3.2 Communication. The communication mechanism implemented in SAM is independent from a specific platform, and conforms to the FIPA model. Agents can send messages to named mailboxes. Those (unique) names can be acquired during communication with other agents or by a naming service offered by generic execution sites. Also, agents can create mailboxes. Those mailboxes can be configured in one of two modes. In store mode, all incoming messages are stored, and the agent retrieve the stored messages by calling a designated primitive. In forward mode, the agent is notified of all incoming messages. A dedicated mechanism ensures this forward even if the agent has left the site. Mailboxes can migrate with their creating agents, following the policy defined by the personnality of the execution site (for example, this is not the case with Jade personalities). This general mechanism enables to implement a variety of synchronous or asynchronous communication methods, such as the method-call mechanism used in Grasshopper.

Finally, let us note that a particular communication mechanism (described in section 4.4) exists between observation agents.

4.3.3 Mobility. On the base of MASIF primitives, we have implemented two kinds of mobility: mobility by cloning, where a clone of the agent moves and simple agent migration.

Migration induces the backup and the restoration of the agent state, but this mechanism is closely related to the runtime of the agent. Thus, as for activity management, mechanisms of code insulation in an appropriate SAM structure are moved to execution unit level, and SAM enables the migration of this structure. So, SAM does not enforce any mobility level and remains generic. Since most agent platforms are implemented in Java, SAM also proposes in a native way the Java object serialization mechanism.

4.3.4 Security. Security is a crucial and difficult problem with mobile code [14]. In SAM we just provide entry points which will enable to develop security policies adapted to the different personalities. Those security policies will be called on the personalities of execution sites when agents try to reach or use remote or local entities. They return booleans indicating whether the operation is authorized. If no policy is defined, the returned booleans are always true.

4.4 Observation agents and test language

The observation notion is linked to the main tester whose role is to stimulate the implementation under test and to observe its reactions for returning a verdict on its conformity. Our idea is to integrate into the tool such entities. We name these entities *observation agents*: those two nouns attest that they have both an observation and an active role.

To that end, we develop a high-level language to describe observation agents. This is similar to the notion of observation language that was proposed for protocol verification in [10] and later implemented in the Veda verification-oriented simulator [12]. Initially, the objective was to replace the human reading of traces, but the concept was enriched following the idea that the observation language used should not be restrained and should allow any operations on the simulation. In the same spirit, we do not see observation agents only as testers. The goal is to make the test tool able to execute tests in a richer environment. For that, the notion of observation agent should exceed the notion of tester and be extended to concepts such as resources or other active entities useful in the development and the enrichment of the environment.

The programming language for observation agents must not restrict the expressivity to the tester description, but may include any other function that a test pilot might consider of interest. For example, we must be able to program entities of different natures, such as testers agents, to guide the test, to check the conformity of the implementation, and give a verdict; resource agents or stubs, to enrich the environment; control agents, to check on-line properties of the implementation; tools agents, programmed by the human tester to analyze the events on test execution. Lastly, the semantics of the language has to be well defined and in direct relationship to the concept of abstract test, which can be considered as a finite state machine.

For conveniency reasons, we decided to extend an existing script language [4] with features of test and object language, such as verdict, method-call, thread, etc. In coherence with the exposed principles, we use the reactive objects studied in [3]. Initiated from the actors world, the reactive objects are autonomous passive or active entities, which are executed in parallel. Based on a semantics of kept events - the transition selected usually depends on a certain stimulus (event input) or boolean expression (guard) -, the reactive approach provides programmers with concurrency, broadcast events, alternative steps, and several primivitives for gaining fine control over the execution of reactive programs.

In this model, reactive agents are executed on a reactive synchronized machine which is an abstraction of an execution unit, controlled by the tool. All reactive machines are synchronized together, in such a way that all observation agents share the same notion of instant. Thus, there is a kind of global logical clock, used by parallel agents to synchronize together, and a new instant can only take place when all parallel agents have finished their execution for the current instant.

The purpose of the reactive machine is to execute the reactive instructions of the observation agents in an environment made of instantaneous broadcast events. Observation agents share the same environment, and communicate using such events. Moreover, new processes or events can be added dynamically in the reactive machine. The observable actions at the SAM level are added in that way, making them instantaneously broadcast to all observation agents. This makes the programming of those agents which have to react to those events quite easy, because the developer does not have to take into account how the events are made known to the testers. Note that synchronization of observation agents is non-trivial since SAM allows for distributed simulation.

Using so tightly synchronized machines would be inefficient in a widely distributed setting, with execution sites far distant from each other, that is in the context of deployment of real multi-agent systems. But this is not our goal here: we just want to test such systems in a controlled way. In that setting where we control the distance between execution sites, the simplicity given by the complete synchronisation between testers and observed events for programming testers seems to us more important that the loss of realism implied by the synchronization hypotheses.

Finally, the formal semantics of the language, based on transition system is very close to abstract test semantics. And the writing of tests is completely independent of the language of the tested system, hence tests can be reused on different implementations of the same specification.

5. RESULTS AND PERSPECTIVES

Development of applications based on mobile agents is still in its infancy, and the software development problems related to this approach still need a fair amount of research to reach the level of maturity achieved in other fields of software development, especially for critical systems. Although testing is often the last part of development to be studied, we consider that it is becoming quite urgent to develop suitable testing approaches to ensure that the applications developed are safe enough.

In this paper, we presented an approach based on a simulation of an underlying platform for mobile agents compliant with the MASIF an FIPA standard. This makes it possible to test in a well controlled environment the behaviour of an application based on a set of mobile processes. Of course, one of the main limits is that it does not test the behaviour of the application on a real environment. Although the tool may be tuned to represent specific characteristics of a real platform (e.g. performance, response time under various loads).

We have implemented those ideas in a first prototype. Our implementation language is Java. The tool enables to execute observation agents written using reactive objects, but also agents designed to execute upon the Grasshopper [1] and Jade [2] platforms. It also offers full support for the MASIF and FIPA standards, offering agent migration, communication, execution and management services.

Mappings to execution platforms proved to be easily written, as soon as the platform is advertised as MASIF-compliant. For example, implementing the Jade mapping took only four days to one of us which had no prior experience with this platform. This mapping is made of 2500 lines of Java code, for 125 ko, whereas the Jade sources use 2 Mo.

For validating SAM, we used all the examples distributed with the Grasshopper and Jade platforms. We were able to execute directly those examples without any modification, even without recompiling. Nevertheless, all migration and communication actions initiated by the agents in those examples were now observable: we wrote observation agents interacting with those examples, and observing them, again without recompiling the examples. This demonstrates how our tool can be used for functional black-box testing of multi-agent mobile systems.

For the future, we plan to demonstrate our approach by collaborating with the developers of multi-agents systems inside FT R&D.[1] SAM will be evaluated as a development tool inside an internal research project.

[1]France Télécom Research and Development

References

[1] C. Bäumer, M. Breugst, S. Choy, and T. Magedanz. Grasshopper — A universal agent platform based on OMG MASIF and FIPA standards. In *First International Workshop MATA'99*, October 1999.

[2] Fabio Bellifemine, Agostino Poggi, and Giovanni Rimassa. JADE — A FIPA-compliant agent framework. In *Proceedings of the 4th International Conference PAAM-99*, London, UK, 1999.

[3] F. Boussinot, G. Doumenc, and J.B. Stefani. Reactive Objects. *Annals of Telecommunications*, 51:459–473, 1996.

[4] Frédéric Boussinot and Laurent Hazard. Reactive scripts. In *International Conference on Real-Time Computing Systems and Applications (RTCSA'96)*, Seoul, October 1996. IEEE.

[5] A. Carzaniga, G.P Pico, and G. Vigna. Designing Distributed Application with Mobile Code Paradigms. In ACM Press, editor, *19th Conference on Software Engineering (ICSE'97)*, pages 22–32, 1997.

[6] G. Cugola, C. Ghezzi, G. Pico, and G. Vigna. Analyzing Mobile Code Languages. *Mobile Object Systems, Lecture Notes in Computer Science*, 1222:94–109, February 1997.

[7] Bruno Dillenseger. Mobilitools: A toolbox for agent mobility and interoperability based on omg standards. In *2nd International Symposium ASA/MA2000*, Zürich, September 2000.

[8] FIPA. FIPA97 Specification. In *Foundation for Intelligent Physical Agents* available from http://www.fipa.org.

[9] A. Fuggetta, G.P. Pico, and G. Vigna. Understanding Code Mobility. In *IEEE Transactions on Softwarw Engineering*, volume 24, pages 342–360, May 1998.

[10] R. Groz. Unrestricted verification of protocol properties in a simulation using an observer approach. In Bochmann & Sarikaya, editor, *In Proceedings of the IFIP WG 6.1 6th Workshop on Protocol Specification, Testing, and Verification*, pages 255–256, Gray Rocks - Montréal, Canada, June 1986.

[11] R. Groz and N. Risser. Eight years of experience in test generation from fdts using tveda. In *In Proceedings of FORTE/PSTV'97*, Osaka, November 1997.

[12] C. Jard, R. Groz, and J.F. Monin. Development of Veda, a prototyping tool for distributed algorithms. *IEEE Transactions on Software Engineering*, 14(3):339–352, March 1988.

[13] M. Marche and Y.M. Quemener. Une approche formelle pour le test de conformité de processus mobile. In *Proceedings of Renpar'12*, Juin 2000.

[14] Jonathan T. Moore. Mobile code security techniques. Technical Report MSCIS -98-28, University of Pennsylvania, Department of Computer and Information Science, May 1998.

[15] OMG. Mobile Agent Systems Interoperability Facilities Specification (MASIF). available from http://www.camb.opengroup.org/RI/MAF/.

[16] Tommy Thorn. Programming Languages for Mobile Code. Technical Report 3134, INRIA, March 1997.

[17] J. Tretmans. Conformance testing with labelled transitions systems: Implementation relations and test generation. *Computer Networks and ISDN Systems*, (29):49–79, 1996.

[18] James E. White. Telescript technology: Mobile agents. Available as General Magic White Paper.

TESTING ACCESS TO EXTERNAL INFORMATION SOURCES IN A MEDIATOR ENVIRONMENT

Zoltán Ádám MANN
Budapest University of Technology and Economics, Hungary
Department of Control Engineering and Information Technology
zoltan.mann@cs.bme.hu

Jacques CALMET and Peter KULLMANN
University of Karlsruhe, Germany
Institute for Algorithms and Cognitive Systems
{calmet,kullmann}@ira.uka.de

Abstract This paper discusses the testing of communication in the increasingly important class of distributed information systems that are based on a mediator architecture.

A mediator integrates existing information sources into a new application. In order to answer complex queries, the mediator splits them up into subqueries which it sends to the information sources, and it combines the replies to answer the original query. Since the information sources are usually remote, autonomous systems, the access to them can be erroneous, most notably when the information source is subject to modifications. Such errors may result in incorrect behaviour of the whole system. This paper addresses the problem of deciding whether an information source as part of a mediatory system was successfully queried or not.

The primary contribution is a formal framework for the general information access testing problem. Besides proposing several solutions, it is investigated what the most important quality measures of such testing methods are. Moreover, the practical usability of the presented approaches is demonstrated on a real-world application using Web-based information sources. Several empirical experiments are conducted to compare the presented methods with previous work in the field.

Keywords: Mediator, information access testing, wrapper verification, information integration, autonomous information sources

1. INTRODUCTION AND PREVIOUS WORK

In the past decades a tremendous amount of data has been stored in electronic form. In recent years, as a consequence of the unbelievable evolution of the World Wide Web, practically any information one can imagine can be found in one format or the other in the WWW.

However, this is not enough for the requirements of the future information society. The problem is not the amount of available information, which is already more than sufficient, but its usability. Information sources (ISs) are designed for their particular purposes, but need to be reused in completely different applications, in conjunction with other pieces of information. This not only holds for the Web but also for a variety of other ISs, such as relational and object-oriented databases, electronic documents, computer algebra systems, specialized software libraries, *etc.*

Mediators. To address the problem of integrating heterogeneous, autonomous ISs, Wiederhold suggested the *mediator* pattern in [16]. The mediator implements the common tasks of splitting complex queries into simpler ones that can be sent to the underlying ISs and combining the replies to answer the original query. The latter also includes the detection and handling of potential conflicts that may arise if two ISs return contradictory results.

The ISs are bound into the mediator architecture via *wrappers*: components that translate queries from the language of the mediator into that of the ISs and the answers from the language or the data model of the IS into that of the mediator. The resulting architecture is depicted in figure 1. More information on mediators can be found *e.g.* in [6, 15].

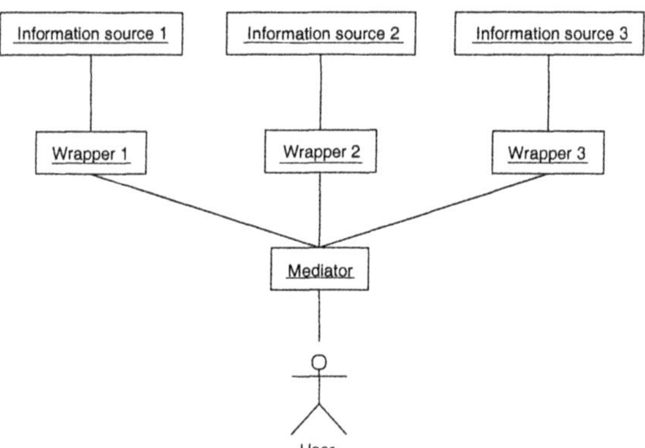

Figure 1 The mediator architecture

The context of the work presented in this paper was provided by KOMET (Karlsruhe Open MEdiator Technology [1]), a logic-based mediator shell developed at the University of Karlsruhe. KOMET uses the declarative language KAMEL (KArlsruhe MEdiator Language), which is based on annotated logic. It provides a framework for the easy construction of mediators, and enables the reuse of existing code.

A particular mediator system, called MetaSearch [2], which is implemented using KOMET, was of special interest. MetaSearch is a meta Web search program that takes queries and delegates them to various Internet search engines such as AltaVista and Google. It then combines the answers of the search engines into one answer page.

MetaSearch is very important for two reasons. First, with the spread of the World Wide Web, the integration of Web-based ISs becomes a major challenge and the most important application for mediator systems, and MetaSearch can be regarded as a prototype of such applications. Second, although MetaSearch is a relatively simple mediator application, it demonstrates very well the features of KOMET and also the problems that arise as a consequence of integrating remote, autonomous ISs.

Since the actual access to the external ISs is performed in the wrappers, they are of special importance from this paper's point of view. In the case of MetaSearch, the conversion from the language of the mediator into that of the IS is simple: it boils down to encoding the query into a URL. The conversion of the answer from the language of the IS into that of the mediator is somewhat more challenging, since the actual answer – the URL, title and excerpt of about 10 relevant pages – is embedded into an HTML page, along with plenty of other data, such as banners and statistics. Therefore the task of the wrapper is to extract the actual answer from the resulting page. In MetaSearch, regular expressions are used for that purpose.

Information access testing. Although regular expressions are not the only possibility for the extraction of information from HTML, this method illustrates the problem well: the information extraction mechanism has to rely on some regularity of the output of the IS. Since the IS is an autonomous system, it may be altered, which may in turn prevent the wrapper from extracting correctly. Thus, the aim of this paper is to investigate the problem of testing communication (*i.e.* access to the external ISs) in the special but increasingly important class of distributed information systems using a mediator-like middleware platform.

There has already been some research on this problem, though not much. The most relevant work is that of Kushmerick [8, 9]. His algorithm RAPTURE uses statistical features, such as length, number of words, number of special characters *etc.* to characterize the extracted text segments. It learns the parameters of normal distributions describing the feature distributions of the extracted pieces of texts. These normal distributions are used to estimate the probability that a new wrapper output is correct.

Much of the remaining scientific work focuses on the automatic creation of wrappers (see *e.g.* [5, 13] and references therein), but there are also some results that can be used for the wrapper testing problem as well. Cohen [3] uses a notion of textual similarity to find "structure" in Web pages: this is useful mainly in wrapper induction but may also be used in wrapper testing and maintenance, because it can detect changes in the structure of the HTML page. Lerman *et. al.* developed DATAPRO [10], an algorithm that uses tokens (words or generalizations of words) to represent text, and learns significant sequences of tokens – sequences that are encountered significantly more often than would be expected by chance. Thus the tuples to be extracted can be characterized by a set of significant token sequences, and a change in them can help discover changes in the HTML layout.

It can be seen that although there are already some promising results, the problem of IA (information access) testing in a mediator environment needs more thorough research because the existing results apply only to a very restricted problem class. The most important restrictions are: (i) only Web-based applications have been investigated; (ii) only errors produced by layout changes have been covered; (iii) only syntactic testing methods for the wrapper output have been proposed. Accordingly, this paper addresses the more general question: how to check whether or not the access to an external IS was correct?

Main results and paper organization. One of the main contributions of the paper is a formal notational framework that enables the definition of the information access testing problem (IATP) in its most general form (section 2). Existing results can be placed naturally in this framework. Moreover, it enables proving the hardness of the IATP (Theorem 1).

Another major problem with the existing results is that although the proposed methods can detect almost every change in the HTML layout, they often give false positives, *i.e.* they relatively often claim correct wrapper outputs to be erroneous. Section 3 investigates how the quality of IA testing can be measured, and demonstrates why the high rate of false positives is intrinsic (Theorem 2).

In section 4, several methods are presented that can be used generally for IA testing in a mediator environment. In particular, the applicability in a Web-based setting is also covered. Section 5 is a case study: it illustrates how the presented methods can be applied in practice, namely in the case of MetaSearch. It is demonstrated with several measurements, how – with appropriate techniques – better testing quality can be achieved. Section 6 concludes the paper.

2. PROBLEM DEFINITION

This section provides a general notational framework for the investigation of the information access testing problem (IATP). Note that the framework will have to cope with the following difficulties: (i) it will have to allow and tolerate some degree of ambiguousness in the replies of ISs; (ii) the testing theory of ISs as systems under test is different from the better understood case of finite state machines (FSM) because of the unavailability of state and specification information.

In order to make the definitions clear, figure 2 shows the whole communication model.

Definition 2.1 (Messages on communication channels) *Let the alphabet of the communication system be the finite set Σ. Thus, messages are elements of Σ^*. ε, the empty string, is also an element of Σ^*. Let ν be a symbol with $\nu \notin \Sigma^*$. ν means 'no message'.*

Note that $\nu \neq \varepsilon$, *i.e.* we differentiate between an empty message and 'no message'.

The following definition describes the interface of ISs. Note that – since ISs are assumed to be completely autonomous – we have no knowledge about their internal state. The only thing we know is that an IS accepts queries, to which it (usually) gives a reply.

Definition 2.2 (Information source) *An information source is a family of functions $I_t : \Sigma^* \rightarrow \Sigma^* \cup \nu$ $(t \in \mathbb{R})$. $I_t(q) = r, r \in \Sigma^*$ means that, at time t, the reply of the IS on query q is r. On the other hand, if $r = \nu$, this means that the IS gave no reply.*

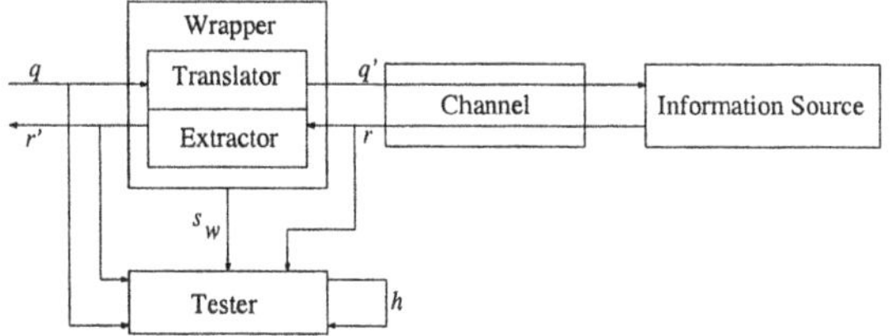

Figure 2 The underlying model

Definition 2.3 (Wrapper) *A wrapper W is a pair of Turing machines, $W = (T, E)$. The translator T implements a function $F_T : \Sigma^* \rightarrow \Sigma^*$,* *translating queries. The extractor E implements a function $F_E : \Sigma^* \cup \nu \rightarrow \Sigma^*$, extracting the replies of the IS.*

Note that, in contrast to ISs, wrappers have a known internal structure (Turing machine). Moreover, they do not change over time. It is also important to note that even if the IS gives no reply, the wrapper has to return something, *i.e.* $F_E(\nu) \in \Sigma^*$. (Although not stated explicitly in the definition, it is assumed that the wrapper can also aggregate and reuse information from its usage history, and thus perform learning.)

Now the task is to implement the IA tester (IAT, or simply: tester), *i.e.* the function that can tell whether the access was correct or not:

Definition 2.4 (Information access tester) *An IAT is a function $V : \Sigma^* \times (\Sigma^* \cup \nu) \times \Sigma^* \times S_W \times H \rightarrow \{correct, incorrect\} \times H$, where $V(q, r, r', s_W, h)$ is the judgement of the tester on the wrapper output r', extracted from the reply r of the IS, given on query q; s_W is any state information of wrapper W, and h is any additional 'historical' information that the tester has collected over time, which is also updated as part of the IAT output.*

It can be seen from this definition that the tester may make use of many observations and different kinds of knowledge; however, it does not have to. As noted in the Introduction, previous work has focused on IA testing using only the wrapper output r'.

The definition assumes that wrappers are not autonomous (as opposed to ISs) so that the IAT has access to their state information. So wrappers are 'observable' Turing machines.

The above definition allows many different testers; the goal is to create the best one in some sense:

Definition 2.5 (Information access testing problem) *Let U be the set of possible testers, $f : U \rightarrow \mathbb{R}$ the objective function. The general IATP consists of constructing the tester V^* which maximizes f on U.*

It would be logical to use the objective function

$$f_0(V) = \begin{cases} 1 & \text{if } V\text{'s judgement is always right} \\ 0 & \text{otherwise} \end{cases}$$

which would mean finding the *perfect* tester. However, this is infeasible:

Theorem 1 *The perfect tester has to be able to tell if the IS or the wrapper has fallen into an infinite loop. Therefore, the perfect tester would solve the Halting Problem of Turing machines, which is not algorithmically solvable.* □

Consequently, we will have to settle for a less ambitious objective. That is, we are looking for methods that work well in most practical cases. To that end, we suggest more realistic objective functions for the evaluation of testers in section 3. Moreover, we have surveyed the typical errors that have to be coped with during the access to external information sources in [12].

Note that the proof of Theorem 1 cannot be made fully precise until the notion of the 'perfect tester' is formalized. This is an important future research issue. Moreover, it might be argued that the IAT already assumes the wrapper output in its input, so there is no need to detect infinite loops. However, this is not true since one of the tasks of the IAT is exactly input handling, *i.e.* deciding if it should wait longer for its input or take it as ν. (Note that it is required that the IAT produce its output after a finite amount of time.)

Finally, one more definition is given. A restricted set of ISs, namely search engines, is of special importance in the paper:

Definition 2.6 (search engine) *A search engine is an IS with* $I_t(q) = (T, U, X)^c$, *where* c *is the number of tuples returned, and each tuple consists of the title* T, *the URL* U, *and the excerpt* X *of a Web page.*

3. QUALITY MEASURES OF IA TESTING

Since it is infeasible to strive for a perfect tester, the aim should be to construct one that is as 'good' as possible. This section tries to formalize the word 'good'. The benefit of this is threefold: (i) the presented quality measures can guide the construction of high-quality testers; (ii) a well-defined comparison of IA testing mechanisms (to be presented in section 4) is made possible; (iii) the introduced formalism sheds some light on common problems with the methods presented in the literature, and it can be proven why this is intrinsic.

If it is infeasible to expect that the judgement of the tester always be correct, it is a natural requirement that its correctness should be as high as possible, in a statistical sense. In order to formalize this, assume that the tester performs N tests, *i.e.* it tests N accesses of a wrapper W to an external IS I_t. The number of flawless accesses is k, the number of accesses during which an error occurred is $N-k$. In each test, the tester must give a judgement whether or not the access was erroneous. The number of tests in which the judgement of the tester is right is denoted by m, thus the number of tests in which the judgement of the tester is false, is $N-m$.

Definition 3.1 (statistical correctness) *The statistical correctness of the tester is* $SC = m/N$.

What does this number express? For instance, is a SC of 0.9 bad or good? Is a SC of 0.999 much better than that of 0.99? The answer to these questions depends on the value of k/N. Generally, it can be assumed that the wrapper works properly most of the time, and errors rarely occur. This implies $k \approx N$. A 'dull' tester that simply judges every access to be correct, has $m = k$ and thus its statistical correctness is $SC_{dull} = k/N \approx 1$!

As can be seen, even a very high value of SC can be bad if it is not significantly higher than k/N. What follows is that SC alone is not expressive enough. The cause of this phenomenon is that one of the outcomes of the test has a much higher probability than the other.

A similar problem arises in the medical sciences, in the context of routine tests for diseases. Since only a small minority of the population is infected, the probability that the patient suffers from a given disease is very low. The problem of evaluating the quality of a particular test methodology is analogous to the problem of evaluating IA testers. To solve this problem, different quality measures are used that are more expressive than SC [4]:

Definition 3.2 (specifity and sensitivity)

$$\begin{aligned} specifity &= Pr(test\ result\ is\ negative|patient\ is\ healthy) \\ sensitivity &= Pr(test\ result\ is\ positive|patient\ is\ ill) \end{aligned}$$

Adapted to the case of IA testing:

$$\begin{aligned} specifity &= Pr(judgement: 'correct'|access\ was\ correct) \\ sensitivity &= Pr(judgement: 'erroneous'|access\ was\ erroneous) \end{aligned}$$

The definition of specifity and sensitivity is symmetric, but the large difference between the probabilities of the possible judgements makes them differently expressive. In order to clarify this, we introduce the reverse conditional probabilities:

Definition 3.3 (negative and positive predictive values)

$$\begin{aligned} NPV &= Pr(access\ correct|judgement\ is: 'correct') \\ PPV &= Pr(access\ erroneous|judgement\ is: 'erroneous') \end{aligned}$$

These are actually the most important quality measures because they show how 'trustworthy' the tester is. That is: if the tester judges the access to be correct/erroneous, what is the probability that the access was really correct/erroneous, respectively?

There is an interesting connection between these values, as captured by the theorem below. First some abbreviations: x = specifity, y = sensitivity, $p = Pr$(the access was erroneous), $q = Pr$(judgement is: 'erroneous').

Theorem 2 *(i) If $x \to 1$ and $y \to 1$ and $p \to 0$ and $q \to 0$, then $NPV \to 1$, but PPV does not necessarily converge to 1.*
(ii) If $x \to 1$ and $y \to 1$, then

$$\frac{\partial PPV}{\partial x} \to \frac{1-p}{p} \quad \textit{and} \quad \frac{\partial PPV}{\partial y} \to 0.$$

As already noted, usually the wrapper functions correctly. It can also be assumed that the judgement of the tester is correct in most cases. This is why the theorem deals only with the case when x and y are high (near 1) and p and q are low (near 0). In this ideal case, one would expect that both predictive values converge to 1. The first claim of theorem 2 shows that this is true for NPV, but not for PPV. If PPV is not high enough, this means that the tester gives many false positives. This is exactly the reason why the testing mechanisms presented in the literature suffer from a relatively large number of false positives. This is an intrinsic property of the IATP. So, an otherwise almost perfect tester guarantees high NPV but not necessarily a high PPV. This also implies that only together can NPV and PPV be used as an expressive quality measure.
The second claim of theorem 2 explains the reason of this phenomenon: in the region where both specifity and sensitivity are high, PPV does not depend on the sensitivity anymore, but it depends heavily on the specifity. (Note that $\frac{1-p}{p}$ is a huge number.) Consequently, if the specifity is a little below 1, the positive predictive value suffers from it severely.

Proof. Using Bayes' theorem,

$$\begin{aligned} NPV &= \frac{Pr(\text{access correct, judgement : 'correct'})}{Pr(\text{judgement : 'correct'})} = \\ &= \frac{\text{specifity} \cdot Pr(\text{access correct})}{Pr(\text{judgement : 'correct'})} = \frac{x(1-p)}{1-q} \to 1 \end{aligned}$$

$$\begin{aligned} PPV &= \frac{Pr(\text{access erroneous, judgement : 'erroneous'})}{Pr(\text{judgement : 'erroneous'})} = \\ &= \frac{\text{sensitivity} \cdot Pr(\text{access erroneous})}{Pr(\text{judgement : 'erroneous'})} = \frac{yp}{q} \end{aligned}$$

The latter does not converge, since the limit would depend on whether p or q converges more rapidly to zero. This proves the first claim. (Note that the problem of a low PPV arises if and only if $p \ll q$, which condition also implies that the tester gives many false positives.)

To prove the second claim, the last expression is transformed so that it contains also x but not q:

$$PPV = \frac{yp}{yp + (1-x)(1-p)} = \frac{1}{1 + \frac{(1-x)(1-p)}{yp}}$$

Obviously, p depends neither on x nor on y. So the partial derivatives are:

$$\frac{\partial PPV}{\partial x} = \frac{1-p}{yp}\left(1 + \frac{(1-x)(1-p)}{yp}\right)^{-2} \to \frac{1-p}{p}$$
$$\frac{\partial PPV}{\partial y} = \frac{(1-x)(1-p)}{y^2 p}\left(1 + \frac{(1-x)(1-p)}{yp}\right)^{-2} \to 0$$

which proves the theorem. □

Beside the requirement that the tester should give correct judgements, there are other, non-functional, requirements that must also be met. To summarize: the 'price' that must be paid for the automatic testing should be kept as low as possible. The most important non-functional quality measures are: efficiency, programming effort (also including maintenance), generality (wrapper-independence), reusability, adaptability, total cost of testing. (A more detailed description can be found in [12].)

4. TESTING METHODS

This section presents various IA testing mechanisms, classified according to the principal concept of their mode of operation. At the end of the section a comparison of the presented methods is given. The practical applicability of the suggested testers will be covered in section 5.

Testing while the wrapper is extracting. The first group of testing schemes test the operation of the wrapper, and not only its output. They can be regarded as white-box test methods. The most important advantage of these methods is that at this point all information is available, whereas if only the output of the wrapper is investigated, the state information of the wrapper (S_W in definition 2.4) is lost. For instance, if the wrapper output is ε, this might be the result of an error but it can also be a valid reply of the IS; if the way the wrapper has worked is investigated, it might be possible to differentiate between these two cases.

The most important disadvantage of such methods is the high wrapper-dependence. Thus, if the wrapper is modified for some reason, the tester also has to be updated. This can increase maintenance costs and decrease reusability significantly.

Testing the output of the wrapper. The methods described in this paragraph make no use of information internal to the wrapper, only its output. This can be thought of as black-box testing. The advantages and disadvantages are exactly the opposite as before: the complete independence of the internal state of the wrapper is advantageous; however, the lack of this information may cause problems. As explained in the Introduction, most existing results use this paradigm for wrapper testing.

The principal idea behind these methods is that the wrapper output takes its values normally from a real subset of Σ^* (denoted by L), *i.e.* certain strings from Σ^* are not plausible. So the task of the tester can be defined as follows: given a wrapper output r, is $r \in L$? The theory of formal languages has invented several methods to represent large, possibly infinite sets finitely and compactly, supposed that the given set is sufficiently structured. For example, a regular grammar, or equivalently, a finite automaton can be used in some cases to encode the set L.

However, the classical results of the theory of formal languages are in many cases insufficient. Most existing work in the literature of wrapper verification focuses on more powerful methods for the testing of the wrapper output (see section 1 and [12] for more details).

Testing using additional ISs. The detection of semantic errors requires additional, more or less domain-specific knowledge. In a mediator system the most natural way to integrate additional knowledge is the integration of new ISs. These ISs can then be used by the tester to determine if the output of the accessed IS makes sense in the given context. Hence, redundancy is achieved, which can generally be used to improve system reliability [14].

Test queries. In testing conventional software systems, regression tests play a vital role [8]. They involve comparison of the output of the system with the known correct output for various inputs – as in black-box testing in general. Unfortunately, this scheme cannot be used directly in the case of the IATP, because it is by no means guaranteed that the IS answers the same query always with the same reply. Hence, this method can only be applied to the very restricted class of static ISs.

However, similar methods can be used more generally. For instance, in order to decide whether an empty wrapper output is correct or a result of an error, a test query can be used for which the IS will surely return a non-empty reply.

It can be generally stated that methods in this category can only be used efficiently in conjunction with other testing methods. However, they are very useful in some cases.

Testing the mediator system. All methods described above can also be used at a higher level, namely to test the whole mediator system instead of just one wrapper. This is in many cases more practical. If q ISs are integrated into the mediator system, this reduces the number of necessary testers from q to 1. Thus, testing is cheaper, more efficient and also more robust because the tester does not have to be modified after every change in the wrappers or the ISs. In many cases, it may not even be feasible to test the replies of each IS because the necessary additional knowledge is not available.

The main disadvantage of such methods is that not necessarily all errors are clear from the output of the mediator system. Thus, some errors can remain undetected, leading to lower sensitivity.

Comparison of the suggested methods. In most applications where communication is textual (*e.g.* in the WWW) the best choice is probably a syntactic test of the wrapper output, because it is relatively simple, it does not depend on the implementation details of the wrappers, and – as a result of the redundancy introduced by textual communication – many errors can be detected with such methods. Unfortunately, these methods can be quite inaccurate in some cases.

If syntactic testing schemes are not enough, more intelligent methods must be used. In this case, the integration of additional ISs should be considered, because this would make it possible to detect semantic errors. However, this will also increase testing costs and overhead significantly.

The other methods (test queries and testing during the operation of the wrapper) are rather special, but there are many cases in which they can be used successfully. Test queries should only be used together with other methods because they can only detect a fraction of all possible errors. Testing during the operation of the wrapper may be very effective; however, it makes maintenance quite hard, so it should only be used if absolutely necessary. If possible, an interface should be defined for the wrapper to communicate its internal state.

Several testing mechanisms have been proposed in this section. However, it is yet to be clarified how this functionality can be best embedded into the mediator architecture. Figure 1 reveals several places suitable for the integration of the tester. Also note that the choice of the tester and the way it should be integrated into the mediator architecture are not completely orthogonal. For a review of the most important possibilities for integrating the testing functionality into the mediator architecture, see [12].

5. CASE STUDY

We implemented several testing methods and conducted several experiments in order to: (i) demonstrate the applicability of the suggested methods; (ii) evaluate and compare the suggested methods; (iii) compare the results with others in the literature.

Implementation. The implementation took place in three steps: (i) an interactive, simplified version of MetaSearch (called ISMS) was created; (ii) several testing mechanisms were implemented; (iii) a batch program was written for the test of the implemented testing methods on a large set of data.

Implementation details of ISMS as well as the experiences made with it are described in [11]. Here we only report on the implemented testing methods and the batch test.

The following testing methods were implemented:

- A syntactic tester for the URLs, using the following regular expression:
```
^((http\://)|(ftp\://))?[-\+\w]+(\.[-\+\w]+)+(\:\d+)?\
(/\~[-\+\.%\w]+)?(/[-\+\.\,\:%\w]+)*/?(\?([-\+\.%\w]+\
=[-\+\.%\w/]+&)*[-\+\.%\w]+=[-\+\.%\w/]+)?$
```
- A syntactic tester for the titles. For this, a very simple but practically well performing method was used: `length(title)<100`.
- A similarly simple, syntactic tester for the excerpt: `0<length(excerpt)<300`.
- A more time-consuming semantic tester for the wrapper output. For this, the Internet itself was used as additional IS. Namely, the tester checks if the extracted URLs point to existing pages.

The third step of the implementation consisted of creating a batch program that evaluated the realized testing methods on a sufficiently large set of real-world test examples. Since wrapper errors are relatively rare, it is by no means easy to collect a set of test cases that contains enough erroneous accesses. Fortunately, Dr. Kushmerick of Department of Computer Science, University College Dublin has made the data he had collected in the period May – October 1998 [8, 9] available. This set of data contains the reply pages of 27 actual Internet sites on a couple of specific queries, collected for 6 months.

For the evaluation of the implemented testing methods, the replies of AltaVista, Lycos and MetaCrawler on the query 'happy' have been selected. In the given period of time there were two changes in the case of AltaVista, one in the case of Lycos and two in the case of MetaCrawler. Accordingly, three wrappers have been constructed for AltaVista, two for Lycos, and three for MetaCrawler. Each page was processed with the corresponding correct wrapper as well as with the other wrapper(s) of the particular search engine. This amounted to about 440 test cases.

Ultimately, we have conducted another set of experiments with a smaller set of current data. The goal was twofold: (i) to check if the results based on the three-year-old data set can be transferred to the current situation; (ii) to identify trends that may have an impact on future IA testing possibilities. In particular, we knew that lots of the URLs returned by the search engines three years ago would be invalid by now, thus corrupting our test results. So we checked how many of the URLs currently returned by the three search engines for the query 'happy' are invalid.

Test results. The results of the batch test are described in full detail in [11]. Five figures were stored for each test case: the number of extracted tuples, and the number of likely errors found by the four implemented testing methods.

The most important conclusion to be drawn from the results is that the implemented, intentionally very simple testing methods can be combined to a virtually perfect tester. Namely, there is a big difference in the behaviour of the utilized methods in the case of correct and incorrect wrapper outputs. In the erroneous case, the wrapper output was either empty, or at least one of the applied methods (but often all of them) judged all tuples to be erroneous. In the case of a correct wrapper output, the number of tuples judged to be syntactically incorrect was at most 40%, and of those judged to be semantically incorrect at most 70%. Moreover, it turned out from our experiments with current data that this last figure is normally much lower, in the range of 0-10%. Thus, there is indeed a wide gap in the behaviour of the testing methods in the correct and incorrect cases.

It is also interesting to investigate how much the individual testing methods contribute to the overall very good performance. Actually, two of the four methods – the syntactic testing methods for the URL and for the excerpt – would have been sufficient to distinguish between correct and incorrect wrapper outputs. But of course other errors are also possible for which the other tests are necessary. Hence, it is important to have at least one testing method for each element of the tuples so that errors concerning only that particular element can be detected.

It has to be noted as well that the principles behind MetaSearch and MetaCrawler are very similar, so that testing the output of MetaCrawler can also be regarded as the prototype of testing a whole mediator system. Hence, it is clear from the tests that the suggested methods are also appropriate for the testing of the whole mediator system.

Another important observation is that the set of changes of the output of search engines in 1998 and in 2001 was very similar. It seems that these modifications are caused by human behaviour, rather than by some particular technology because the latter changes rapidly. Consequently, similar changes are likely to occur in the future as well. This makes it possible to construct testers that can be used robustly for many years.

6. CONCLUSION

In this paper, we have presented the general information access testing problem (IATP) that arises in mediator systems, when making use of the integrated external, autonomous information sources. A formal framework was presented that allows the investigation of the problem in a setting as general as possible. This generalizes past results from the literature [3, 7, 9, 10]. We have proven that the general IATP is not solvable algorithmically in its most natural form, so we presented quality measures that make it possible to quantify imperfect, but in most cases properly working testers. We have investigated the connection between the most important quality measures, namely specifity, sensitivity and positive and negative predictive values.

In the other, more practically-focused part of the paper, possible solutions were suggested. Moreover, to illustrate the practical applicability of the presented algorithms, some testing schemes have been evaluated on MetaSearch, a simple, but real-world example mediator system.

The most important contributions of the paper are: (i) a general framework for the IATP; (ii) existing results can be transferred to and explained in the new framework; (iii) with careful redundancy techniques better results can be achieved; (iv) the framework allows the proof of intrinsic properties of the IATP with mathematic rigor; (v) the mathematical methods can be combined with an engineering approach to obtain the most important rules for the construction of efficient, economic testers; (vi) the framework shows many future research directions. In particular, the work presented in this paper could be applied to similar environments, where statistical testing is the only solution, raising the problems of significance of the test, quality and coverage of the test, and correctness of the test.

References

[1] J. Calmet, S. Jekutsch, P. Kullmann, and J. Schü. KOMET – A system for the integration of heterogeneous information sources. In *10th International Symposium on Methodologies for Intelligent Systems (ISMIS)*, 1997.

[2] J. Calmet and P. Kullmann. Meta web search with KOMET. In *International Joint Conference on Artificial Intelligence, Stockholm*, 1999.

[3] W. W. Cohen. Recognizing structure in web pages using similarity queries. In *AAAI-99 (Orlando)*, 1999.

[4] Cornell University, College of Veterinary Medicine. Diagnostic accuracy. `http://web.vet.cornell.edu/CVM/Imaging/notes_diagnosis.htm`.

[5] T. Goan, N. Benson, and O. Etzioni. A grammar inference algorithm for the world wide web. In *Proc. of the 1996 AAAI Spring Symposium on Machine Learning in Information Access (MLIA), Stanford, CA*. AAAI Press, 1996.

[6] Intelligent Information Integration, Inofficial home page. `http://www.tzi.org/grp/i3`.

[7] C. A. Knoblock, K. Lerman, S. Minton, and I. Muslea. Accurately and reliably extracting data from the web: a machine learning approach. *Data Engineering Bulletin*.

[8] N. Kushmerick. Regression testing for wrapper maintenance. In *Proc. of AAAI-99 (Orlando)*, pages 74–79, 1999.

[9] N. Kushmerick. Wrapper verification. *World Wide Web Journal*, 3(2):79–94, 2000. (Special issue on Web Data Management).

[10] K. Lerman and S. Minton. Learning the common structure of data. In *AAAI-2000 (Austin)*, 2000.

[11] Z. Á. Mann. Dynamische Validierung von Zugriffen auf externe Informationsquellen in einer Mediatorumgebung. Master's thesis, University of Karlsruhe, Institute for Algorithms and Cognitive Systems, 2001.

[12] Z. Á. Mann. Validating access to external information sources in a mediator environment. Technical report, `http://www.cs.bme.hu/~manusz/work/mediator-2001/techrep.pdf`, 2001.

[13] I. Muslea, S. Minton, and C. Knoblock. Hierarchical wrapper induction for semistructured information sources. *Journal of Autonomous Agents and Multi-Agent Systems*, 2001.

[14] B. Randell, J.-C. Laprie, H. Kopetz, and B. Littlewood, editors. *Predictably dependable computing systems*. Springer-Verlag, Berlin, 1995.

[15] V. S. Subrahmanian, S. Adalı, A. Brink, R. Emery, J. J. Lu, A. Rajput, T. J. Rogers, R. Ross, and C. Ward. HERMES: A heterogeneous reasoning and mediator system. Technical report, University of Maryland, 1995.

[16] G. Wiederhold. Mediators in the architecture of future information systems. *IEEE Computer*, 25(3):38–49, March 1992.

SESSION III

INDUSTRIAL SESSION I

COMPLIANCE OF WIRELESS APPLICATION PROTOCOLS

Ousmane Koné
LaBRI/CNRS - INPL***
* *351, Cours de la Libération F-33405 Bordeaux*
** *2, Avenue de la Forêt de Haye F-54516 Nancy*
kone@labri.fr - okone@ensem.inpl-nancy.fr

Abstract The work presented in this paper contributes to WAP testing effort, by proposing an approach to compliance tests development. Here, this approach is illustrated with the design of compliance or interoperability tests for the WSP-protocol operating over a WTP-service.

Keywords: Compliance, Interoperability, Wireless Systems, WAP, Internet, WWW.

1. INTRODUCTION

Wireless Application Protocols (WAP) constitute reference standards for the new architectures combining mobile telephony and Internet. In order to achieve reliability and interoperability, WAP implementations must be tested against these standards. According to the WAP forum, the testing process would follow two tracks/phases: track one, *Certification testing*, focused on WAP application level, and track two, *Compliance testing*, concerned with protocol level. To date, the main developments have been concerned with track one and since last year, more than 60 products from industry (mobile equipments and servers) have been WAP-certified. But we are not aware of developments on compliance issues which are the concern and contribution of our paper.

Some results of our work will be used in connection with a French RNRT project [11], in which we have been asked to propose test platforms for experimenting new industrial applications in wireless environment. Here, a testing approach to compliance of WAP sublayers, is proposed and illustrated with WSP (Wireless Session Protocol) layer.

Section 2 recalls some main issues related to WAP systems compliance. Section 3 provides a brief description of our testing approach. In section 4, we comment the results of this approach to the design of tests against WSP operating over a Wireless Transaction Service.

2. WAP SYSTEMS AGAINST COMPLIANCE

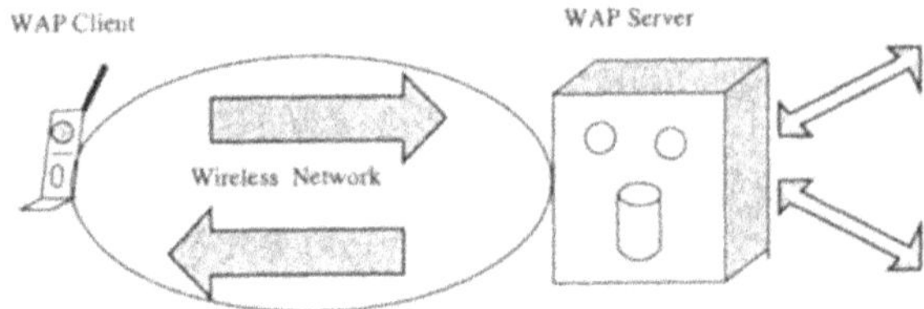

Figure 1. Wireless Network

Within the WWW, a computer program can ask another one to execute some request. The first program is called *client* and the second one is called *server*. In a similar manner, WAP is aimed at enabling wireless terminals to access Internet-like services (figure 1). WAP features are organized into different layers (figure 2). The **Application layer** provides the wireless terminal with a uniform environment enabling access to standard telephony and WWW services. This application environment includes a WML browser. The **Session service** provides application layers with a consistent interface for maintained session. We will be back to this layer in section 4. The **Transaction layer** handles the execution of transactions requested by upper layers, in a transparent manner. etc.

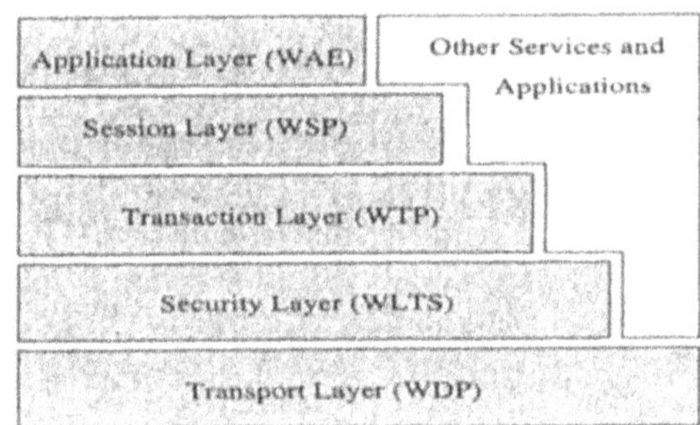

Figure 2. WAP protocol stack

For interoperability reasons, WAP systems must respect the above standard. To date, WAP forum has concentrated its efforts on the development of a certification program, which consists of validating WAP products application environment. The ICS (Implementation Conformance Statements) constitute reference documents on the basis of which manufacturer products are certified for conformance. Certification testing is carried under the responsability of an organization sanctioned by WAP forum as the "Certification Authority". The components involved in a test campaign are WAP-certified equipments, and the framework and process for delivering certification labels are defined by WAP forum. From November 2000 to November 2001, certification labels have been delivered for more than 6 WAP servers and more than 55 WAP terminals (clients). But there are few developments published on the testing of underlying protocol operations. Compliance involves protocol *inter-operations*, in the sequel, we will interprete *compliance testing* as some *interoperability testing*, and vice versa.

3. TESTING APPROACH OVERVIEW

The test development approach adopted follows a generic methodology that we named TOP [5, 1, 6], and which handles interoperability test automation from specifications to test execution via a CORBA platform. For space reasons, we will not racall all aspects of TOP in this paper. We invite the reader to report to the above references for details. In the following, we consider some key issues of standard testing activity:
(•) *Test architecture:* The test architecture represents the configuration in which a test experiment is undertaken. (•) *Test case generation:* A test case (≡ test sequence) is a sequence of interactions to be submitted to implementation under test. (•) *Test deployment:* Test deployment is concerned with effective execution of test cases within a given test architecture. Even if the literature is poor in this field, test deployment remains an important aspect of testing activity.

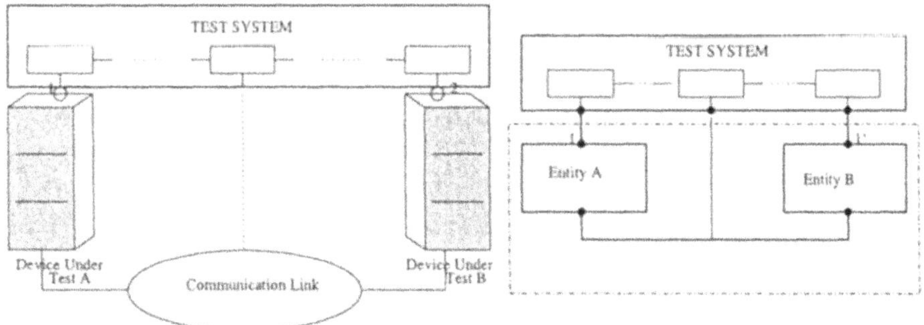

Figure 3. Functional views of the Test Architecture

Test Architecture and Deployment. Figure 3 depicts functional views of the architecture we use for interoperability. The test system interacts with the DUTs (Devices Under Test), through the Service Access Points (also corresponding to PCOs: Points of Control and Observation) labeled with 1 and 2 (1 and 1' in the right part). An optional interaction point enables it to access the PDU (Protocol Data Unit) at lower communication level. Notice that this architecture is similar to the one proposed by the ATM forum for interoperability. The monitor point of ATM forum corresponds to the optional interaction point in figure 3. In our approach, implementations can be stimulated, directly with the test cases executed by the test system through PCOs, or via upper layer running-applications (figure 4). In both cases, the test sequences computed constitute reference traces that can be checked during or after test execution (kind of passive testing). But those architectures, including the ones defined in standard ISO-9646 [3], describe only functional configurations. In this case, they do not provide information to concrete design of PCOs for the interaction between the test system and DUTs. This aspect is left to test laboratory and test execution concern. In our methodology, we have designed a portable test platform for handling test deployment issues [6]. The platform is featured over the CORBA standard, which facilitates test deployment for a wide range of DUTs. We do not develop test deployment aspects in this paper.

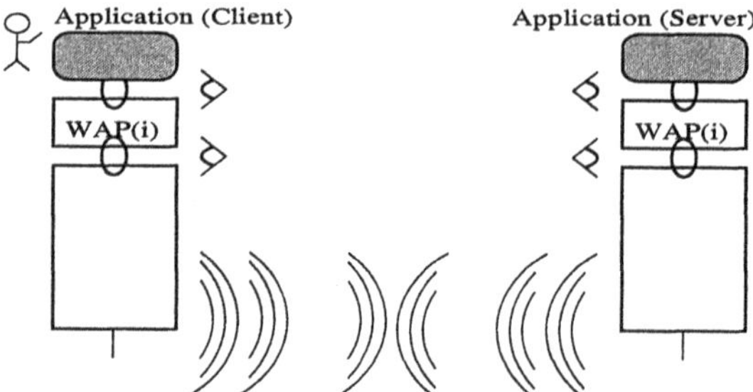

Figure 4. Towards an experimental test configuration

Test case generation. Unlike usual techniques to interoperability test sequences generation [2, 10], our test generation tool implements an *on the fly* exploration technique, which is recognised to be efficient against complex specifications [4]. It directly extracts test paths by analysing the sub-specifications (model of entity A and model of entity B). The algorithm implemented works with input/output automata modelling the specifications and the TPs (*Test Purpose* $\stackrel{\text{def}}{=}$ *A behavioral property to be tested*). It has been implemented in the so-called TESCOMS tool by our students, with C++ language. The tool has been successfully used before, with specifications like ATM sublayers, and we are currently using it for computing WAP specifications.

This section summarized the main steps of our testing approach: `(Specifications)` → [TESCOMS] → `(Test case)` → [TBROKER] → ... ... → [TBROKER] → `(Test Deployment/Execution)`. Below, we consider the case study with WSP.

4. COMPLIANCE TESTS SUITE PRODUCTION

Following the general recommendations of WAP forum, on certification and compliance testing process [8], we have shown in previous works, the feasability of automatic tests computation for WAP. Here we focus on reporting our test production experiment against the session layer.

Specification and Test Purpose issues. WSP [9] enables client and server applications to exchange contents through a maintained communication session. Here, we consider the connection-mode protocol only, as the connectionless one is fairly simple. WSP is mainly featured to establish and release a session between a client and a server, exchange contents of the two applications, suspend and resume the session. In the specification, service primitives are of the form `S-Service-type`, (e.g. `S-Connect-req`), where `S` is the label of the session layer, `Service` indicates the name of the service. The type is also indicated. Protocol inter-operations are performed through the use of a transaction service (`TR`). For remembering the WAP stack, look again at figure 2. The PDUs exchanged between the WSP peer-entities are encapsulated in the `TR` primitives: `TR-Service(PDU)` denotes the encapsulation of a given `PDU` in a `TR-Service` primitive. In the standard, the session protocol is described with a set of state tables that we exploited and translated directly in terms of input/output automata and SDL specifications. Of course, we will not include the specification model (equivalent of about 3000 lines of SDL code) in this paper.

The reference document we used for selection of test purpose, was the WAP ICS [8]. WSP implementation features are organized into groups of functionality: `Session creation`, `Session suspend/resume`, `Push facilities`, etc. In this paper, we will not include all the test cases considered. We will present a couple of examples to illustrate the experiment results: the session creation - the session release.

The test suite / Session Creation - Session Release. These features fall in the category of mandatory services to be implemented by both WAP clients and servers.

Test method: The session creation starts with an S-Connect-req, and ends with an S-Connect-cnf. The session release starts with an S-Disconnect-req (initiated, in this example, by the server) and ends with the notification of the disconnection.

The test purpose is defined with a finite automaton: The syntax used requires one transition per line. Each line describes an interaction as well as the implementation which executes it. In the first line of the example below, "1" represents the identifier of the WAP-client implementation. In the second line, "2" represents the identifier of the WAP-server implementation. The last state encountered (TP7 in the example) is implicitely an accepting state.

Test Purpose: Identifiers WSP_CO_C001, WSP_CO_C002 of the ICS proforma.

```
TP1 ? 1.S-Connect-req 1 TP2
TP2 ? 2.S-Connect-res 2 TP3
TP3 ! 1.S-Connect-cnf 1 TP4
TP4 ? 2.S-Disconnect-req 2 TP5
TP5 ! 1.S-Disconnect-ind(DISCONNECT) 1 TP6
TP6 ! 2.S-Disconnect-ind(USERREQ) 2 TP7
```

The output below represents the test case produced by the TESCOMS test generation tool. The comments of the form [XXX XXX XXX] represent internal identifiers related to the global state which may be actually reached during the computation of the concurrent input system: In the first line example, NULL represents the starting state of the client side, the second NULL represents the starting state of the server side, and TP1 represents the beginning of the test purpose. Between these identifiers are displayed (with tabs) the actual interaction to be executed.

Test case dynamic behavior:

```
[NULL NULL TP1]
 1:    ? 1.S-Connect-req 1
[NUCIA1 NULL TP2]
 2:     ! TR-Invoke(Connect) 1
[CONNECTING NUCIA1 TP2]
 3:      ! TR-Invoke.ack 2
[CONNECTING NUCIA2 TP2]
 4:       ! 2.S-Connect-ind 2
[CONNECTING CONNECTING TP2]
 5:        ? 2.S-Connect-res 2
[CONNECTING CIC2A1 TP3]
 6:         ! TR-Result(ConnectReply) 2
```

```
[CICEA1 CONNECTING-2 TP3]
 7:          ! TR-Result.ack 1
[CICEA2 CONNECTED TP3]
 8:           ! 1.S-Connect-cnf 1
[CONNECTED CONNECTED TP4]
 9:           ? 2.S-Disconnect-req 2
[CONNECTED CENUA1 TP5]
10:            ! TR-Invoke(Disconnect) 2
[CENUC1 CENUA2 TP5]
11:             ! 1.S-Disconnect-ind(DISCONNECT) 1
[NULL CENUA2 TP6]
12:             ! 2.S-Disconnect-ind(USERREQ) 2
[NULL NULL TP7]
```

Test case analysis: [1:] A Connection request is received by implementation 1 (the client session entity). [2:] The client invokes the transaction layer for sending its Connect PDU. [3:] Upon reception of that PDU, the server (session entity) acknowledges it through the transaction layer. [4:] The server sends a Connection indication to the upper layers. [5:] Then it receives the response notifying that the application accepted the connection. [6:] This notification is sent to the client, as a result of its Connect request. [7:] The client acknowledges the result. [8:] The client session user is sent a confirmation notifying that the connection has been established. [9:] The server side receives an Disconnection request. [10:] Then the request is hold by the transaction layer. [11,12:] The upper layers are notified that the session has been released.

Analysis of the produced test suite. Table 1 recaps the features covered by the overall WSP computed test suite. In this table, the column "Function" represents service functionalities. For each function, we present the PDUs involved in the operation of the function, or the related capabilities. Some of the functionalities specified in the standard are mandatory while the other ones are optional. Most of the mandatory features have been computed (80%). Capabilities represent a set of service facilities and parameter settings related to the operation of the service provider. There are different kinds of facilities defined in the standard, but the service provider may recognise optional/additional facilities. Some examples of facilities are *Aliases, Extended methods, Protocol options.* The basic methods of WAP correspond to the ones defined in the HTTP/1.1 standard, and the *Extended methods* correspond to those beyond HTTP/1.1. *Proprietary methods* fall in this category. During the connection, the peer entities can perform a *Capabilities negociation* in order to agree on a common communication profile. The Connect PDU can be used to specify the required capabilities of the initiator, and the ConnectReply PDU would contain the capabilities acknowledged by

Table 1. Analysis of dynamic behaviour computed

Function	PDU/Capabilities	Mandatory Feature	Tests computed
Session Creation	Connect PDU	Yes	Yes
Capabilities Negotiation	Connect PDU, Connect Reply PDU	Yes	No
Session Release	Disconnect PDU	Yes	Yes
Session Suspend, Session Resume	Suspend PDU, Resume PDU	No	Yes
Push	Push PDU	No	Yes
Confirmed Push	ConfirmedPush PDU	Yes	Yes
Extended Methods	Proprietary Methods	No	No
Methods GET, POST	Get PDU, Post PDU, Reply PDU	No	Yes
Methods DELETE, HEAD, OPTION, TRACE	Get PDU, Reply PDU	No	Yes
Method PUT	Post PDU, Reply PDU	No	Yes

the responder. Since all the actual capabilities are not provided in the current standard, and as these capabilities depend on the actual WSP service users, we did not look into this aspect. For the time being, we have treated the connection procedure (session creation PDUs) that conveys users defined facilities. 100% of the standard defined PDUs and also 100% of the standard defined ASPs are involved in the test suite. This guarantees that each elementary protocol operation can be experimented by the computed test suite.

In the overall test suite, some portions of tests suite are replayed. For instance, all the `Method Invocation` facilities have basically the same operation scheme. At the WSP level, methods can be invoked by three basics PDUs, namely the `Get PDU`, `Post PDU` and the `Reply PDU`. The current `Method` reference is encapsulated in these PDUs.

5. CONCLUSIONS

The work presented is a contribution to the testing of protocol interoperations against compliance with WAP standard. Of course, for space reasons, we could not include in this paper all the test cases designed. We illustrated our work with WSP, which is the first layer below application level. Almost all the mandatory functionalities have been experimented in dynamic test generation. We did not complete the aspects related to capability negociation, which are rather a concern of actual telecommunication service provider. Furthermore, the number of possible facilities is unknown a priori. A preliminary static interoperability review of actual WAP-applications communicating through the WSP service may allow for the selection of a subset of relevant facilities to be experimented.

Our testing approach, suitable for layered protocols, can be experimented with other lower layers of WAP stack, with few limitations. For the time being, we are interested in concrete experimentation/deployment of the produced test cases. Most of telecommunications operators have already done some developments related to the WAP technology, and we have obtained, for free, a prototype of WAP client, and a WAP server (with full source code in C language). We are currently using these implementations to conduct concrete test experimentations.

References

[1] X.Balliet, N.Eloy. Development of a distributed test system with CORBA. Co-authored Master's thesis. ENSEM, Polytechnic Institute Nancy, March 2000.

[2] A.Fukada et al. A conformance testing for communication protocols modeled as a set of DFSMs with common inputs. In. Testing of Communicating Systems Vol. 10. Chapman & Hall, 1997.

[3] ISO/IEC 9646, Information Technology – Open Systems Interconnection-Conformance testing methodology and framework - Part 1-5. 1991.

[4] O.Koné. A local approach to the testing of real-time systems. *The Computer Journal*, British Computer Society, Oxford Press. Vol. 44 N.5, 2001.

[5] O. Koné, R. Castanet. Test generation for interworking systems In. *Computer Communications*, Elsevier Science Publishers, Vol. 23 N.7, 2000. pp 642-652.

[6] O.Koné. The TBROKER platform for the interoperability of communications systems. 5th IEEE/Worldses Conference on Communications. Crete, July 2001.

[7] Wireless Application Protocol. Architecture Specification, WAP forum, April, 1998. URL: `http://www.wapforum.com`

[8] Wireless Application Protocol. Conformance Statement, Compliance Profile and Release List. WAP forum, April 1998. URL: `http://www.wapforum.com`.

[9] Wireless Session Protocol Specification. WAP forum. URL: `http://www.wapforum.com`, 1999

[10] M.Malek, S.Dibuz. A pragmatic method for interoperability test suite derivation. Proc. EUROMICRO Conference. Sweden, August 1998.

[11] Réseau National de Recherche en Télécommunications. URL: `http://www.telecom.gouv.fr/rnrt`.

A FLEXIBLE TRAFFIC GENERATOR FOR TESTING PABX AND CALL CENTER PERFORMANCE

Georg Rößler

Tenovis GmbH & Co. KG,

Kleyerstraße 94, D-60326 Frankfurt am Main, Germany, Georg.Roessler@tenovis.com

Thomas Steinert

Univ. of Stuttgart, Institute of Communication Networks and Computer Engineering,

Pfaffenwaldring 47, D-70569 Stuttgart, Germany, steinert@ind.uni-stuttgart.de

Abstract Testing PABXs and call centers under high load is of paramount importance because customers rely on these systems for safety and business critical applications. A traffic generator for high traffic volumes is presented in this paper. The two key characteristics of the traffic generator are the generation of traffic with configurable statistical properties and its flexibility in many aspects, ranging from the number and kind of emulated users to the user behaviour models and signalling protocols. This extraordinary flexibility could only be achieved by a pure software approach. The architecture clearly separates the basic runtime system and support functions which are implemented in the traffic generator core from user models and signalling protocols which the traffic generator reads and executes during tests.

Keywords: Environment simulation, ISDN-PABX, call center, performance testing

1. MOTIVATION

Todays enterprise telecommunications infrastructure consists of interconnected systems ranging from networked PABXs (Private Automatic Branch Exchange) to server computers and client PCs. The applications running on these systems provide a large range of services to users, for example computer-supported telephony for increased productivity and convenience; call centers with sophisticated rule-based call distribution schemes; location tracking of medical personnel using mobile phones in hospitals for optimal dispatching of emergency calls. These examples illustrate the enormous increase of the system complexity compared to the stand-alone PABX system which once was the backbone of the enterprise telecommunications infrastructure.

Because of the safety and business critical applications, the systems must exhibit outstanding reliability. This reliability must also be guaranteed during high load or overload situations. Careful system design and performance analysis give confidence that a system can handle the traffic volume it has been designed for and that it performs well in overload phases. However, it is absolutely necessary to verify the expected performance through tests before it is deployed on customer sites.

In our context, the focus for load tests is on signalling traffic in the PABX as well as on the interaction between PABXs and servers. The main traffic sources are still in the telephone part of the system, hence the load generator aims at the emulation of telephone users attached via terminals or trunk lines. This paper describes a load generator which we call LGen. It is designed to fulfill two main requirements. The first requirement is that LGen can generate high traffic volumes with configurable statistical properties. The second requirement is flexibility such that it can easily be adapted and extended to varying and newly emerging test situations.

The next section explains the requirements to LGen in more detail. Then the system concept and its structure are described. The subsequent section presents example tests which have been carried out.

2. REQUIREMENTS TO THE LOAD GENERATOR LGen

The first requirement is that the generated traffic has to be statistically correct which means that call interarrival times, call holding times, etc. have to follow given distributions. Additionally, the generated traffic has to react correctly on varying system behaviour, e.g. repeat call attempts after call blocking due to overload. Further, LGen has to provide burst call arrivals as they appear in call centers when phone numbers are presented in TV commercials. LGen has to be parameterizable in order to simulate different load conditions. Both the distributions and their parameters must be configurable. Finally, the generated traffic has to reach an offered load of at least 30000 BHCA. This load is high enough to saturate a single module of the Tenovis Integral 33 PABX [1].

The desired flexibility implies that user behaviour and signalling protocols must not be hard-coded in LGen. Instead, this behaviour has to be provided by separate description files which LGen reads and executes.

Call patterns and timing behaviour have to be easily configurable. Otherwise, testers find it difficult to use the test system. Also, number and kind of emulated telephone users and trunk lines should be easily configurable. This permits LGen to adapt to different PABX configurations with little effort.

In a first step, fixed digital terminals for standard subscribers and for call center agents as well as digital trunk lines have to be supported. Later, mobile DECT (Digital Enhanced Cordless Telephone) subscribers have to be added. Both telephony and user movement which causes roaming and handover for DECT phones have to be emulated.

Statistics on events and durations have to be collected. These statistics are particularly important for long tests and tests sequences. Tracing of events and protocol data units (PDUs) with configurable filter conditions is required. The primary application area of LGen is in the laboratory during development and integration testing. It is an advantage, however, if LGen can also be applied for tests on customer systems, in particular for call centers (during off-peak hours).

3. LOAD TEST SYSTEM

LGen is implemented in software running on standard workstations. The following section presents the general principle of performing load tests with LGen. Section 3.2 presents the realization of LGen.

3.1 General principle

Figure 1 shows a typical test configuration for testing the Integral 33 system from Tenovis. An Integral 33 module comprises a Generic Control Unit (GCU) on which runs the switching software, a switching fabric, and several line cards called Interface Control Units (ICUs).

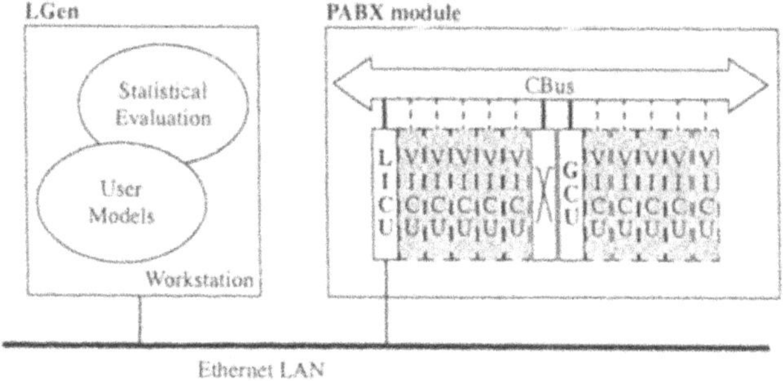

Figure 1. Typical test configuration of the load test system

In the PABX, the test focus is on the software running on the GCU. Usually, subscriber and trunk lines are connected to ICUs. They exchange signalling messages with the GCU via the CBus which is a proprietary communication system for message transfer.

For load tests with LGen, the real ICUs are removed and replaced by virtual ICUs (VICUs). The key characteristic of a VICU is that the GCU software receives the same messages as if a real ICU was present, although the ICU slot is empty. Note that it is possible to replace only some real ICUs by virtual ones and to keep some real ICUs in the module and to include them in the tests.

The so called LAN ICU (LICU) plays an important role for the representation of VICUs. The main task of the LICU is to forward signalling messages from the LAN to the CBus and vice versa. The LGen software generates the signalling messages - as if real users were present - and sends them through a TCP connection to the LICU. The LICU simply transmits the messages on the CBus. For CBus messages from the GCU, the LICU uses the same TCP connection to send them to LGen.

An LICU is capable to represent multiple VICUs at the same time. This is possible because the LICU can be configured to receive CBus messages for multiple destination addresses simultaneously. The source addresses for CBus messages are provided by the sender of messages.

The second task of the LICU is to relieve LGen from handling the commissioning phase for VICUs. A set of simple control messages between LGen and LICU has been defined for that purpose.

While in Figure 1 only one PABX module is depicted, it is possible to run tests with multiple modules of a PABX (or even multiple PABX systems) from a single LGen. It is sufficient to put an LICU in each module where VICUs are simulated to generate traffic.

3.2 Realization

This section presents the realization of LGen and, furthermore, shows the possibilities of this approach. For a detailed description of the structure and especially the traffic generation principle we refer to [2].

Figure 2 shows the building blocks of the software structure of LGen. The communication between them is based on LGen internal messages. This allows to decouple the execution of the different signal processing entities and, thus, to process the messages concurrently in multiple threads. The model applied is very similar to the "peer model" (also known as "workcrew model"). This principle allows to distribute the load to different threads, so that LGen adapts to the underlying hardware platform, e.g. a multiprocessor workstation, in an optimized way.

Furthermore, all software modules of LGen are designed in that way, that no searching routine for e.g. the determination of the destination of a message takes place during a test. Only a calendar module performs a search routine, but its algorithms do not depend on the number of entries. Therefore, LGen scales not only with the underlying hardware platform but also with the number of emulated users.

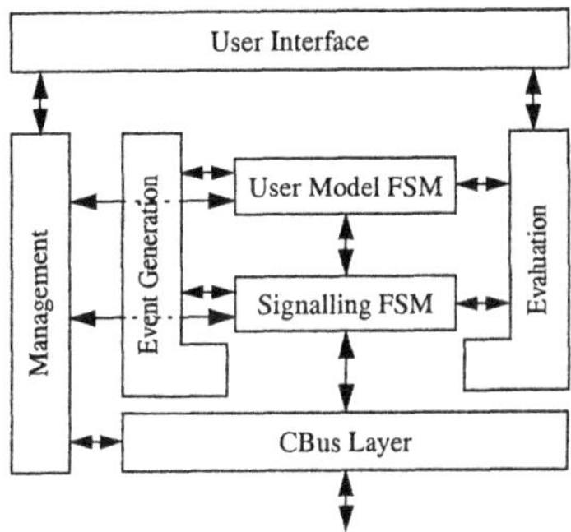

Figure 2. Software structure of LGen

The traffic generation principle of LGen is based on the emulation of the behaviour of single users by so called "User Models". The superposition of the signalling traffic of a multitude of these User Models represents a realistic traffic mixture. For describing a User Model an FSM approach was chosen, where the functional behaviour of an emulated user is separated from its temporal behaviour. The functional behaviour is defined by the **User Model FSM** and determines what an emulated user does, e.g. how he reacts on a refused connection establishment. The temporal behaviour is defined by means of **Event Generators** and determines, when a user does something, e.g. when he will try again to establish a connection. This allows to use one User Model FSM for different temporal behaviours e.g. to emulate a standard user and a business user with the same User Model FSM only with different behaviour concerning the time. There are quite a number of publications about augmented FSMs describing both functional and temporal behaviour, e.g. [3] gives a nice overview. Except a paper by Lemppenau and Tran-Gia [4] describing also a system for traffic generation most of the publications focus on performance analysis and not on the emulation of behaviour in real-time.

A User Model FSM controls a **Signalling FSM** which realizes layer 3 of a signalling system by means of Service Data Units (SDUs). SDUs sent by the User Model FSM trigger actions of the Signalling FSM, those received by the User Model FSM indicate the current state of the Signalling FSM. By this approach the User Model FSM creates an abstract view of the underlying signalling protocol.

To generate traffic a User Model has to perform spontaneous actions. Therefore the principle of Event Generators was introduced: Event Generators generate input signals for User Model FSMs which we call Events. The interarrival times of these Events are statistically distributed according to adjustable distribution density functions. Upon reception of an Event a User Model FSM performs a state transition where further signalling actions like sending an SDU to trigger the setup of a signalling connection take place. Figure 3 shows the relation between User Model FSM, Event Generator and Signalling FSM.

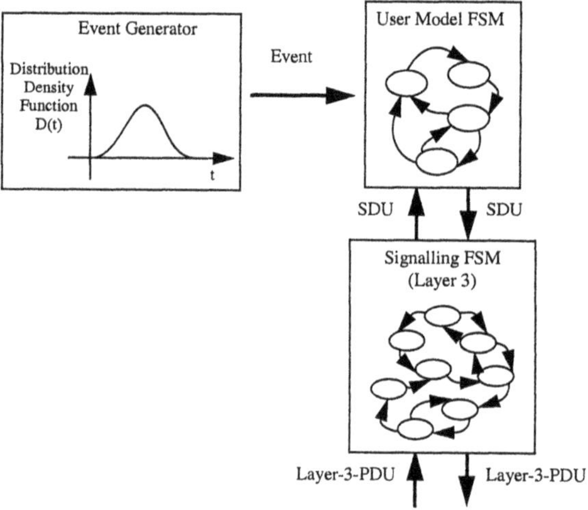

Figure 3. Relation between User Model FSM, Event Generator and Signalling FSM

For the **Evaluation** of a load test measurement variables concerning signalling connections, like e.g. "Setup Answer Delay" or "Number of Accepted Setup", are collected. Furthermore, it is possible to record a message trace of the exchanged signalling messages, which allows to examine them in detail.

For the specification of a User Model FSM a subset of the Specification and Description Language (SDL) defined by the ITU-T is applied. In the configuration phase LGen creates a data structure corresponding to the specified User Model FSM relating its SDL statements to implemented and compiled C functions. During a load test the data structure is interpreted and the corresponding functions are executed. This principle combines the flexible method for specifying a communication process by means of SDL with the capabilities of a programming language and the performance of a speed optimized program.

The same principle is also applied for Signalling FSMs which are realized according to the respective standards. Only the interface to the upper layer, the User Model FSM, is adapted for the needs of LGen by communicating via protocol independent SDUs. Signalling FSMs send layer 3 PDUs as a reaction on a time out, an SDU or a PDU. At the **CBus Layer** these PDUs are integrated into CBus Messages and sent to an LICU of a PABX module. In the other direction layer 3 PDUs which are extracted from CBus Messages received by the CBus Layer are sent to the corresponding Signalling FSM.

This approach allows to integrate several signalling protocols into LGen. So far the ISDN-D-channel protocols according to ITU-T Q.931 and to TN-1R6 which is a Tenovis specific proprietary advancement of the german ISDN-D-channel protocol 1TR6 and a signalling protocol for DECT are realized. Therefore, LGen is capable to emulate various user types as standard users at ISDN terminals, ACD (Automatic Call Distribution) users at call centers, digital trunk lines and DECT mobile users. Furthermore, for each user type multiple temporal configurations can be applied in a load test.

An important requirement of LGen is the generation of traffic bursts. This is already integrated in the standard way of defining the traffic characteristics: A group of emulated users which will be activated at the same time has to be configured in that way that it generates a call within a short time frame after activation. This results in a signalling traffic peak after the activation of this group of users.

4. EXAMPLE TESTS

A first series of load tests concentrated on the PABX. The expected switching performance and the system stability under high load and overload could be confirmed. A selection of these tests is repeated with each new software release. The fact that LGen can produce high load and keep it constant gave the opportunity to validate the system dimensioning rules as they are implemented in a configuration tool.

In an ideal system, each call contributes a fixed amount of CPU occupation. In real systems, however, operations like searching for a particular call context to which a signalling message belongs may take longer when many calls are active at the same time. A series of tests demonstrated a linear relation between the offered traffic and the observed CPU load of the GCU. Thus the real system can be regarded as an ideal system in this respect.

The next step was towards call centers and other CTI-based systems. Testing these systems is the main application area of LGen. The focus for these tests is on the interaction between servers and the PABX and on the applications running on dedicated servers. The call distribution application is a key element of a call center. The call distribution schemes are implemented in customer specific call flow scripts which the application interprets. In the more sophisticated call flow scripts, the resulting system load usually increases faster than the offered traffic. This phenomenon is mainly caused by additional activities, for example automatic announcements about possibilities to leave a voice message or about the expected waiting time, for callers who have to wait before they can be connected to an agent. An important question in this case is which load a call center can handle, in particular if the offered load exceeds the customer expectations such that many callers have to wait.

In a further step, LGen was extended for emulation of DECT mobile users. Emulating DECT users for load tests is interesting because the high user density together with the narrow cells results in potentially high roaming and handover rates. Inside buildings, base stations are usually installed only a few tens of meters apart on each floor. Moreover, in DECT the phones send roaming requests when they detect that another base station is more suitable for them, whereas in public cellular mobile networks like GSM it is usually the network that triggers the roaming. With LGen scenarios like many DECT users leaving a meeting at the same time and thus creating many roaming events could be tested. The special caching mechanisms which have been implemented to cope with mass roaming situations have been found to work well.

5. CONCLUSION

LGen has proven to be a valuable tool for testing enterprise telecommunications systems. Call rates of more than 100000 BHCA can be generated on a Sun UltraSPARC 1 workstation. The high performance is due to the system design for efficient execution of user and signalling models. This illustrates that the flexibility has been achieved without negative impact on the performance.

References

[1] http://www.tenovis.com/tenovis_international/Details/Integral33.htm

[2] T. Steinert, G. Rößler: Generation of realistic signalling traffic in an ISDN load test system using SDL User Models, Proceedings of FORTE/PSTV 2000, Pisa

[3] Mitschele-Thiel, Müller-Clostermann: Performance engineering of SDL/MSC systems, Computer Networks 31 (1999)

[4] Lemppenau, Tran-Gia: A Universal Environment Simulator for SPC Switching System Testing, Proc. 11th International Teletraffic Congress (ITC), Kyoto 1985

SESSION IV

INTEROPERABILITY TESTING

INTEROPERABILITY TEST GENERATION FOR COMMUNICATION PROTOCOLS BASED ON MULTIPLE STIMULI PRINCIPLE[3]

Soonuk Seol[†], Myungchul Kim[†], and Samuel T. Chanson[††]
[†]*Information and Communications University, Korea*
{ suseol, mckim }@icu.ac.kr
[††]*Hong Kong University of Science & Technology, China*
chanson@cs.ust.hk

Abstract This paper presents a method for generating interoperability test suites for the class of communication protocols such as the ATM/B-ISDN signaling protocol and TCP that are modeled as communicating nondeterministic finite-state machines. To our knowledge, no test generation method exists for protocol interoperability testing that supports multiple simultaneous inputs to the implementations. In other words, it has been assumed that communicating systems adhere to the single stimulus principle in generating test cases. In practice, however, there exists the possibility that additional messages will be sent to a machine while the previous message is still being processed, and/or simultaneous messages will be sent to several machines at the same time (e.g., TCP's simultaneous open/close). To cope with these situations, we have developed an interoperability test suite derivation algorithm based on formal models. Experimental results show that our method is applicable to practical systems and can generate validation-equivalent interoperability test suites in terms of transition coverage.

Keywords: Interoperability testing, protocol testing, test case generation, validation, single stimulus, multiple stimuli, transition coverage, stable state, TCP, ATM

1. INTRODUCTION

To increase the confidence that protocol products conform to international standards, various protocol testing methodologies have been developed and applied. In particular, conformance testing that checks whether an implementation is correct with respect to the relevant standards

[3] This work has been supported by KOSEF (No. 995-0900-007-2).

has been standardized by ISO [1] and ITU-T [12] and applied to protocols such as N-ISDN and ATM/B-ISDN. Nevertheless, it is well known that conformance testing has limitations in ensuring interoperability. Thus, even two conforming implementations may fail to interoperate [2, 3]. The reasons include ambiguity of protocol standards, incompatible option settings and incomplete conformance testing [4].

There has been some research work on interoperability testing in the literature. Rafiq and Castanet [2] dealt with interoperability test suite generation based on reachability analysis. However, a rigorous definition of interoperability was not used and the work considered only the case where lower testers exist between two Implementations Under Test (IUTs). Vermeer and Blik [5] described experiences with interoperability testing of the FTAM protocol. The work used a single tester between two IUTs and thus had limited capability. Arakawa et al. [3] derived a conformance test suite and an interoperability test suite separately and later manually combined them to reduce the number of conformance test cases. Kang and Kim [6] developed a method for systematically dealing with symmetric communication protocols and used an interoperability test architecture that did not observe the interface behavior between two IUTs. Shin and Kang [4] proposed and applied a test derivation method suitable for testing interoperability for the class of communication protocols such as the ATM/B-ISDN signaling protocol. Seol et al. [7] later enhanced the algorithm in [6, 4] and applied the algorithm to the ATM/B-ISDN signaling protocol and TCP with analysis on transition coverage. Kang et al. [8] developed a coherent framework of interoperability testing and a systematic interoperability test suite derivation method based on the framework.

Quite a number of methods and tools for test case generation get inputs in the form of deterministic, nondeterministic, or extended Finite State Machine (FSM) specifications. However, these methods are generally applicable only when the protocol consists of a single FSM. For communication protocols, most interoperability test suite derivation methods are based on some form of reachability analysis and the protocols are modeled by communicating finite state machines. To our knowledge, the single stimulus principle has always been explicitly or implicitly assumed. These models therefore do not support multiple stimuli. The single stimulus principle means that only a single stimulus can be given at each stable state. A stable state for concurrent systems or communicating protocols is defined in [9] as the system state (i) that is reachable from the initial state adhering to the single stimulus principle, and (ii) from which no change can occur without another stimulus. Systems adhering to the single stimulus principle are said to be running in a slow environment [10]. In a slow environment, inputs can be sent from the environment to the system only when all the queues and all the channels are empty. According to the single stimulus principle, simultaneous stimuli and stimuli during transitions are not considered.

When protocol implementations interact with one another, it is possible that additional messages are sent to the implementation(s) while the previous message is still being processed and/or simultaneous messages are sent to each implementation at the same time. For instance, TCP allows simultaneous open and simultaneous close of a TCP connection. Therefore, checking multiple stimuli in interoperability testing is important because multiple stimuli are an essential part of many protocol behaviors and their implementation seems to be especially error-prone.

In this paper, we propose a new method to support concurrent behavior of protocols in generating test cases for interoperability testing. The rest of this paper is organized as follows: Section 2 presents some related work. In Section 3, we define formal models for communication protocols and interoperability test cases. Section 4 explains our approach to interoperability testing and the procedure for generating interoperability test suites. In Section 5, we present the results of applying our proposal to the TCP and ATM/B-ISDN signaling protocols with transition coverage analysis. Finally, Section 6 summarizes the contributions of the paper and suggests further research directions.

2. RELATED WORK AND MOTIVATION

In this section, we present some existing methods that are related to our work and discuss their limitations due to the single stimuli assumption.

Luo et al. [10] proposed a method of generating test sequences for concurrent programs and communication protocols modeled as communicating nondetermini-stic finite state machines (CNFSMs). The method first reduces a system of CNFSMs into a single NFSM by reachability analysis. The NFSM is then transformed into a trace-equivalent observable NFSM from which test sequences are generated. Basically, a global state denotes contents of channels, input queues, and states in each machine. As mentioned in their paper, it is obvious that the number of states in a global state machine becomes infinite in case of unlimited channels and/or queues. For that reason, they made the assumptions that queues and channels are bounded, and that the system runs in a slow environment. The first assumption is reasonable since unbounded queues or unbounded channels cannot be implemented in practice. The second assumption, however, is not reasonable for those protocols that allow multiple and simultaneous messages.

Paula Lima and Cavalli [11] proposed a pragmatic approach to generating test sequences for embedded components of complex systems. Embedded testing and interoperability testing are similar in that internal actions are usually invisible and thus hard to control. Their method provides means to support multiple outputs (i.e., when one signal from the environment stimulates several simultaneous outputs) and non-determinism of components. A drawback of their method is that it limits the number of external inputs between stable states to one. In other words, an input can be given to the system only if the previous input has been completely processed and the system is not undergoing any state change at the time.

Recently, Kang et al. [8] proposed a framework for interoperability testing of communication protocols. They developed an interoperability test derivation method based on stable states, and applied their method to the ATM signaling protocol. This method also has the same drawback as the other methods mentioned above. As their method adheres to the single stimulus principle so that multiple stimuli and stimuli during transitions between stable states cannot be handled.

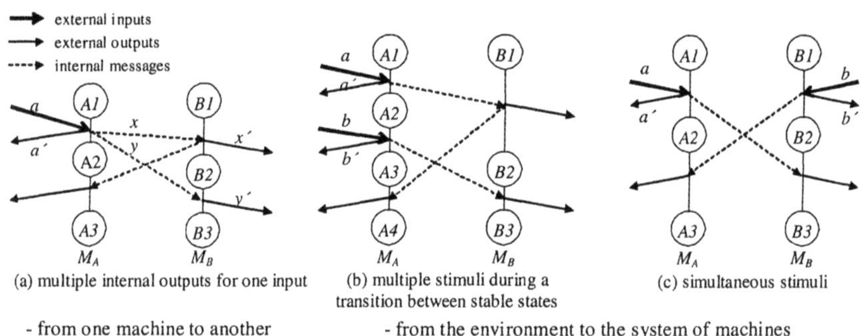

Figure 1. Multiple stimuli.

In practice, multiple messages between communicating entities often occur. Figure 1 shows three cases of multiple messages in MSC-like charts. There are two machines which exchange messages with each other and with the environment. In this paper, we shall call the former messages internal messages and the latter external messages. Case (a) involves multiple stimuli from one entity to the peer entity for a given external input while cases (b) and (c) involve multiple stimuli from the environment to the system of machines. In (a), the machine MA produces two internal messages x and y arising from the external input a. Note that multiple output messages can be produced not only from an external input but is possible also from an internal input. In (b), external input b is given while the previous input a is still being processed. This case is an example of multiple stimuli during a transition from one stable state to another. Note that the global states (A1, B1) and (A4, B3) in Figure 1(b) are stable states. A similar case is shown in Figure 1(c) where one input goes to MA and another input goes to MB at the same time. This is known as simultaneous stimuli which is a special case of multiple stimuli. Simultaneous stimuli can be seen in TCP's simultaneous open and close behaviors. These cases can often happen in the real world and may also occur in faulty implementations. Therefore, interoperability testing should test for these behaviors as well.

3. FORMAL MODELS

This section defines formal models for communicating entities and for interoperability test cases. The specifications and implementations of communicating entities can be modelled using a special type of FSMs known as input output state machine (IOSM). IOSM is defined as follows:

Definition 1. An IOSM is a 5-tuple ($\mathbf{S}$, S_0, $\mathbf{L_{in}}$, $\mathbf{L_{out}}$, $\mathbf{Tr}$) where:

(1) $\mathbf{S} = \{ S_0, S_1, \ldots, S_{n-1} \}$ is a set of states;
(2) $S_0 \in \mathbf{S}$ is the initial state;
(3) $\mathbf{L_{in}} = \{ v_1, v_2, \ldots, v_m \}$ is a set of input symbols;
(4) $\mathbf{L_{out}} = \{ u_1, u_2, \ldots, u_k \}$ is a set of output symbols;
(5) $\mathbf{Tr} \subseteq \{ S_s \text{—} v/U \rightarrow S_d \mid S_s, S_d \in \mathbf{S} \wedge v \in \mathbf{L_{in}} \wedge U \in \mathbf{P}(\mathbf{L^*_{out}}) \}$ is a set of transitions where $\mathbf{L^*_{out}}$ denotes the set of sequences of symbols in $\mathbf{L_{out}}$ and $\mathbf{P}(\mathbf{X})$ denotes the power set of the set $\mathbf{X}$.

Bold letters in Definition 1 represent sets. $\mathbf{L_{in}}$ is divided into two sets $\mathbf{L_{in,E}}$ and $\mathbf{L_{in,I}}$ that are, respectively, the set of external input symbols and the set of internal input symbols. Similarly, $\mathbf{L_{out}}$ is divided into two sets $\mathbf{L_{out,E}}$ and $\mathbf{L_{out,I}}$ that are, respectively, the set of external output symbols and the set of internal output symbols. For example, symbol a in Figure 1(a) is an external input symbol and a' is an external output symbol. Symbols x and y are internal output symbols for machine M_A and, at the same time, are internal input symbols for machine M_B. "S_s—$v/U\rightarrow S_d$" is a transition where S_s, S_d, v, and U are, respectively, the starting state, the destination state, an input symbol and a sequence of output symbols. For a transition tr in $\mathbf{Tr}$, the '.' notation is used to refer to one of the elements of the following sets such as S_s, S_d, v, and U. For example, $tr.S_s$ represents the starting state of the transition tr. In case of a deterministic IOSM, there is at most one transition in $\mathbf{Tr}$ for each input symbol while there is at least one transition in a completely defined IOSM.

Definition 2. For every transition tr ($\forall tr \in \mathbf{Tr}$) whose starting state is S_i ($tr.S_s = S_i$), the state $S_i \in \mathbf{S}$ is said to be:
(1) *controllable* iff $tr.v \in \mathbf{L_{in,E}}$;
(2) *uncontrollable* iff $tr.v \in \mathbf{L_{in,I}}$;
(3) *semi-controllable* iff $\exists tr_j.v \in \mathbf{L_{in,E}}$ and $\exists tr_k.v \in \mathbf{L_{in,I}}$ where $j \neq k$.

We classify states in an IOSM into three types according to Definition 2. If a state can be changed only by external inputs, the state is said to be *controllable*. Such a state is controlled only by the testers' inputs. If all possible inputs at a state are internal ones, the state is said to be *uncontrollable*. If some possible inputs at a state are internal and others are external, the state is *semi-controllable*. This classification is illustrated in Figure 2. In IOSM M_A, a part of which is depicted in the box in Figure 2, state *A1* is controllable, *A3* is uncontrollable, and *A2* is semi-controllable. There are two transitions from state *A2* as depicted in the box in Figure 2. One transition goes to state *A3* with external input y and the other goes to state *A4* with internal input c. Let us trace the behavior of multiple stimuli in this system. When the system's global state is (*A1*, *B1*) which is a stable state, an external input x is given. Then, M_A goes to state *A2*, sending an external output x' and an internal output a, and M_B replies with an internal message c. Before the message c reaches M_A, another external message y (multiple stimuli from the environment) is given. This is because the state *A2* of M_A is a semi-controllable state. If M_A receives the internal message c in state *A2*, it will go to state *A4*, but it will go to state *A3* if it receives the external input y. Although the system is in a transient global state (*A2*, *B2*), the next stable state of the system is unpredictable since the transient global state includes a semi-controllable state. In general, if a machine in a system is in a semi-controllable state and an internal signal comes from a peer communication machine, the existing test generation methods cannot examine the external inputs since the methods adhere to the single stimulus principle.

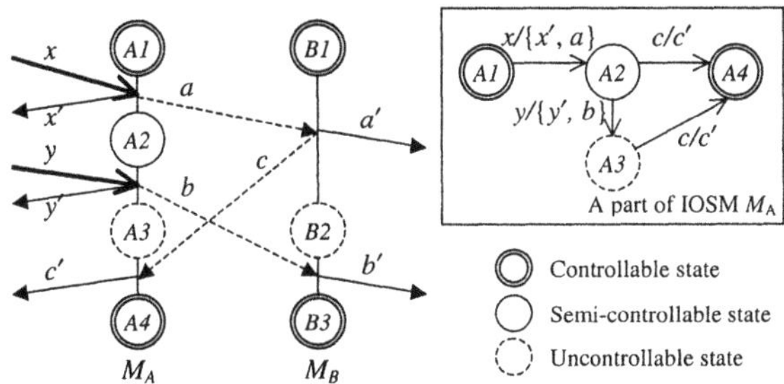

Figure 2. Three types of states in an IOSM.

Now we define a behavior model for two IOSMs communicating with each other and the environment. Let Π be the composition of the two IOSMs, one, M_A, for the specification A and the other, M_B, for the specification B. Then Π is defined as follows:

Definition 3. The composite IOSM Π is a 5-tuple ($\mathbf{S}_\Pi$, $S_{\Pi 0}$, $\mathbf{L}_{\Pi,\mathbf{in}}$, $\mathbf{L}_{\Pi,\mathbf{out}}$, $\mathbf{Tr}_\Pi$, Q_Π) where:

(1) $\mathbf{S}_\Pi = \{ S_{\Pi 0}, S_{\Pi 1}, \ldots, S_{\Pi n-1} \}$ is a set of global states, and $S_{\Pi i} = (S_A, S_B)$, where S_A and S_B are states of M_A and M_B, respectively;

(2) $S_{\Pi 0} \in \mathbf{S}_\Pi$ is the initial state. Namely, $S_{\Pi 0} = (S_{A0}, S_{B0})$;

(3) $\mathbf{L}_{\Pi,\mathbf{in}} = \{ v_{\Pi 1}, v_{\Pi 2}, \ldots, v_{\Pi m} \}$ is a set of input symbols. These messages are external inputs of each machine. Namely, $\mathbf{L}_{\Pi,\mathbf{in}} = (\mathbf{L}^{\mathbf{A}}_{\mathbf{in,E}} \cup \mathbf{L}^{\mathbf{B}}_{\mathbf{in,E}})$;

(4) $\mathbf{L}_{\Pi,\mathbf{out}} = \{ u_{\Pi 1}, u_{\Pi 2}, \ldots, u_{\Pi k} \}$ is a set of output symbols. These messages are external outputs of each machine. Namely, $\mathbf{L}_{\Pi,\mathbf{out}} = (\mathbf{L}^{\mathbf{A}}_{\mathbf{out,E}} \cup \mathbf{L}^{\mathbf{B}}_{\mathbf{out,E}})$;

(5) $\mathbf{Tr}_\Pi \subseteq \{ tr_{\Pi 0}, tr_{\Pi 1}, \ldots, tr_{\Pi t-1} \}$ is a set of sequences of transitions, and a sequence of transitions $\{ tr_\Pi \} \Leftrightarrow tr_0, tr_1, \ldots, tr_{l-1}$ where $tr_i \in (\mathbf{Tr_A} \cup \mathbf{Tr_B})$;

(6) $Q_\Pi = (Q_A, Q_B)$ is a pair of directed channels where Q_A is the channel from M_B to M_A, and Q_B from M_A to M_B; both channels are represented by queues.

A global state and directed channels (modelled by queues) in a composite IOSM Π determine the system state of the IOSM Π. Here, the system state is used to describe the state of the system as a whole while a global state is used to depict each local state of the IOSMs in the system. Note that work in [8, 10] defined a global state as one describing the entire system, including information for input queues and/or channels.

An IOSM receives messages from either the environment or its channel queue. Then, the two IOSMs and the two directed channels constitute a composite IOSM Π as shown in Figure 3. Note that in this model IOSM Π does not have any queue for inputs from the environment. This is the same as a single IOSM because its formal model does not define any queue. Since each state in an IOSM consumes one message at a time, messages following the current message do not affect the next state. We assume that internal outputs are instantly placed in the channel queue directed to the receiving IOSM. This implies *first-come first-served* (FCFS) message queuing and handling. A message leaving one machine before another message will arrive at the other machine and served before the other message.

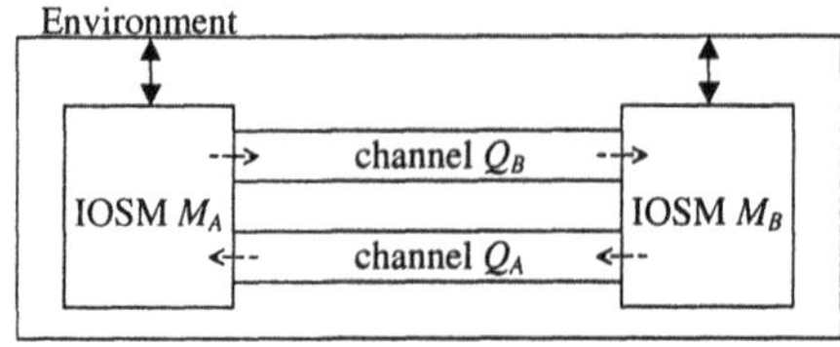

Figure 3. A composite IOSM Π.

A global state is classified into one of two types depending on the channel contents.

Definition 4. The global states of two IOSMs are classified into two types.
$\forall S_\Pi = (S_A, S_B) \in \mathbf{S}_\Pi$,
(1) A global state S_Π is said to be *stable* iff Q_A and Q_B are both empty.
(2) S_Π is in a *transient* state otherwise.

When a system is in a stable state, the system will change its state due to external inputs only. Both local states in a stable state cannot be uncontrollable states, otherwise the system is in a deadlock state because both machines will wait for messages from each other indefinitely. When a system is in a transient state, the system will change its state soon. However, the existing test generation methods do not allow for the system to receive additional external inputs. Our method, on the other hand, examines all possible external inputs. Namely, when one of the two local states in a transient global state is semi-controllable, we examine the cases where the IOSM receives an external input in the semi-controllable state as well as the cases where it consumes an internal message from its receiving channel.

Finally, we define an interoperability test suite in Definition 5. Each machine in a system consumes one input (either internal or external) at each state, that is, one transition at a time for each IOSM. Therefore, an interoperability test case can be represented by a sequence of transitions in either IOSMs in the system. An interoperability test suite is defined in terms of interoperability test cases. Note that a test case whose length is 1 is simply a conformance test case.

Definition 5. An interoperability test suite **IOPTS** $\subseteq$ $\mathbf{Tr}_{\Pi}$ is defined as follows:
IOPTS = { $iopt_0$, $iopt_1$, ..., $iopt_{n-1}$ } is a set of interoperability test cases where an interoperability test case is defined as a set of sequences of transitions,

$$\{ iopt \} \Leftrightarrow tr_0, tr_1, \ldots, tr_{l-1} \text{ where } tr_i \in (\mathbf{Tr_A} \cup \mathbf{Tr_B}), 0 \leq i \leq l\text{-}1, \text{ and } l \geq 2.$$

The interoperability test case illustrated in Figure 2 can be represented as follows. The length of this interoperability test case is 4. The starting stable state is (*A1*, *B1*) and the destination stable state is (*A4*, *B3*).

A1-x/{x',a}->A2, A2-y/{y',b}->A3, B1-a/{a',c}->B2, B2-b/b'->B3, A3-c/c'->A4

4. OUR PROPOSED APPROACH

This section describes our approach to generate interoperability test cases based on the formal models defined in Section 3. First, we explain the overall procedure of our approach and the associated assumptions. Next, we select the test architecture that achieves the desired test coverage. Finally, we discuss how to generate interoperability test cases based on the multiple stimuli principle. For the purpose of analysis, we divide the multiple stimuli into two sets classified in Figure 1 and considered in Section 4.3 and 4.4, respectively.

4.1 An overview

In order to derive test cases, we first need to derive IOSMs from the given protocol specifications. We assume that there is no autonomous transition, e.g., a timer. This is because even though we are able to generate test cases involving time constraints, it is difficult to apply them to real test environments. The interoperability test derivation algorithm generates test cases from the IOSMs by constructing an interaction graph. The algorithm starts from the initial stable state consisting of each IOSM's initial states and at each step examines all possible external inputs even in transient states, until a stable state is reached. In the meantime, new paths are generated based on the multiple stimuli principle, and newly found stable states are added to the associated state space. This procedure is repeated for every new stable state until all stable states are covered. One can apply our algorithm for deriving interoperability test cases based on the single stimulus principle as well, especially when resources (such as available points of control and observation) are limited. The input-enumeration procedure used in our approach is similar to what is known as state-perturbation [15]. However, the goal of our procedure is to build a reachability tree and then generate interoperability test cases based on its stable states, while the goal of state-perturbation is to build a reachability tree for validating protocols between interacting processes without the concept of stable state. Moreover, generating interoperability test cases mainly focuses on inputs and outputs to and from the systems of machines, which are regarded as black- or grey-boxes. However, the model (labelled transition systems) used in paper [15] is focused on internal interactions between systems of machines only.

4.2 Test architecture

To cater to the multiple stimuli principle, we need a test architecture with a tester between the two IUTs as well as one at each end as shown in Figure 4. The arrows in Figure 4 represent points of control and observation (PCOs) with both observability and controllability functions. It is assumed that there is a communication channel through which the testers coordinate with each other. Tester C should be able to hold messages passing through it for a while. In this way, simulating multiple stimuli is feasible. In the case of TCP/IP, for example, tester C will be configured with two network interface cards for each IUT. The tester duplicates and drops all the messages between the two IUTs using libpcap [14], a library for system-independent packet capture, and then sends the messages according to the interoperability test cases, coordinating with the other two testers in doing so.

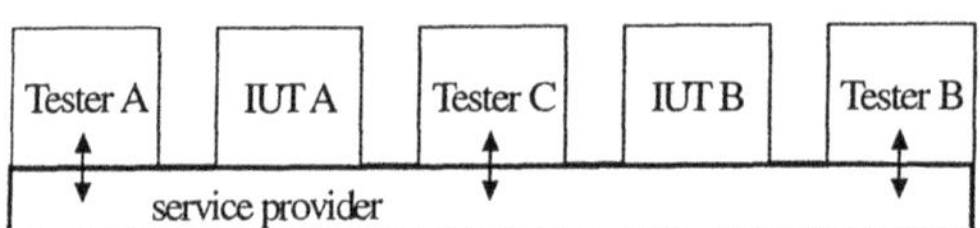

Figure 4. Interoperability test architecture.

4.3 Multiple stimuli from one machine to another

Figure 5 shows the channel status (modelled by queues) for every transition execution in deriving an interoperability test case in the given example. Starting with an external input *ex*, the algorithm pushes every internal output generated by the input into the channel Q_{AB}. Next it moves to the peer machine M_B and processes all the messages in the channel and pushes all internal outputs produced during the process into the channel Q_{BA}. This procedure is repeated until both channels are empty. Note that the order of messages, a, b, c (or, 0, 1, 2, 3) remains unchanged since first-come first-served scheduling is used. Moreover, protocol concurrency is still maintained, e.g., $tr_b \mid tr_1$, $tr_c \mid tr_2$, and $tr_c \mid tr_3$.

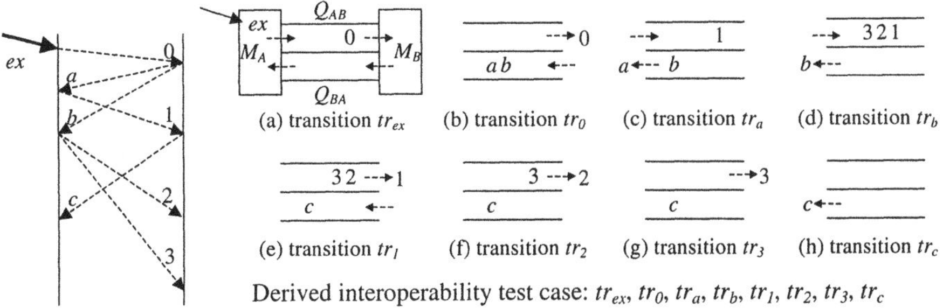

Figure 5. Derivation of interoperability test case for multiple internal outputs.

4.4 Multiple stimuli from the environment

To support multiple messages from the environment, an additional step is needed. Before the algorithm picks up an element from a channel, it examines whether the current local state of the machine is semi-controllable or not. If so, a new path is generated for all possible external inputs in this semi-controllable state. At this point, information of the current global state (which is a transient state) and all queues will be copied and the algorithm will generate test cases for each path recursively.

The procedure of generating interoperability test cases explained so far can be formalized into the algorithm given below. Lines 1 to 10 describe the main (control) part of the algorithm. This part initializes variables and calls the *interaction_sequences*() function for every stable state in the **NEW** set that has been initialized with the initial stable state (S_{A0}, S_{B0}). The function described in the rest of the algorithm generates all possible transitions based on the multiple stimuli principle. From lines 14 to 24, it checks the termination condition by examining the queue contents and updating the **NEW**, **IOPTS**, and $\mathbf{Tr}_\Pi$ sets, or calling itself recursively. From lines 25 to 37, it examines all possible transitions whose inputs are either external inputs or the current message from the queue, and then calls itself recursively with appropriate variables for this test case. Finally, the rest of the function checks whether or not the current interoperability test case has encountered a specification error, namely, there are no transition for the current message (so-called *implicit signal consumption).* This algorithm is implemented in the C language with about 1000 lines of codes. The execution time of the program is negligible (80 milliseconds for generating 1012 test cases from 150 transitions).

```
1:  LΠ,in:=L^A_in,E∪L^B_in,E; SΠ0:=(SA0,SB0); SΠ:={ SΠ,0 }; TrΠ:={}; IOPTS:={}; NEW:=SΠ
2:  while NEW≠∅ do begin
3:      set gs to any global state in NEW
4:      delete the global state from NEW
5:      for each possible external input symbol v in global state gs
6:          prepare two empty queues QA and QB, and an empty transition list iopt
7:          push v to corresponding queue, QA or QB
8:          interaction_sequences( QA or QB, QB or QA, gs, iopt, NEW )
9:      end for
10: end while
11:
12: procedure interaction_sequences( var Q1, var Q2, gs, var iopt, var NEW )
13: begin
14:     if Q1 is empty then begin
15:         if Q2 is empty then begin
16:             if iopt has more than one transition  then
17:                 insert this new interoperability test case iopt to IOPTS
18:             if iopt do not end with an error code then
19:                 insert this new global state gs to NEW
20:             insert iopt to a set of global transitions TrΠ
21:         end
22:         else interaction_sequences( Q2, Q1, gs, iopt, NEW )
23:         return
24:     end
25:     else begin
26:         in := pop(Q1);  atLeastOne := false
27:         for each possible transition tr from the current global state gs
28:             change gs according to the input in the transition, tr.v
29:             copy Q1, Q2, and iopt to newQ1, newQ2, and newiopt, respectively
30:             if the input tr.v (≠ in) is external  then
31:                 insert current input in to the back of newQ1
32:             if the transition tr has internal outputs then
33:                 push all the outputs to newQ2
34:             append the transition tr to newiopt
35:             interaction_sequences( newQ1, newQ1, gs, newiopt, NEW )
36:             atLeastOne := true
37:         end for
38:         if atLeastOne := false then begin
39:             report there is a specification error
40:             append an error code to iopt to stop expanding the current path
41:             interaction_sequences(Q1, Q2, gs, iopt, NEW )
42:         end
43:     end
44: end procedure
```

Algorithm 1. Interoperability test suite derivation

5. APPLICATIONS

In this section, we apply our method to the ATM/B-ISDN signaling protocols and TCP. Figures 6 and 7 show the IOSMs of these protocols (for more details, refer to papers [7, 8]) respectively.

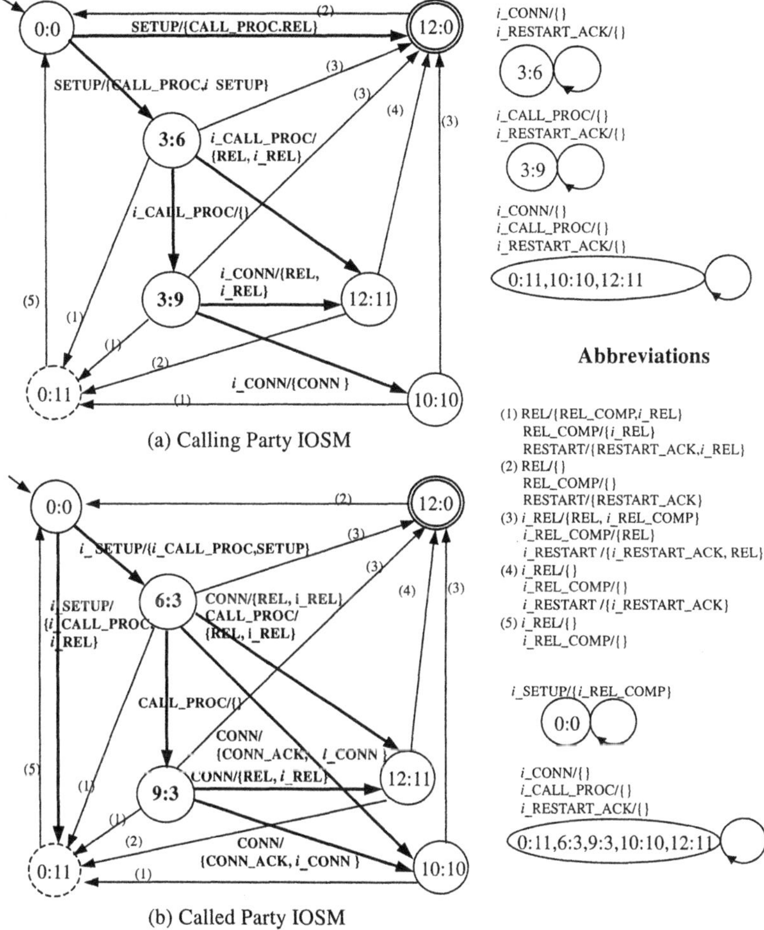

Note 1) The Input alphabet and the output alphabet of the Calling Party IOSM and the Called Party IOSM are the same, i.e. {SETUP, CALL_PROC, CONN, CONN_ACK, REL, REL_COMP, RESTART, RESTART_ACK, *i*_SETUP, *i*_CALL_PROC, *i*_CONN, *i*_REL_COMP, *i*_RESTART, *i*_ RESTART_ACK}.

Note 2) PNNI specifies three alternative ways to handle unexpected messages: i.e., ignore the received message, send STATUS and clear the call. Except in 0:0 and 12:0 above, it is assumed (for simplicity) that unexpected messages are ignored.

Note 3) Dot ('.') notation denotes that messages are set one after another successively. For instance, {*i*_CALL_PROC.*i*_REL} means that *i*_CALL_PROC is sent followed by *i*_REL.

Figure 6. The IOSM of ATM signaling protocol.

Given the IOSMs, the input data for our method can be derived systematically. An IOSM is described in a file, in which each line represents a transition in the IOSM. For instance, "[1]0:0 3:6 SETUPb CALL_PROC *i*_SETUP" is the transition whose starting state is 0:0, destination state is 3:6, input message is SETUPb, and output messages are CALL_PROC and *i*_SETUP. For convenience of reference, index numbers are given to the original data file. The postfix is used to specify specific IOSM, e.g., SETUPb is an external message being sent to IOSM M_B. The prefix '*i*_' is used to denote internal messages.

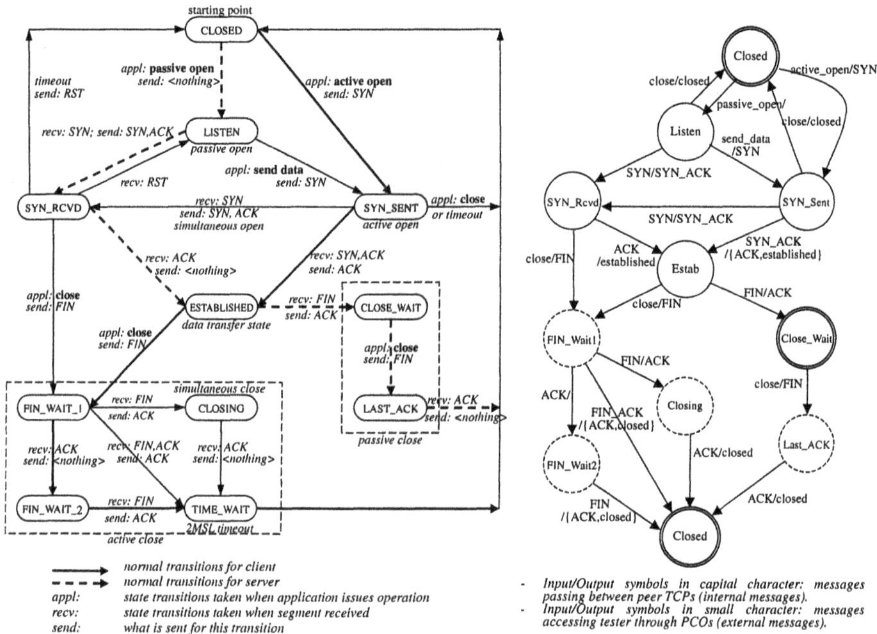

Figure 7. The TCP IOSM and its simplified one.

The results of applying our method to the two protocols are summarized in Table 1. In the case of ATM signaling protocol, a total of 1012 test cases were derived. 16 cases among them are only for one IUT and thus they are for conformance testing since there is no interaction between IUTs. Another 6 cases address specification errors for requesting the IUTs to receive unspecified input messages. Note that our method can also be used in detecting specification errors in the design phase.

The number of interoperability test cases based on the single and multiple stimulus principle are 54 and 990 respectively. Without taking into account of multiple stimuli, we have derived exactly the same 54 test cases reported in a previous work [8].

Figure 8 shows two examples in the derived interoperability test cases. An interoperability test case consists of several transitions in given IOSMs. Each transition has a unique *id*. Minus sign is used to denote the transitions of one IUT and plus sign to denote the transitions of the other one. Illustrated in Figure 8(a), the interoperability test case, <-1, 4, -12, -61, 5, 16, 8, -60, -8>, involves multiple stimuli. This test case is based on the specification and represents one of the correct behaviors of the protocol. Depicted in Figure 8(b), the interoperability test case, <-1, 75, -12, -9, -999.>, reveals specification error.

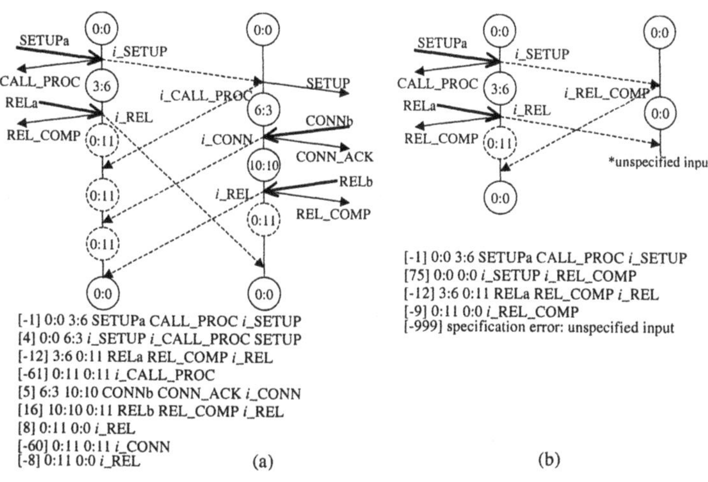

Figure 8. Examples of interoperability test cases.

Table 1 summarizes the results of our applications to the TCP and ATM signaling protocols. The test cases are classified into test cases for checking specification errors, conformance test cases, and interoperability test cases. It is shown that our method generates more test cases than existing methods [7, 8] in order to support multiple stimuli. For example, in the case of the ATM signaling protocol, we have derived 990 interoperability test cases while 54 were derived by the method [7] that assumes the single stimulus principle. Therefore, it is clear the existing methods cannot detect faults due to multiple stimuli.

Table 1. Test case generation for the IOSMs of TCP's connection establishment phase and ATM signaling protocol

TCP's connection establishment phase (Each IOSM consists of 19 transitions)		
used principle	single stimulus principle	multiple stimuli principle
test cases	20	74
test cases due to specification error	4	54
conformance test cases	8	8
interoperability test cases	8	12

ATM signaling protocol (Each IOSM consists of 75 transitions)		
used principle	single stimulus principle	multiple stimuli principle
test cases	70	1012
test cases due to specification error	0	6
conformance test cases	16	16
interoperability test cases	54	990

Table 2 gives the transition coverage for the IOSMs of TCP's connection establishment phase and the ATM signaling protocol. It is shown that our method, which is based on the multiple stimuli principle, has higher transition coverage than the existing methods, which are based on the single stimulus principle. Our method traverses 5 more transitions of TCP and 9 more transitions of ATM than the existing methods in [7, 8]. Our coverage is exactly the same as that covered by validation[4] techniques. A SDL commercial tool [13] was used to obtain the result on validation reported in Table 2. In other words, our method can generate interoperability test suite whose transition coverage is equivalent to that of validation.

Table 2. Transition coverage

methods	the existing methods [7, 8] (single stimulus principle)		our method (multiple stimuli principle)		validation	
protocols	TCP	ATM	TCP	ATM	TCP	ATM
traversed tr.	13 (68%)	39 (52%)	18 (95%)	48 (64%)	18	48
untraversed tr.	6 (32%)	36 (48%)	1 (5%)	27 (36%)	1	27

Table 3. Untraversed transitions

	the existing methods [7, 8]		our method	
protocols (untraversed tr.)	TCP (6)	ATM (36)	TCP (1)	ATM (27)
wrongly specified	1 (5%)	13 (17%)	1	13
over-specified	0 (0%)	14 (19%)	0	14
limitation of the method	5 (26%)	9 (12%)	0	0

[4] Validation is based on the state space exploration technique. It automatically checks a distributed system's design for errors and makes it possible to prove a system will work before implementation. Validation executes all possible combinations of events that can happen, and reports any indication that something has gone wrong.

Table 3 shows the reasons why some transitions are not traversed. First, some transitions are wrongly specified and will never be executed due to absence of transitions that send the corresponding signals. For instance, some transitions in Figure 6 need an input signal i_RESTART, but there is no transition that sends the required signal. Note that a wrongly specified transition may give rise to subsequent untraversed transitions. Also, some transitions are over-specified. Over-specified transitions are superfluous and are unnecessary for our purpose. They include self-transitions whose start state and final state are the same. Actually they are sometimes used for error handling. Since checking correct behavior is the objective of our method, such transitions are considered as over-specified in this paper. Finally, some transitions are not traversed due to the limitation of the method used. As shown in the table, our method can traverse all the transitions that cannot be handled by the existing methods.

6. CONCLUSION AND FUTURE WORK

We have proposed a new method for generating interoperability test suites that support multiple inputs to the system under test. This means the method adopts the multiple stimuli principle rather than the traditional single stimulus principle used in existing methods. To do this, we have developed appropriate formal models on which the interoperability test suite derivation algorithm is based. We have applied our method to the ATM signaling protocol and also to a part of TCP. Experimental results have shown that our method has higher transition coverage than the existing methods: 26% higher for TCP and 12% higher for ATM. Our transition coverage is equivalent to that managed by the validation technique. As future work, the derived test cases will be applied to production protocols for interoperability testing in a real-life environment.

REFERENCES

[1] ISO/IEC 9646-1, "Information Technology – OSI Conformance Testing Methodology and Framework. Part 1: General Concepts", 1994.

[2] Rafiq, O. and Castanet, R., "From Conformance Testing to Interoperability testing", Proceedings of the 3rd International Workshop on Protocol Test System, 1990.

[3] Arakawa, N., Phalippou, M., Risser, N. and Soneoka, T., "Combination of conformance and interoperability testing", Formal Description Techniques, V (C-10) M. Diaz and R. Groz (Eds.), Elsevier Science Publishers, 1993.

[4] Shin, J. and Kang, S., "Interoperability Test Suite Derivation for the ATM/B-ISDN Signaling Protocol", Testing of Communicating Systems, Vol 11, Kluwer Academic Publishers, pp. 313-330, 1998.

[5] Vermeer, G. S. and Blik, H., "Interoperability Testing: Basis for the Acceptance of Communicating Systems", Protocol Test System, VI, Elsevier Science Publishers, 1994.

[6] Kang, S. and Kim, M., "Interoperability Test Suite Derivation for Symmetric Communication Protocols", IFIP Joint International Conference on Formal Description Techniques (FORTE X) and Protocol Specification Testing and Verification (PSTV XVII), pp. 57-72, November 1997.

[7] Seol, S., Kim, M., Kang, S. and Park, Y., "Interoperability Test Suite Derivation for the TCP protocol", IFIP Joint International Conference on Formal Description Techniques for Distributed Systems and Communication Protocols (FORTE XII) and Protocol Specification Testing and Verification (PSTV XIX), 1999.

[8] Kang, S., Shin, J. and Kim, M., "Interoperability Test Suite Derivation for Communication Protocols", Computer Networks, 2000.

[9] Arakawa, N. and Soneoka, T., "A Test Case Generation Method for Concurrent Programs", Protocol Test Systems, IV, Elsevier Science Publishers, 1992.

[10] Luo, G., Bochmann G., and Petrenko, A., "Test Selection Based on communicating Nondeterministic Finite-State Machines Using a Generalized Wp-Method", IEEE Transactions on S.E., Vol 20, No. 2, pp. 149-162, February 1994.

[11] Lima Jr., L. Paula and Cavalli, A., A Pragmatic Approach to Generating Test Sequences for Embedded Systems, IWTCS, 1997.

[12] ITU-T X.290 Series, Conformance Testing Methodology and Framework, 1994.

[13] "Telelogic SDT 3.2 Manuals", Telelogic, September 1997.

[14] The Tcpdump Group, "libpcap", available at http://www.tcpdump.org.

[15] Zafiropulo P., West C.H., Rudin H., Cowan D.D., and Brand D., "Towards Analyzing and Synthesizing Protocols (Computer Networks)", IEEE Transactions on Communications, vol.28, no.4, pp.651-661, April 1980.

AUTOMATED GENERATION OF INTEROPERABILITY TESTS*

Cédric Besse*, Ana Cavalli*, Myungchul Kim**, Fatiha Zadi*
*_Institut National des Telecommunications_
9 rue Charles Fourier
F-91011 Evry Cedex, France
Email : {Cedric.Besse,Ana.Cavalli,Fatiha.Zaidi}@int-evry.fr
**_Information and Communications University_
Hwaam-dong 58-4, Yusung-gu
Taejon 305-732, Korea
Email : mckim@icu.ac.kr

Abstract In this paper we present two methods for automated interoperability tests generation. The tests are applied to different entities implementing the same protocol and are peer-to-peer tests. They can be executed on test architectures either including only Points of Control and Observation (PCOs), or including both PCOs and Point of Observation (POs) to facilitate the diagnosis after the test execution. Both methods are applied in a case study to the interoperability test of the TCP/IP protocol. The protocol used for the experiment is TCP-Reno, which is specified in SDL. It is one of the most commonly referenced implementations. In the paper we present the tests sequences obtained and compare the experimental results of both methods.

Keywords: Conformance testing, interoperability testing, automated test sequences generation, fault coverage, SDL, TCP/IP protocol.

1. INTRODUCTION

Conformance testing of a protocol component means to test the conformance of the component to its specification, but this is not enough when this component needs to interact and communicate with other components. Moreover, with the development of networks and, particularly of the Internet, a large family of protocols and new services are

*This work has been partially supported by Korean Science and Engineering Foundation and ARIEL-Confrence des Grandes Ecoles, France (No. 995-0900-007-2).

coming up. If two or more components that are a part of different communicating systems must interact between them to perform a task, it must be validated that they can interact as expected. The evaluation of this interoperability is one of the essential aspects of the correctness of the integrated systems.

Interoperability tests need to be performed to evaluate the interoperability of the integrated components that can be implemented by different providers. In addition, although each component is usually considered as a black-box, a finer degree of observability is needed to enable a diagnosis, which determines the causes of non-interoperability, after tests execution.

Several methods have been proposed on interoperability testing [13, 9, 11, 4]. One of the main issues in these works is the definition of a test case selection criterion that guarantees the coverage of faults related to components interoperability. Some of these works only provide testing of the control part of a system under test [13, 11].

The aim of the work presented in this paper is to provide an answer to the previous issues. We first propose two methods for automated the interoperability test generation. The tests are peer-to-peer tests. The first method is based on an algorithm designed originally for automated test generation for embedded components of a complex system [5]. It uses the interactions of the embedded component as a guide for test sequence generation. We have adapted this algorithm for interoperability test generation: we now use the interactions between the interacting entities as a criterion for the selection of test cases and as a guide for the test sequences generation. Thus we do not generate redundant tests. The second method we present is based on an algorithm designed originally for the optimization of test suites [2]. The algorithm is based on the coloring of some transitions of the original specification. Each transition representing an interaction of an entity corresponds to several transitions of the global graph. We assign the same color to all such transitions. In this way, we define a criteria for the selection of interoperability tests: we produce a minimum set of paths that covers all the colored transitions. In addition, both methods take data into account when generating tests (test sequences include parameters values).

There are a number of test architectures for interoperability testing [4]. Some of them include Points of Control and Observation(PCOs) only and some of them include both PCOs and Point of Observations (POs). Tests generated by the methods presented in this paper can be applied to both test architectures. However, we consider the test architectures that include both PCOs and POs, which have more observability, in order to facilitate a fault diagnosis.

We have applied both methods to generate interoperability tests of the TCP/IP protocol. The protocol used for the experiment is TCP-Reno [10], which is specified in SDL [7]. It is one of the most commonly referenced implementations. These implementations can be supplied by different providers. As a result of our work we can generate two sequences of tests, generated by the two proposed methods. The generated test sequences can be used for interoperability testing between two entities of the TCP/IP protocol. Note that for TCP/IP tests peer-to-peer are end-to-end tests, which means that they perform testing of entities that are at the extremities of the network and need to exchange information.

The sequences of tests obtained by the two methods are different. We have analyzed and compared the results, and then found that the two methods are complementary. The first method that uses interactions as a guide for simulation provides better results in testing control parts. The second method that uses a coloring technique permits an easier data differentiation, particularly in branches where decisions are embedded. This complementarity constitutes for us a proof of the interest of our methods: users can choose one of the best fitted to their needs.

The rest of the paper is organized as follows. In Section 2, some basic definitions are given. This section also introduces the criteria used for test selection to guarantee interoperability fault coverage and diagnosis. Section 3 presents the two methods for generating interoperability tests. Section 4 gives an outline of TCP/IP protocol and presents its SDL specification. Section 5 presents the experimental results of the application of the two methods. Finally, Section 6 gives the conclusion and perspectives of this work.

2. RELATED WORK

Conformance testing cannot guarantee that two components or more will interoperate properly within a communicating system. Specific interoperability testing strategies have to be developed, once conformance testing techniques have been applied and conformance has been stated.

Some works have been performed in regard to interoperability, in order to furnish either a formal framework, or experimental results. The authors of [13] were the first to propose a solution for interoperability tests generation. Their work lies on the generation of the reachability graph of the communicating system. [4] has formalized the relation of interoperability by adapting the existing conformance relations. [11] proposed algorithms to generate a test suite. For this purpose, their composition algorithm considers stable states and only tests the control part of the system. These previous methods can be classified in methods based on reachability analysis. Thus, they are faced to the well-known problem of state space explosion, for real or simply realistic case studies. Other methods have been also proposed, such [3, 16]. All of these methods are based on experimentations, and no coherent framework is proposed. [9] based their work on interoperability by proposing a test generation technique from the joint behaviour of end-users interfaces. This method, in order to avoid the problem of combinatorial explosion, classifies the edges concerning interoperation as black edges and those concerning local activities as white edges. Then, they propose an efficient algorithm to retrieve the significant transitions, in other words the black edges.

Another drawback of all the previous methods is that they only consider the control part of the protocol. In our case, we deal with control and data parts. The generated tests comprehend parameters values in messages and consider variables in graph generation.

3. BASICS

3.1 Extended Finite State Machines

Protocols can be properly modeled by extended finite state machines [12]. In this paper, we have chosen this formalism to describe the studied systems and the test generation algorithms.

Definition. An *extended finite state machine* (EFSM) is a quintuple $M = (I, O, S, \vec{x}, T)$ where I, O, S, $\vec{x}$, and T are finite sets of input symbols, output symbols, states, variables, and transitions, respectively. Each transition t in the set T is a 6-tuple:

$$t = (s_t, q_t, a_t, o_t, P_t, A_t)$$

where s_t, q_t, a_t, and o_t are the current state, next state, input, and output, respectively. $P_t(\vec{x})$ is a predicate on the current variable values, and $A_t(\vec{x})$ specifies an action on the variable values.

Initially, the machine is in an initial state $s^{(0)} \in S$ with initial variable values: $\vec{x}^{(0)}$. Suppose that the machine is in state s_t with the current variable values $\vec{x}$ and an outgoing transition t from s_t. Upon input a_t, if $\vec{x}$ is valid for P_t, i.e., $P_t(\vec{x}) =$ TRUE, then the machine follows the transition t, outputs o_t, changes the current variable values by action $\vec{x} := A_t(\vec{x})$, and moves to state q_t.

3.2 Fault Coverage

The definition of a test case selection criterion that guarantees a fault coverage related to components interoperability is one of the main issues in research work related to interoperability testing. In this paper we propose the following test selection criterion: we select in the protocol specification the transitions that represent an interaction between protocol entities under test. This selection is performed in the first method by considering the set of transitions, which are involved in entities interoperability, as test purposes. These transitions will be used as a guide for simulation. In the second method the selection is performed by coloring the interoperability transitions. In other words, for interoperability tests generation the coverage criterion is reduced to cover some parts of the specification that are related to the communication between interworking entities. In the work presented in this paper, interoperability concerns the test of distinct communicating entities of the same layer.

Another important issue to perform interoperability testing is that since some of the interfaces of the components under test are not directly accessible, interactions through these interfaces can only be observed. To take into account this issue, we use a test architecture (see figure 1) with Points of Control and Observation (PCO) and Points of Observation (POs) below each protocol entity. The POs allow to observe interactions we cannot directly access to. In particular for the TCP/IP protocol it is possible to observe execution traces. Both methods presented in this

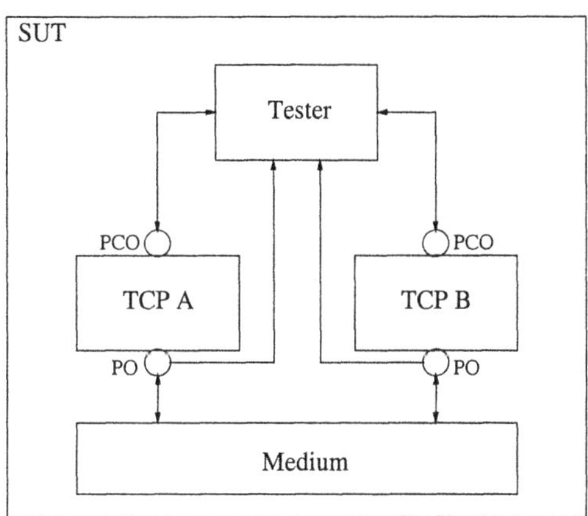

Figure 1. Test architecture

paper allows to detect all output faults in covered transitions. The first method generates a test sequence that covers all the trasitions that represent entities interactions. The second method generates a set of paths that also covers these transitions.

4. TWO DIFFERENT METHODS FOR AUTOMATED INTEROPERABILITY TESTS GENERATION

In this section, we present for the two methods the algorithms for interoperability test sequences generation.

4.1 Method 1: Interoperability based on interactions as test purposes

As mentionned in section 3 our test purpose covers all the interactions from the entity A to the entity B in the case of a communication protocol. Indeed we will focus on the interactions between two protocol entities. The test purposes cover all the interactions. Note that we obtain a test case for each interaction.

The algorithm presented in this section is based on the generation of partial reachability graphs [5]. It offers an alternative to the second method presented in this paper, which is based on the generation of a global reachability graph. Sometimes it is not possible or impractical to construct such a global reachability graph due to the state-space explosion problem. To overcome this problem we propose a technique which avoids the construction of the complete system reachability graph. Figure 2 presents the algorithm. The technique we propose conducts, at any moment, a local search from the current state in a neighborhood of the reachability graph (step 2 of figure 2). If an untested part is found, we test that part (steps 3 to 7) and continue the process from there (step 8). Otherwise we move randomly to the frontier of the neighborhood searched (steps 10 to 13) and continue the process from there (step 14). A condition for the application of the algorithm is the definition of the tests purposes we want to test. A pre-defined limitation for the search must be defined by the user. For example, it can be a depth limit. Due to this limit we avoid the construction of the complete reachability graph. In fact it's just a bet on non-locality, we want to move to untested parts of the specification, and thus to avoid to be trapped in certain part of the specification. The algorithm terminates when all the interactions present in the set are found. Moreover, the exhaustive search can be a depth-first, breadth-first or bounded depth-first.

```
Algorithm
  inputs. two CEFSMs A and B that are in their initial states, as well
          as the variables values.
  predicate. set of interactions to cover, interact_seq_set.
  an interaction is a global transition where both entities exchange
  messages
  output. interoperability test case
  1. while interact_seq_set ≠ ∅ do begin
  2.     From the current state conduct an exhaustive search
  3.     if one of the interact_seq_set = true
  4.         then
  5.             Stop the exhaustive search;
  6.             Keep track of the path from the current node to the
                 interaction reached (extend the current sequence
                 with the path from the root to the interaction we got);
  7.             Remove the true interaction from interact_seq_set;
  8.             Go to the new current node (reached after the
                 interruption of the exhaustive search on the found
                 interaction).
  9.         else
  10.            We stopped the exhaustive search on a pre-defined limit;
  11.            Consider one spanning tree of the partially deployed
                 FSM;
  12.            Examine all the leaf nodes of the tree, and select
                 one uniformly and randomly;
  13.            Include the path from the root to the selected leaf in
                 the test sequence;
  14.            Go to the new current state.
  15.    end if
  16. end while
  17. Return the test sequence.
```

Figure 2. Description of the algorithm used by method 1

4.2 Method 2: Interoperability based on the coloring of the interactions

We presented in [2] an automatic and optimized technique for test generation of communication protocol control and data portions with the goal of minimizing the number of tests with a guaranteed fault coverage. This coverage corresponds to a set of entities that we want to cover (transitions of the specification, variable values, etc). Different colors are assigned to such entities, to cover interactions transitions. Each interaction transition is involved in a number of transitions of the global reachability graph. Those colors remain in the reachability graph of the protocol produced by simulation. The algorithm then finds a minimal number of paths from the source node of the graph covering each one a maximum number of uncovered colors. Each path is counted as one sequence, and the set of tests has to cover all the colors.

The algorithm is in fact applied to a Direct Acyclic Graph (DAG), obtained from the colored reachability graph. Construction of the DAG consists in shrinking each Strongly Connected Component (SCC) of the graph into what becomes a node of the DAG. That node contains all the colors of the SCC, and be referred to as an SCC-node of the DAG. Once paths are generated, these are completed to take into account all the colors of each SCC-node involved in a path. It is done by finding in the corresponding SCC a colors tour, which is added to the path.

Algorithm

input. a colored DAG $G =< V, E >$ with V and E respectively sets of vertices and edges of G, and the source node v_0.

output. an approximate maximal color path from v_0.

1. topologically sort nodes in V: $v_0, v_1, \ldots, v_{n-1}$;
2. **for** $i = n-1, \ldots, 0$ /* bottom-up */
3. $\quad\kappa(v_i) = \emptyset$; /* $\kappa(v_i)$: computed color set of chosen path from v_i */
4. $\quad p(v_i) = \text{NULL}$; /* $p(\cdot)$: pointer to next node on chosen path */
5. $\quad$ let outgoing edges from v_i be: $(v_i, w_1), \ldots, (v_i, w_r)$;
6. $\quad$ **for** $j = 1, \ldots, r$
7. $\quad\quad$ **if** $|c(v_i) \cup c(v_i, w_j) \cup \kappa(w_j)| > |\kappa(v_i)|$
8. $\quad\quad\quad \kappa(v_i) = c(v_i) \cup c(v_i, w_j) \cup \kappa(w_j)$,
   $\quad\quad\quad p(v_i) = w_j$;/* pick up winner */
9. $path = v_0$; /* $path$: constructed max-color path */
10. $v = v_0$; /* construct path top-down */
11. **while** $p(v) \neq \text{NULL}$
12. $\quad v = p(v)$; /* get to next node on path */
13. $\quad path = path \circ v$;
14. **return** $path$;

Figure 3. Description of the algorithm used by method 2

Given a colored DAG G, each node v and edge (u, v) is associated with a set of colors: $c(v), c(u, v) \subseteq C$. We want to find a path (test) from the source node v_0, covering a maximal number of colors. Since the graph G is a DAG, we topologically sort the nodes [8], and compute a desired path bottom-up in a reverse topological order as follows.

Note that $c(\cdot)$ denotes the color set associated with a node or edge, which is given by the testing criteria and is fixed. We denote $\kappa(v_i)$ is the color set of the max-color path from node v_i, constructed by the algorithm. When we process a node v_i at Line 3-8 and consider all the outgoing edges (v_i, w_j), we take the union of the colors of node v_i, edge (v_i, w_j), and $\kappa(w_j)$. We compare the resulting color sets from all the outgoing edges from v_i and keep one with the largest cardinality. Line 9-13 collect nodes top-down from v_0 along the constructed path. Since we examine each edge once and take unions of and compare color sets of no more than k colors, the time and space complexity of the algorithm is $O(km)$ where m is the number of edges of G.

This **Maximum Color Path** algorithm has to be modified to be used for interoperability testing. We assign a color to all the transitions of the specification. This allows us to keep a trace of the part of the specification we have to pass through to obtain the required interoperability test sequences, and measure the algorithm efficiency in terms of coverage. We give a **priority** to each color that is either an input or an output of one of the interoperating systems. The major effect on the algorithm is that the set of tests has now to cover not all the colors, but **at least** all the colors with priority.

In such a manner, we generate interoperability tests. The algorithm used by this method is presented in Figure 3.

5. THE TCP/IP PROTOCOL

The TCP protocol is a highly reliable host-to-host protocol in packet-switched computer communication networks, and in interconnected systems of such networks [14]. For the description of the protocol we have used the SDL langage, standardized by ITU-T [7], which is widely used for the specification of protocols. As it is mentioned in [10], the SDL specification of the TCP includes the description of the protocol architecture. This architecture is organized in three layers: application, communication and network layers. The application layer includes a socket layer with two different variants: Client and Server. They are described as SDL blocks that represent the behavior of the environment and some applications. The SDL description follows the TCP Transition Diagram presented in [14]. The states represented in the SDL specification are the same as that in the TCP Transitions Diagram. **Experiments**
The experiments are performed on the TCP-Reno specification. As the complete reachability graph of the specification is too big, and considering the fact that we are especially interested in the part of the system that describes the interworking between the two TCP A and B, at the TCP Layers, we have reshaped the specification, moving Socket and Client Layers outside the system, so that Socket Layer becomes the new

system environment, in accordance with the test architecture presented in section 3.

5.1 Method 1 experiments

In this section we describe the results obtained after applying method 1 to the TCP-Reno specification. To use this method we need to set some prerequisites. First of all we have to select the test purposes, as mentioned in section 3.2. We want to test the interactions between TCP A and TCP B. With this method we can define test purposes, which in that case are the interactions that we want to test. In the following we explain how to define the test purposes.

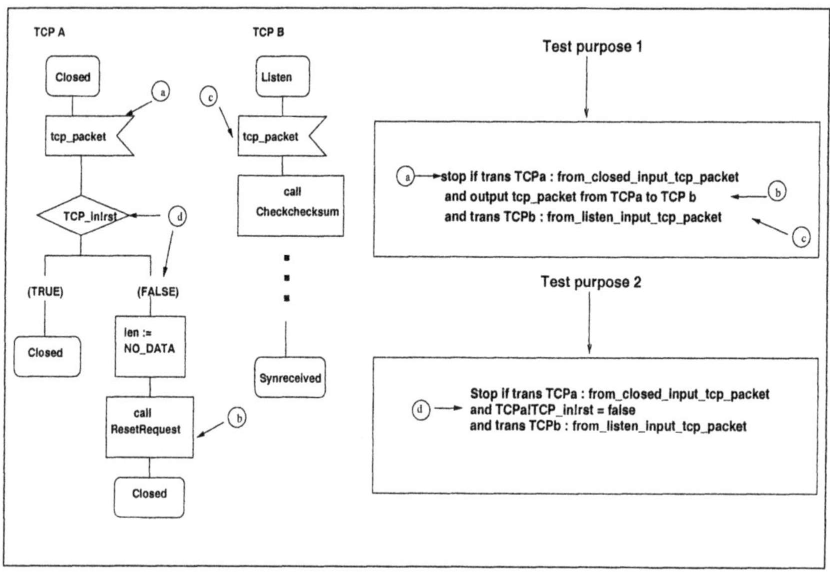

Figure 4. Test purposes definition

Description of test purposes based on interactions between TCP A and TCP B

Figure 4 illustrates how to select the test purposes: on the left side you can find the graphical SDL of the two TCP entities and on the right side the test purposes. To express the test purposes the algorithm uses a special syntax close to the SDL syntax. The algorithm has been implemented in such a way that it manages the simulator of ObjectGEODE, and we use some features of this tool to write the test purposes. The interested readers can refer to [5] for a more detailed description of the implementation of this algorithm.

Concerning the test purposes, to facilitate the understanding of their meaning, we describe them in the following using natural language. The test purpose 1 in figure 4 represents each part of an interaction that we want to test. The test purpose 1 exhibits an end-to-end interaction between the two distinct entities. The test purpose 2 shows how it is possible, using this formalism, to distinguish two decision branches on the variables. These two test purposes express the same interaction to test. This interaction is the following: TCP A is in state *Closed*, when it receives a *tcp_packet* (a in figure 4), it tests the *rst* flag (d), if it is equal to false, TCP A calls the procedure *ResetRequest* (b), which sends *tcp_packet* to TCP B. TCP B receives this packet in state *Listen* (c) and calls the procedure *checkchecksum*, which allows to check the correctness of the *tcp* header.

The application of the method to the specification of TCP-Reno produced the following results. We covered **36** interactions concerning the two different TCP entities. Indeed we obtain test sequences that represent a path from one of entity to the other, it is what we call an end-to-end interoperability test sequence.

To illustrate this application we present in the figure 5 one of the test sequences that we have obtained. This one is a simplified version of the original sequence, that illustrates the connection establishing. The TCP connection is done with a three-way handshake. In this example TCP A is the initiator of the connection, at the beginning it is in *passive* (listening) state, it receives an *active open* request from the environment (the socket layer). At the same time the TCP B receives a *passive open* with an unspecified foreign socket (represented by the *upo* signal). This specification and most APIs (Application Programming Interface) do not provide a way to treat this. Thus TCP B must leave the foreign socket and wait for a connection to arrive, it moves then to the state *Listen*. TCP A sends a TCP segment with the flag *SYN*, it means that the synchronization flag is set. TCP A remembers it has sent this initial *SYN* packet by entering the *Synsent* state. In response TCP B after receiving this TCP segment enters the state *Synreceived* and responds with its own TCP segment and acknowledging receipt of the initial *SYN* packet by putting the *ACK* flag. In figure 5, the *tcp_packet* fields flag *SYN* and *ACK* are equal to true. TCP A acknowledges receipt of the *SYN* from TCP B and enters the state *Established*. And when TCP B receives this it enters also the *Established* state. This test sequence has been obtained by the concatenation of the two test purposes, the first one to obtain the interaction between the peer TCP in their *Closed* states, and a second one for the interaction between the *Synsent* state (TCP A) and *Synreceived* state (TCP B).

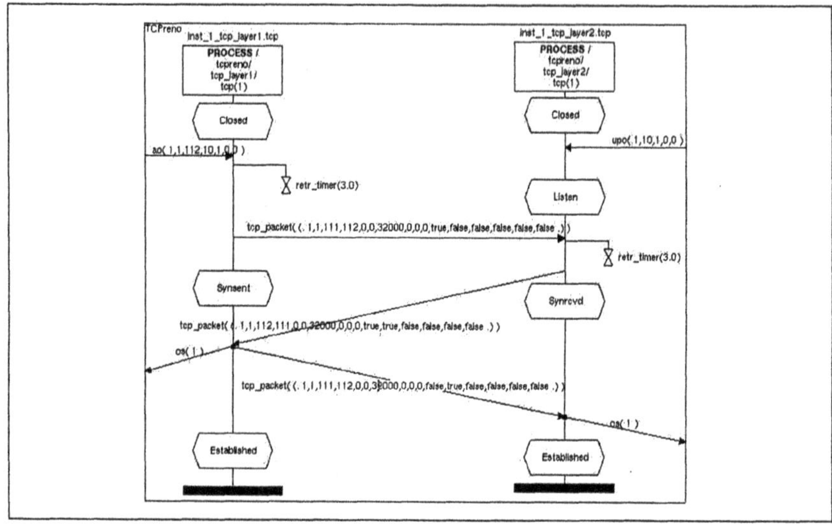

Figure 5. A generated simplified test sequence for the connexion establishing

Fault diagnosis

The PCOs that appear in figure 1, permit to detect the output faults. Indeed the testers according to the response of the system under test can establish a verdict. Moreover, if a fault occurs during the interaction of the TCP entities, thanks to the POs, we will be able to detect this fault and to have a finer verdict.

5.2 Method 2 experiments

All transitions are colored and to obtain interoperability test sequences priority is given to the transitions representing the exchanges between TCP A and TCP B. A reachability graph with good cover rates of transitions and states can be generated by an exhaustive simulation, see Table 1.

We obtain a minimal reachability graph, from which we apply the maximal color path algorithm repeatedly until all the transitions with priority are covered. The results are shown in Table 2.

In total, to cover the **36** colors with priority deployed in the graph, **11** paths are generated.

Table 1. Exhaustive Simulation of the TCP specification

# of States	14008
# of Transitions	46695
Maximum depth reached	21
Maximum breadth reached	3146

Table 2. Final results for the minimal reachability graph

# of Nodes	1926
# of Edges	14767
# of Maximum Color Paths	11

As illustrated by table 3 the first path covers **16** colors, among which are **5** colors with priority. The next three paths cover **5** colors with priority, the next one **4**, and so on. Given the large number of nodes

Table 3. Created paths

Path	# of covered colors	# of colors with priority	Length
0	16	5	18
1	6	5	17
2	6	5	17
3	6	5	17
4	5	4	17
5	4	4	16
6	4	2	17
7	3	2	18
8	4	2	17
9	1	1	17
10	1	1	17

and edges in the minimal reachability graph, our algorithm efficiently constructs a rather small number of tests, **11**, that cover the required parts of the specification.

The figure 6 presents the MSC obtained from the path number 0. This path correspond to a connection establishment phase presented in figure 6, initiated by TCP A. This can be expressed as follows. An *active open* is sent by the Socket_A layer to TCP A, that synchronizes its sequence number with TCP B sequence number, and wait for a connection acknowledgement from TCP B. Once it is obtained, TCP A sends its acknowledgement to TCP B and asks the Socket_A Layer for a socket to be opened (*open socket* signal) on its side. TCP B then receives TCP A acknowledgement and sends an *open socket* signal to the Socket B Layer.

At this point of the path execution, connection is fully established between TCP A and TCP B (both TCP are in the *Established* state). The end of the path corresponds to the beginning of a connection termination phase.

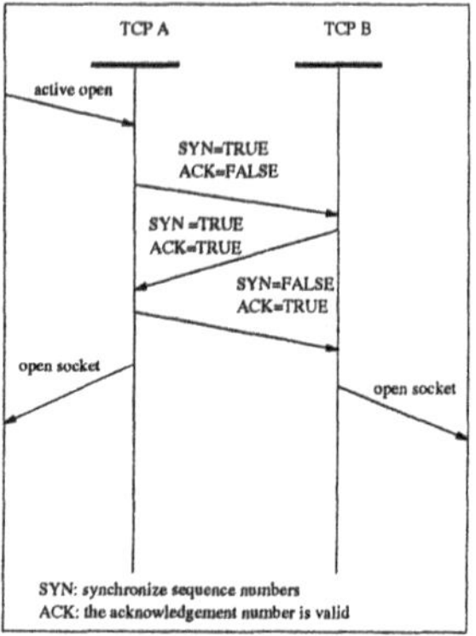

Figure 6. Connection establishment phase

5.3 Comparison of the obtained results

In this section, we compare the results of the two methods. Both methods have similar goals, i.e. obtain tests for the interoperability parts of the specification and both have been applied successfully. Nevertheless there are some differences between the two methods. Indeed, some interactions found in method 1 cannot be detected using method 2, and reciprocally some interactions found by method 2 cannot be detected using method 1.

Method 2 can easily distinguish interactions according to variable values, because we can assign different colors to different branches of a transition, as a decision based on data values might modify the parameters of a sent signal. Most of the time is spent on the generation of the reachability graph. Once the graph is obtained, the paths are automatically and quickly generated by an algorithm developed at INT and integrated to our tool TESTGEN. The cost is fairly high in term of resource consuming, as we first compute the whole reachability graph to obtain the DAG.

On the other hand, applying method 1, we do not have to obtain a global reachability graph. Method 1 requires to spend more time to express test purposes as they are until now handcrafted, whereas they can be generated automatically in method 2. Both methods demand a relative knowledge of the protocol to test. This is more significant in method 1, since writing test purposes can be more complex than the coloring of transitions. Once the interactions are located and formally expressed, we can focus the efforts on the complexity of test generation. We mean the launching of the tool developped at the INT, for each interaction. Finally, we can say that method 1 is time consuming in term of the characterization of interactions to test, but not in term of execution. In term of resource consuming, we can say that this cost is very low in method 1, as we only compute at each step a partially reachability graph and we do not keep in memory track of this graph.

Comparison can also be made between length of the tests. A sequence of 1,500 transitions (joining all the sequences) is obtained using method 1, whereas method 2 generates 11 paths, each one having about 17 transitions, for a total of 188 transitions. This awesome difference (about 8 times less transitions) is caused because paths construction is intended to maximize the number of interactions in it. On the contrary, a sequence in method 1 only contain one interaction.

The coverage of the 36 transitions covered by both methods, is complete with respect to the interoperability requirements presented in the specification. In fact, these 36 transitions represent all the interactions between TCP A and TCP B on a total number of 282 transitions for the whole specification.

6. CONCLUSION

To summarize, the contribution of our work consists in the development of two methods for interoperability tests generation and their application to a real protocol, TCP/IP. This application illustrates their suitability. Both methods have been applied in a test architecture that enables to control and to observe the entities interactions. This is an important factor for the faults diagnosis.

The two methods use the same basic idea for generating interoperability test sequences: to select in the protocol specification the transitions that represent an interaction between the protocol entities under test. The experiments showed that both methods are complementary, one is well adapted to test more different control parts and the other permits an easier data differentiation. We have also compared the length of the test sequence and the concatenation of the set of paths.

Both methods have been integrated in a tool set for automated test generation, TESTGEN [6, 5], that we have developed in our research group at INT.

The outcomes of this work will be used in a future work related to the development of a platform for the interoperability testing of services and protocols, with an application to the wireless access to Internet.

References

[1] *RFC 793: Transmission Control Protocol*, September 1981.

[2] C. Besse, A. Cavalli, and D. Lee. An automatic and optimized test generation technique. applying to TCP/IP protocol. In *ASE'99 (14th IEEE International Conference on Automated Software Engineering)*, october 12-15 1999.

[3] Grard Bonnes. IBM OSI Interoperability Services. In *Protocol Test Systems, III*. North-Holland, 1991.

[4] R. Castanet and O. Kone. Deriving coordinated testers for interoperability. *Protocol Test Systems*, VI (C-19):331–345, 1994. Elsevier Science Publ B. V.(North-Holland).

[5] A. Cavalli, D. Lee, Ch. Rinderknecht, and F. Zadi. Hit-or-Jump: An Algorithm for Embedded Testing with Applications to IN Services. In *Formal Methods for Protocol Engineering And Distributed Systems*, pages 41–56. Kluwer Academic, October 1999.

[6] A. R. Cavalli, B. Chin, and K. Chon. Testing methods for SDL Systems. In *Computer Networks and ISDN Systems*, volume 28, pages 1669–1683, 1996.

[7] CCITT, ITU-T General Secretariat, Geneve, Switzerland. *Recommendation Z.100: Specification and Description Language (SDL)*, 1992.

[8] T. H. Cormen, C. E. Leiserson, and R. L. Rivest. *Introduction to Algorithms*. MIT Press, 1990.

[9] N. Griffeth, R. Hao, D. Lee, and R. K. Sinha. Integrated system interoperability testing with applications to VOIP. In *FORTE/PSTV'00*, October 2000.

[10] J. Hintelman and R. Westerfeld. Performance analysis of tcp's flow control mechanisms using queueing SDL. In *In Proc. of SDL Forum'97*. Elsevier, September 1997.

[11] S. Kang and M. Kim. Interoperability test suite derivation for symmetric communication protocols. In *FORTE/PSTV'97*, 1997.

[12] D. Lee and M. Yannakakis. Principles and Methods of Testing Finite State Machines - A Survey. *Proc. of the IEEE*, 84(8):1090–1123, August 1996.

[13] O. Rafiq and R. Castanet. From conformance testing to interoperability testing. *The 3rd Int. Workshop on Protocol Test Systems*, 1990.

[14] W. R. Stevens. *TCP/IP Illustrated*. The protocols. Addison-Wesley, 1994.

[15] Verilog. *ObjectGEODE Simulator, Reference manual*, 1997.

[16] G.S. Vermeer and H. Blik. Interoperabillity testing : Basis for the acceptance of communication systems: Theory and practice. In *Protocol Test Systems, VI (C-19)*. North-Holland, 1994.

KEYNOTE SPEECH II - ABSTRACT

APPLYING FORMAL METHODS IN MOBILE PROTOCOL TESTING

Experiences and Challenges

Ari Ahtiainen
Nokia Research Center, Helsinki, Finland
ari.ahtiainen@nokia.com

Abstract The introduction of 3rd Generation mobile systems underlines the need for interoperability and conformity to internationally standardized protocols in order to fulfil the promise of worldwide availability of services. Although the systems specifications for 3rd Generation radio technologies and UMTS networking protocols have grown in size and complexity the mobile networking community is now equipped with the experiences of making the GSM system a worldwide success. Adoption of conformance testing based on formal methods like TTCN has helped the GSM operators and users to utilize the openness of the protocol interfaces as well as increased the productivity of testing in the network manufacturers' laboratories. The power of TTCN based testing methodology has been proven during the continuous evolution of GSM specifications, which has justified the investments into formal modelling and validation as part of the industrial testing practices. The first part of the presentation summarizes these lessons from testing of GSM networks. The 3rd generation system has brought the wireless and IP protocol engineering communities closer to each other. Although they represent somewhat different approaches on protocol specification and testing, they do share the overall goal of making the 3rd generation system protocols well specified and interoperable. The second part of the presentation considers these challenges from the industrial practices point of view.

SESSION V

INDUSTRIAL SESSION II

EXPERIENCES OF TTCN–3 TEST EXECUTOR DEVELOPMENT

János Zoltán Szabó
Ericsson Research
Conformance Center, Ericsson Ltd.
H-1037 Budapest, Laborc u. 1., Hungary
Szabo.Janos@eth.ericsson.se

Abstract The new generation of communication protocols requires new test methods. The third version of Tree and Tabular Combined Notation (TTCN–3) embodies such a method. Because of conceptual changes, the existing TTCN–2 test environments cannot be reused; completely new tools shall be built on new bases. This paper shares our experiences gained during the design and usage of a TTCN–3 test executor developed for Ericsson interim use. The system architecture and basic ideas of implementation are described in details. We also present some case studies to demonstrate how efficiently the TTCN–3 language and the test executor can be used in real-life testing projects.

Keywords: TTCN–3, test execution, conformance testing

1. INTRODUCTION

Tree and Tabular Combined Notation version 3 (TTCN–3) [1] is a new test description language standardized recently by ETSI. TTCN–3 is the successor of TTCN–2 [2], which is widely used for conformance testing of telecommunication protocols based on OSI basic reference model. The designers' goals were to extend the new language's application area, simplify its syntax and, of course, provide backward compatibility. TTCN–3 has numerous new features compared to TTCN–2, such as dynamic creation and re-configuration of parallel test components and procedure call based interfaces. The new constructs make the language capable of performance testing in addition to conformance testing. TTCN–3 can be applied not only for testing communication protocols, but distributed systems and APIs as well. The Machine Processable (MP) format of TTCN–2 went under significant changes and became TTCN–3 Core Language (CL) [3]. Instead of textual representation of strictly defined tables, TTCN–3 CL rather resembles a high-level programming language. Based on the CL several graphical presentations can be defined. Currently there are two standardized presentation formats: the Tabular Presentation Format (TFT), which provides partial compatibility with TTCN–2 and the Graphical Format for TTCN–3 (GFT).

The main goal of our project was to design and develop a software toolset that can execute TTCN–3 Abstract Test Suites (ATSes) on a generic hardware platform (e.g. on a PC or workstation). The work was started in early 2000, in parallel with the development of TTCN–3 language itself. Our prototype development was based on draft standards of TTCN–3 CL published by ETSI. We decided to develop a compiler that translates TTCN–3 Core Language to C++ source code, which has to be extended with a library and some modules written by the user. These pieces of code together form the source code of the Executable Test Suite (ETS).

Our motivations for making a TTCN–3 executor were complex. First of all, in the beginning not only the syntax but the static and operational semantics of TTCN–3 were not settled yet. The implementation of such tool could detect most of the inconsistencies and ambiguities in the language. On the other hand, our goal was to establish an efficient, high performance test execution platform that allows the use of TTCN–3 on its new application areas, including load testing. Finally, the existence of a tool encourages the usage of the language. Thus the new users can gain TTCN–3 knowledge very early by writing, checking and executing many kinds of test suites for various protocols without waiting for commercial tools to appear on the market.

This paper is organized as follows. The next section outlines the system architecture of our TTCN–3 executor. Section 3 describes the mapping of most important TTCN–3 language elements in details and Section 4 presents some case studies, that is, some applications of our test executor in real testing projects. Finally, the conclusion is drawn in Section 5.

2. THE STRUCTURE OF TTCN–3 TEST EXECUTOR

The schematic block diagram of our TTCN–3 test executor can be seen on Figure 1. The test executor itself consists of two major parts: a *TTCN–3 compiler* and a so-called *Base Library*. The third part (*Test Port*) is a C++ program module written by the user. This section presents these blocks in details.

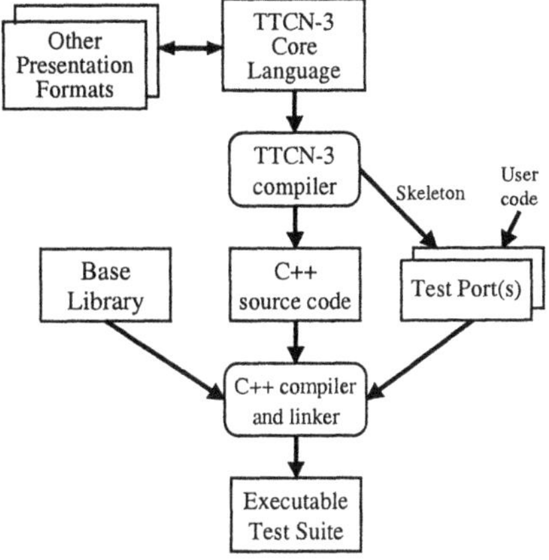

Figure 1. Block structure of the TTCN–3 executor

2.1 TTCN–3 to C++ compiler

The task of the compiler is to transform TTCN–3 CL modules into C++ source code that can be further translated to get an ETS. It has two functional units: The parser part (so-called *front-end*) reads the TTCN–3 input, checks its syntax and breaks it into data structures. The code generator part (*back-end*) synthesizes target (C++) code based on these structures. The parser and the code generator are tightly merged on the level of source code, but their functionality clearly separates.

The front-end is an LALR(1) syntax checker based on the well-proven GNU tools. *Flex* was used for building the tokenizer and *bison* for the grammatical analyzer.

The back-end is written in C language as parser actions. The translation is performed on the fly whenever the right side of a grammar rule becomes available on the top of the parser's stack. The relation between the TTCN–3 language elements and their C++ code equivalents is outlined in Section 3.

The compiler is stateless, which means, when translating a CL element it does not remember the previously passed parts of its input. Thus, the C++ equivalent of a TTCN–3 construct depends only on the original construct and not on any other definitions. The simplicity and the short development time are the most important advantages of this approach. However, the compiler is unable to detect semantic errors in its input and can generate inconsistent target code, which can make the localizing of TTCN–3 errors extremely difficult. Besides, the TTCN–3 interleaved constructs can not be translated in this stateless manner at all.

2.2 TTCN–3 Base Library

The Base Library holds the common parts of C++ code that is used in all ETSes and hereby simplifies the back-end of the compiler. These basic definitions are written once, but they might be used in all modules of the ETS.

The C++ classes representing timers and built-in TTCN–3 data types, the snapshot handler and logging functions as well as the supporting routines of parallel test execution are implemented in the Base Library.

2.3 Test Ports

The purpose of Test Ports (TPs) is to adapt the test executor to a given protocol, that is, to facilitate the communication between the test executor and the SUT. Test Ports are C++ program modules whose skeleton is generated by the compiler from CL port and type definitions. The user shall write the body of the functions using the primitives of TP Application Programming Interface (API). The TPs are also responsible for the encoding and decoding of PDUs.

Although TPs have similar functionality as SUT Adaptors in the reference model of TTCN–3 Run-time Interface (TRI) [4], they are based on different concepts. Instead of TRI's global approach, the Test Ports perform the adaptation locally – they are coupled with TTCN–3 test components. This eliminates the bottleneck of a centralized API and makes our test executor capable of performance testing as well. Unlike TRI, the adaptors of different protocols are clearly separated in our model, which makes the re-use of existing TPs easier in new test configurations. Based on the socket-related operations of UNIX operating systems, our API provides proper ways for the scheduling of the incoming data processing.

In our API each TP is a class, which implements a TTCN–3 port type. The port instances of TTCN–3 test components are represented by the objects of TP class. All SUT related TTCN–3 port operations – except receiving operations – (start, stop, send, map, etc.) are mapped to member function calls of TP classes. While sending, the outgoing PDU is passed to the appropriate member function as parameter in the internal data representation format of the test executor.

The handling of incoming data is based on an event handler mechanism. Each TP class is provided with an event handler function that can be configured by API primitives to trigger after certain amount of time or incoming data on given socket file descriptors. When the test execution is blocked waiting for a new snapshot (e.g. because it has reached an alt statement), the snapshot manager of Base Library calls the TP event handler functions whenever a trigger condition is fulfilled. The event handlers can append the decoded PDUs to the port input queue by special primitives.

3. TRANSLATION OF TTCN–3 LANGUAGE ELEMENTS

Our compiler translates each CL element into one or more C++ definitions depending on its kind. The mapping of some TTCN–3 constructs is very simple, but the translation of others is a bit sophisticated. Our translation scheme exploits the object-oriented and the non-object-oriented features of C++.

Each TTCN–3 module is translated into a pair of C++ header and source files and consequently into one object file. In case of modular test suites the resulting object files shall be linked together, that is, the module hierarchy of ETS reflects to the original structure of ATS. In order to support forward referencing, that is, the usage of a definition that is given later – which is allowed in TTCN–3 but not in C++ – the target header and source files are split up into sections. For example, type definitions, function prototypes, global variables are placed into different sections. The number and ordering of sections are fixed, but the ordering of definitions within a section does not matter.

Data types. Both pre-defined and compound TTCN–3 data types are mapped to C++ classes. The classes for predefined types are implemented in the Base Library, while the equivalent classes for user-defined compound types are generated by the compiler using the classes of field types. The C++ equivalents of TTCN–3 constants and variables are objects of their respective type. The built-in TTCN–3 data operations are implemented using the operator overloading feature of the C++ language, and therefore the translated TTCN–3 expressions look very similar to the original. We had to use the same field accessing mechanism in classes representing record, set and union types because the stateless compiler is unable to distinguish them in the source code.

Templates. The templates of each TTCN–3 type are represented by a C++ class that can carry all possible patterns of that type. There is a one-by-one relation between the value classes and the template representation classes (TRCs): the TRCs of built-in TTCN–3 types can be found in the Base Library while the TRCs of compound types are generated by the compiler based on the TRCs of field types. Each TRC has a type field, which indicates what pattern construct (specific value, complemented list, any value, etc.) is selected. The classes are equipped with member functions that can set the appropriate pattern type and value. The match and valueof operations (which are used in sending and receiving port operations as well) are also implemented in member functions of TRCs.

Our experiments showed that the most frequently used template constructs are the specific values, the any value (?) and the any or omit (*) symbols. That is why the TRCs were designed to be optimal in terms of speed and memory usage with these conditions.

TTCN–3 template instances are mapped to the objects of TRCs. Simple templates become static global objects while parameterized ones are mapped to C++ functions returning an instance of the appropriate TRC. Therefore the formal and actual template parameter lists in C++ resemble their TTCN–3 source. The modified templates are produced by copying and overwriting the ancestor.

Special constructs. TTCN–3 timers are implemented as a C++ class in Base Library. The time is measured internally by UNIX system calls, without user libraries such as Platform Adapters of TRI [4]. The compiler generates the queue handler functions of ports, but the handling of port connections is the same for all port types and therefore it is implemented in the Base Library.

Behaviour definitions. TTCN–3 behaviour definitions, such as functions, test cases, control parts are mapped to C++ functions. The mapping of control constructs, variable instantiations and assignments is almost trivial. Thanks the OO-like notation style of TTCN–3, the translated function bodies look very similar to the original. External functions can be easily implemented in C++ language.

Alternatives, Named alts. The C++ equivalents of TTCN–3 alt constructs are not obvious. Each branch of an alternative consists of three parts: a boolean guard expression, a guarding port or timer operation and the body. The translator routine of the compiler takes a sequence containing the translated form of the previous three parts and produces a single continuous C++ function block, which is equivalent with the original TTCN–3 alt construct.

Unlike the boolean approach of TTCN–3 operational semantics, the receiving and timeout operations can return one of three possible values. YES is returned if the operation was successful. MAYBE indicates that the operation was not successful just now, but it can be succeeded in the future after some delay. NO is returned for an unsuccessful operation that can never be succeeded no matter how much time we wait. For example, a receive operation returns YES if the first incoming value matches the given template and NO if not. MAYBE is returned if the queue is empty.

The equivalent code block of alt constructs works according to the following algorithm. To avoid unnecessarily repeated guard evaluations, the C++ code defines a local flag variable for each branch to store the last result of guard evaluations. The algorithm iterates through the branches in an infinite loop and sets the flags according to Table 1.

Result of guard expression	Result of guard operation	New value of the flag
true	YES	YES
true	MAYBE	MAYBE
true	NO	NO
false	not evaluated	NO

Table 1. Rules for setting the alternative flags

If one flag becomes YES, the body of that branch will be executed and the alternative is finished. If all branches were visited and no successful one was selected, the algorithm checks the flags. If there will never be a suitable branch for selection, that is, all flags are set to NO, the test executor signals a dynamic testcase error. Otherwise, it blocks until something happens to ports or timers and it takes a new snapshot. Finally, the investigation of branches continues from the beginning, but only the guard operations are evaluated. Once a flag is set to NO, the guards of its branch will not be investigated again.

The TTCN-3 named alts are macros without own scope, thus they are translated to C preprocessor macros. These macros contain parts of the previous algorithm's body. The compiler translates expand statements to the expansion of these macros and the code of alt construct is glued together from its parts. Of course, this translation scheme can be applied on recursively nested alt constructs. The stand-alone receive or timeout statements are dealt with very similarly.

4. CASE STUDIES

This section shows some applications that demonstrate how our test executor can be used in real-life testing projects. Although our system has been used in more than ten – smaller or bigger – testing projects, only the results of the most significant five conformance test suites are presented.

The first ATS covers the basic functionality of Internet Protocol version 6 (IPv6) [5] as well as its mobility extensions. The second test suite was written for testing the Management Information Base of IP routers supporting Simple Network Management Protocol (SNMP) [6]. The third example is an extensive conformance test suite for the IP based routing protocol Open Shortest Path First (OSPF) [7]. The fourth case study was developed for conformance testing the Robust Header Compression (ROHC) protocol [8], which can significantly reduce the overhead of IP headers for mobile terminals transmitting voice over IP. In our last example TTCN-3 was used both for conformance and performance testing of BRAIN Candidate Mobility Protocol (BCMP), which is a new IP micro mobility protocol.

Table 2 shows the sizes and characteristics of our example test suites. The translation and execution times were measured on a desktop PC with Intel Pentium III 450 MHz CPU and Linux operating system. We used GCC 3.0 as C++ compiler without optimization switches.

Projects	IPv6	SNMP	OSPF	ROHC	BCMP
Number of TTCN-3 modules	12	4	12	5	6
Total number of lines in ATS	12833	6395	17372	5777	3896
Number of data types	62	20	35	103	48
Number of templates	59	11	57	100	26
Number of test cases	205	10	181	44	41
Translation time (s)	587.9	68.4	164.0	139.1	50.3
Size of binary ETS (kbytes)	10867	804	2912	1807	710
Execution time (μs/operation)	162	217	515	1249	40

Table 2. Comparison of TTCN-3 test suites

The translation times include all steps required for getting the complete binary ETS from the TTCN-3 ATS. The most significant part of this time is spent on translating the generated C++ modules to binary code while the translation from TTCN-3 to C++ takes less than one second in all cases. The binary ETS includes the appropriate Test Ports and the Base Library as well. The relatively long compilation time and large ETS for IPv6 test suite is a result of the extensive use of named alts and expand statements.

The run-time performance of an ETS depends on the complexity of tested protocol. The most significant indicator is the time required for communication operations. The last row of Table 2 shows the average execution times of typical send operations, which include template building and evaluation, data encoding and sending on a physical interface. The main reason for the lower performance of the ROHC test suite is that it uses a relatively slow serial link as output device while the others send their data through a 10 Mbps Ethernet card. By publishing these results we want to set up some benchmarks for tool vendors and users to compare the forthcoming commercial TTCN–3 executors with.

5. CONCLUSION

This paper is the result of the development of a TTCN–3 test execution environment. It presents the system architecture of our test executor and outlines some implementation details. Our intention was also to share the experiences obtained within one year, during the usage of the tool and TTCN–3 language in different areas of testing. The run-time performance indicators of our executable test suites are also shown. We believe that our tool is fast enough for running performance tests on complex protocols as well.

In the future, we want to implement the missing or newly introduced TTCN–3 features in our tool, such as call based ports or regular expressions. On the other hand, we want to include semantic analysis and code optimization in our compiler. In addition, we do not agree completely with the frequent changes of TTCN–3 syntax and semantics that cause incompatibilities. This often requires the re-design of not only some parts of the test executor but the existing test suites as well.

References

[1] J. Grabowski, A. Wiles, C. Willcock, D. Hogrefe, On the design of the new testing language TTCN–3. In: Testing of Communicating Systems, volume 13, Kluwer Academic Publishers, 2000.

[2] Information technology – Open Systems Interconnection – Conformance testing methodology and framework; The Tree and Tabular Combined Notation (TTCN) (Ed. 2++). ETSI TR 101 666 Version 1.0.0, May 1999.

[3] Methods for Testing and Specification (MTS); The Tree and Tabular Combined Notation version 3. TTCN–3: Core Language. ETSI ES 201 837-1 Version 1.1.2, June 2001.

[4] T. Vassiliou-Gioles, S. Schulz, The TTCN–3 Runtime Interface (TRI); Concepts and Interface Definition of the TRI, ETSI Standard Draft, v4.2, September 2001.

[5] S. Deering, R. Hinden, Internet Protocol Version 6 (IPv6) Specification. RFC2460, IETF Network Working Group, December 1998.

[6] J.D. Case, M. Fedor, M.L. Schoffstall, C. Davin, Simple Network Management Protocol (SNMP), RFC1157, IETF Network Working Group, May 1990.

[7] J. Moy, OSPF Version 2, RFC2328, IETF Network Working Group, April 1998.

[8] C. Bormann et al, RObust Header Compression (ROHC): Framework and four profiles: RTP, UDP, ESP, and uncompressed. RFC3095, IETF Network Working Group, July 2001.

Making TTCN-3 testing a success

Key issues for an efficient tool environment

Wolfgang Sachse
Danet GmbH, Mobile Communications Technology
Gutenbergstrasse 10, D-64331 Weiterstadt, Germany
wolfgang.sachse@danet.de

Abstract: Now that the TTCN-3 standard has matured, first tools are appearing on the market. But the enhanced capabilities of TTCN-3 can only be fully exploited in a smart, flexible and open test environment.

This contribution from a test tool manufacturer's point of view highlights some of the key features and tool aspects that users of TTCN-3 should consider when setting up their test environment.

Key words: TTCN-3, tools, compiler, TRI, ASN.1

With TTCN-3, the 'Testing and Test Control Notation' of ETSI (European Telecommunication Standardisation Institute), a new global standard for a test specification language has turned up. TTCN-3 is not only 'just another revision' but a completely modernised edition of the well-proven test language which is now aiming at an additional deployment in the datacom domain. ETSI members have expressed their support by deciding early that TTCN-3 will be used for the development of test specifications for the voice-over-IP protocols SIP and OSP.

Its predecessor, TTCN-2++, is widely used in the telecommunications area for black-box system testing and conformance testing. Its particular merits are the integration in a framework of testing methodology and supporting standards, the independence from vendors and test systems and the availability of test suites, e.g. for DECT, UMTS and Bluetooth technologies.

TTCN-3 was meant to keep all of these advantages, and substantial effort was made to make the new version fit for additional testing applications by adding support for e.g. distributed systems, client server architectures (e.g. CORBA-based), and type/value systems (IDL and other programming languages). Also, the readability has been enhanced by creating a textual presentation format, called 'Core Notation', that looks like a 'normal' programming language. Other notations to specify tests comprise a tabular and graphical format. Now it is up to the test community to take advantage of the powerful new test capabilities that TTCN-3 is offering.

But all the benefits and the strength of such a powerful language can only be realised when it is supported by smart and efficient tools that allow users to concentrate on their basic tasks and to reach their goals in all phases of the testing process quickly.

The requirements for a TTCN tool environment are manifold as there are different types of users focusing on several different aspects. Therefore, beside the basic technical merits, the usability aspects and the openness and flexibility of a tool solution are very important for success and acceptance of the new test methodology. Based on Danet's rich experience over the past decade with its own TTCN test solution, called TTCN Toolbox, a closer look on some tool aspects and key requirements for a TTCN-3 test solution is taken in the following sections.

A general comment about suitable test solutions would be that not only the technical merits and features of the TTCN compiler are key issues, but also seamless tool integration and ease of use account for a good overall TTCN-3 testing solution.

Test Development	Test Generation	Test Execution	Result Analysis	Test Reporting
• Test conception • Create Test Environment • Develop own test suite • Edit and modify existing test cases • Convert 'old' TTCN-2 test cases to TTCN-3	• Semantic and syntax checks • Support for TTCN-3 base features • Support for test interface libraries • Generate and compile executable code	• Assign parameter values and test ports • Select test cases for execution • Provide run-time options • Run and supervise test campaign • Display results	• Display trace files • Visualise trace data graphically • Provide good support for fault-finding • Support for message decoding • Support for debugging	• Provide statistic data • Generate test reports and statements • Generate alarms • Provide access to network management systems
TTCN-3 Test Suite →	Executable Test Code →	Test Results →	Information →	Test Reports

Figure 1. Test phases overview.

As depicted above, the testing process can be divided into five major phases that all require support by tools aiding the user and off-loading him from routine or unnecessary tasks.

The first major step is the **Test Development** phase where the test environment is created and the test cases are written. In particular, the question of how the test cases 'talk' to the implementation under test is of interest as here the testing infrastructure needs to be implemented. This communication might be implemented using simple mechanisms like a TCP connection or a serial link, in more complex cases an interface towards CORBA or proprietary protocol stacks might be required. Here it is important that the TTCN tool environment supports all those possibilities using an open mechanism that allows to make use of a well defined interface and providing sample implementations. ETSI has defined TRI, the 'TTCN-3 Runtime Interface' along with TTCN-3 to facilitate a standardised communication mechanism. Therefore it is a must for a TTCN test solution to provide a communications library based on TRI and to actively support users.

The second important point in the Test Development phase, of course, is the generation of a test suite and the test cases contained. Since many users still have a large stock of 'old' test cases that they want to continue to use and because TTCN-3 differs much from the TTCN-2 notation, it is crucial to provide a migration tool that automatically converts TTCN-2 test suites into TTCN-3. All further work can then be based on those migrated test cases, thus protecting the investment in previous test case development.

For modifying and writing own test cases, editing capabilities should be available. TTCN-3 now supports a textual presentation format that is easily readable for humans, looking mostly like C-code. This so-called 'Core Notation' is the common exchange format for TTCN-3. Therefore an integrated text editor (with syntax highlighting and further language support) is highly desirable. Beside the 'traditional' tabular presentation format which requires a specialised editor, TTCN-3 test specifications can also be 'designed' in a graphical presentation, called Test Sequence Charts, TSC. Whatever presentation format is used for the test case development, it is important that the use of editors is well integrated into the tool solution, even if third-party products are employed. A good integration provides for 'hyperlinking' from e.g. the TTCN compiler's error window or from the post-execution trace display back to the source code representation of the referenced object.

The second major step in the test process is the **Test Generation** phase where the TTCN-3 source code is translated into executable test programs. In this step, the power and features of the TTCN compiler define the quality of the test solution. The obvious issues, namely supported functionality and technologies are rather easy to decide: if a particular requirement cannot be met, the solution is not suitable. This already starts with the simple question of supported platforms: Does the tool solution run in the preferred (or intended) environment? Can test code be generated for UNIX, Windows, real-time environments or, using cross-compilers, for rather 'exotic' test environments? Other relevant aspects in this area are the support of TTCN-3 language elements and supporting technologies. For example, a comprehensive TTCN-3 solution in the telecom domain must support the data description language ASN.1 (X.680, '97) with the associated encoding rules (BER, PER, X.690). Particularly for a deployment in the datacom and CORBA world, IDL should be supported. Also ETSI's Test Synchronisation Protocol, TSP.1 would be desirable feature, particularly for testing in a distributed environment.

Apart from those rather easy-to-decide features, the implementation details of the TTCN-3 code generator significantly determine the quality and strength of the whole test solution. Flexibility and openness definitely enhance a test tool as these offer additional influence on the system's behaviour.

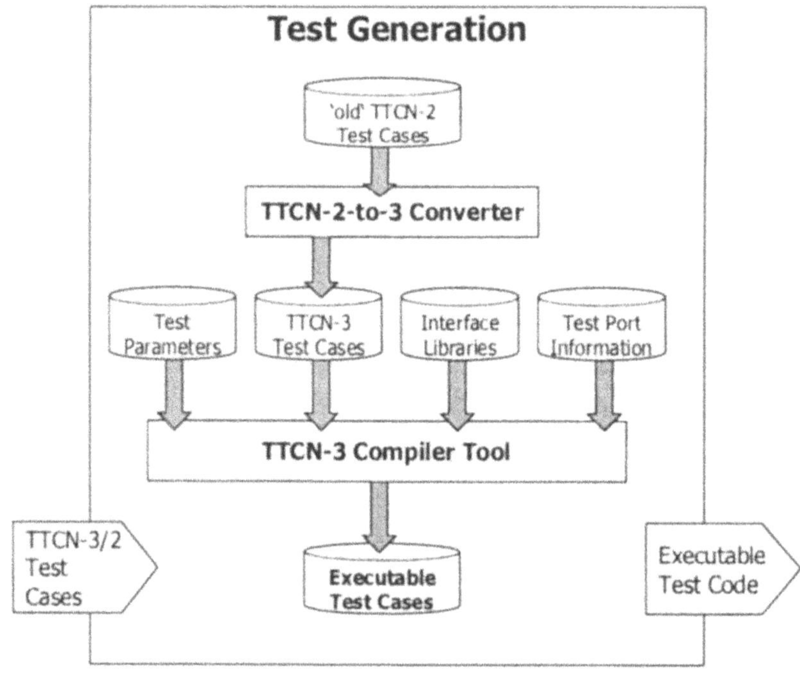

Figure 2. Test Generation phase.

In a first step of the Test Generation phase, test suites are parsed and analysed for syntactical and semantic correctness. A good compiler should check a test suite very rigidly because any faults or 'flaws' not discovered at this level may lead to very hard-to-find errors during the test execution phase. At worst, a test case may not perform its intended purpose at all!

Generally, not only for performance reasons, the translation from TTCN-3 to executable code is performed by translating TTCN-3 into an intermediate 'standard' language. In Danet's TTCN Toolbox, for example, C++ code is generated here. Using this two-step approach has several advantages: code can be compiled for virtually any target platform, existing libraries (e.g. for interface adaptations, available external functionality) can be linked to the test programs and standard compiler control and code optimisation tools can be used to fine-tune the generated code.

The speed of the test generation process and the size of the generated executables, however, should not be underestimated as these factors heavily influence the turn-around times perceived by the test case developer. Incremental compilation (only re-compiling recent changes in TTCN test modules), selective compiling (only compiling relevant test cases) and the possibility to use dynamically linked libraries improve the tool usability and user acceptance significantly.

Another advantage of the described two-step code generation process is the possibility to re-use the generated intermediate C++ code for other purposes. For example, complete (!) functions for message de- and encoding are generated automatically based on the protocol knowledge the compiler got from the test specification. Also, adding additional protocol knowledge facilitating de-/encoding of under-defined message codings should be supported by a good tool solution. This would also allow to implement coders for proprietary encoding rules (such as CSN.1). Beside the automatic generation of de-/encoders, available external protocol-specific coders should be appliable.

Last but not least in the Test Generation phase, the administration of the generated code needs to be performed. Where shall the test programs be put, into a database, in a file system, in a repository? Since these requirements cannot be met at the same time in a standard product, the tool vendor should be able to offer customised solutions upon request.

The third major step in the test process is the **Test Execution** (or test campaign) phase where the user wishes to run the previously generated test programs, either to verify them (test case developer) or to perform the actual testing tasks (tester). But before running a test case, the user needs to assign parameters and test ports, based on the current test environment's settings. Also, some options for the execution of the test campaign may be required to set. These tasks should be supported by dedicated tools in the TTCN-3 test solution.

Since at compile time only the test parameter names and types are known, but not their values, this assignment needs to be made just before run-time. This should be performed using a test suite parameter editor provided by the test campaign manager. Also the assignment of logical test ports (from the test suite's point of view) to their physical implementations needs to be supported by a tool.

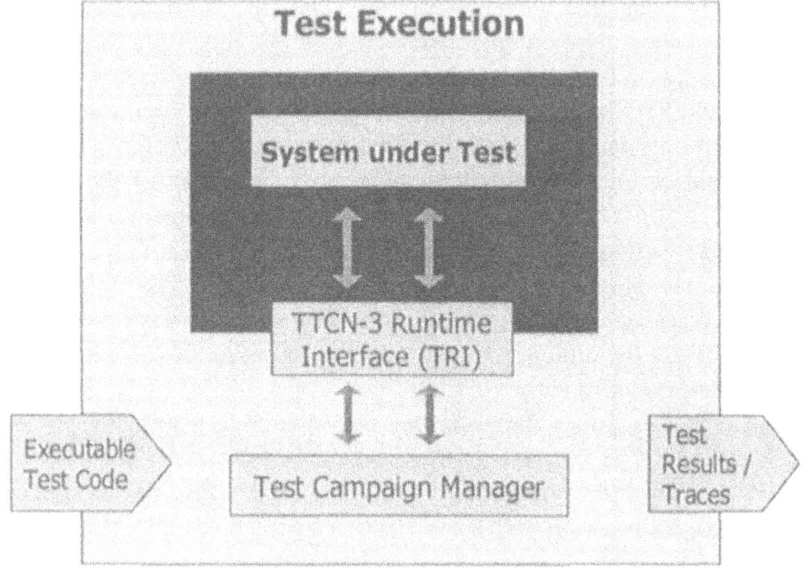

Figure 3. Test Execution phase.

For the definition of a test campaign and the selection of contained test cases, a good representation of the test suite's structure and possibilities to interactively select test cases would be very helpful. Alternatively, making use of the new 'control' structure of TTCN-3 that allows to influence the test execution in a script-like way is a desirable feature of a flexible test solution. Some features supporting e.g. 'timed' execution of a test campaign and the display of verdicts and the current status of the execution are improving the use of the test campaign management.

The fourth major step in the test process is the **Result Analysis** phase. This phase becomes particularly important for test cases that did not 'pass' as expected. Then a tool-based analysis of the results obtained from the test execution should support the user to pinpoint the problem.

A well-structured trace display function on TTCN level gives a good overview and provides information about the overall behaviour of the test case. It shows all relevant dynamic actions of all test components of a test case and provides the user with additional, useful information by fully decoding messages and showing variable assignments. Very helpful is the ability to 'hyperlink' from a line in the trace window directly to the associated TTCN source code statement, highlighted by the TTCN editor. This provides a means for quick turn-around times and efficient fault-finding facilities. Complementary to the textual traces is a graphical representation of the trace information in sequence diagrams, e.g. as Message Sequence Charts, MSC. This way of displaying the trace information is more intuitive for human users and also offers a better overview of the events during a test case's run.

Apart from comprehensive tracing facilities, a good result analysis tool should offer support to locate a problem and assist a user in finding the cause for a 'deviation' from the expected result. Hence, after guiding the user to such a location of interest, additional information displaying the actual and the expected result will reveal what exactly caused a particular verdict.

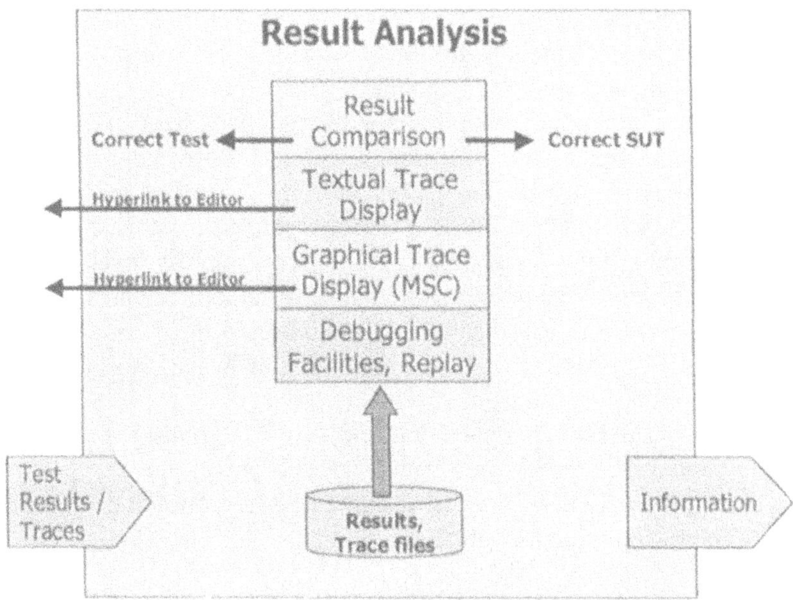

Figure 4. Result Analysis phase.

Debugging facilities may prove useful to identify hard-to-find problems with a test suite, especially when applied by advanced users. To get around the real-time problems of low-level debugging, 'recording' a test case's dynamic behaviour and subsequently re-playing this trace data back to the test program is a smart solution. This allows to simulate the behaviour while offering extensive off-line debugging facilities and avoiding timer problems.

The last major step in the test process is the **Test Reporting** phase which mainly comprises functions for automated post-processing and evaluation of test execution results. Unlike in the previous phases where the test tool's functions are mostly supporting user interactions, the reporting phase mostly off-loads the user from tiresome routine tasks. Particularly for conformance testing and similar test applications, the generation of standard reports and the documentation of test results is a must. In test environments for monitoring purposes, it is vital to automatically generate alarms based on particular test results. Hence, interfaces to network management systems (in the case of telecom applications) or other alarming services are additional benefits.

Regarding the documentation support, a good and flexible tool should provide access to the information gathered during the test campaign in an open format. This information may comprise the test case execution information, obtained verdicts, information about the test configuration, the traces files, the test suite parameters and other collected or logged data. By importing, post-processing and transforming this information into custom reports, most user's demands for result documentation and management information systems should easily be met.

Going a bit further than just providing the raw data that can be processed into reports or templates in a second step, the test tool vendor may offer to generate the required reports directly in a customer-specific format.

So, after all, what makes TTCN-3 testing a success? As one can see from the above considerations, a good TTCN-3 test solution is much more than just a few 'ticks' in a buzz word feature list. It is the tool vendor's experience and the user feedback, together with a flexible and open architecture that define the quality of the overall test solution and hence, the user's testing success.

Based on Danet's experience with its TTCN Toolbox product, also customer support and the 'surrounding' services offered to the user contribute to the success of a TTCN-3 test environment, apart from the pure technical merits of the test solution, of course.

TESTING AUTOMATION WITH COMPUTER AIDED TEST CASE GENERATION

Tapio Heikkilä, Petri Tenno and Jarmo Väänänen
NetHawk Solutions Oy, Elektroniikkatie 2 A
FIN-90570 Oulu, FINLAND
tapio.heikkila@nethawk.fi

Abstract This paper considers techniques to increase the level of automation in testing object oriented software systems. The focus is in utilizing software requirements specifications; for this a computer aided test case generation tool prototype is introduced. The tool uses software requirements specifications in the form of system level message sequences (UML collaboration models) and constraint descriptions of the input and output variables (attribute constraints in UML class models).

Key words: software testing, test case generation, testing automation, UML

1. INTRODUCTION

Software testing provides a great potential for improving the efficiency of software development. Software testing means a wider set of systematic methods and techniques for organizing the tests, test system, and carrying out the actual tests. While looking for methods of improvement, a process oriented development does not alone lead us to desired results but automation with appropriate strategy and software tools are implied.

Here we consider techniques to increase the level of automation in testing object oriented software systems. In the following chapters software development and testing processes are reviewed and possibilities to automate the testing are discussed. We propose to utilize software requirements specifications for improving the efficiency of testing GUI based software. For this a computer aided test case generation tool prototype is introduced, to be used together with a commercial GUI test driver. The tool has been developed initially for improving the efficiency within internal software development of the NetHawk group (NetHawk, 2001). The test case generation tool uses software requirements specifications, given in the form of system level message sequences, expressed as UML collaboration models, and constraint descriptions of the input and output variables, expressed as attribute constraints in UML class models. We consider certain testing techniques, originating in the equivalence partitioning principle (Kit, 1995) as the basis for test case design for system testing. Our target is to provide a software tool to increase the level of automation in the testing, especially by decreasing the level of manual programming of testing scripts. However, we are not targeting to full automation, neither in the sense of having automated all possible test cases nor in the sense of having a tool without human interaction during test planning and design. We assume to be dealing with component based software, e.g., with a user interface composed of GUI components, because the test case execution mechanism is based on a GUI test driver integrating to the software under test through the windows API, typical for GUI components.

2. SOFTWARE DEVELOPMENT AND TESTING PROCESSES

A clear and sound software process model is necessary for systematic software development, including testing. The process model can interconnect the oftware development activities into the testing activities by a revised waterfall model, i.e., the V-model (Fewster and Graham, 1999) or even adding the storage & retrieval of the re-usable components; X-model, (Hodgson, 1990) into the process model. V- and X- models cover the whole software process but are abstract in the sense that they do not provide details about the stages of development, and further on, the entry criteria (or inputs) and exit criteria (or outputs) of the different phases. There are a number models focusing on these details, especially for object oriented development using Unified Modeling Language (UML) as a representation framework, though without the dynamics and synchronization of the development and testing activities. Although using UML as a notational framework, their development phases do have different types of UML models as outcomes. In our case we have followed the Real-Time UML. Real-Time UML is dividing the development into three phases (Douglass, 1998)

1. *Requirements Analysis*: Context modelling, Use Case modelling, Scenario modelling
2. *Analysis*: Defining object structure, Defining object behaviour

3. *Design*: Architectural design (system and processor wide design), Mechanistic design (inter-object design), Detailed design (intra-object design)

We are considering here the system testing phase, which needs information from requirements analysis and analysis.

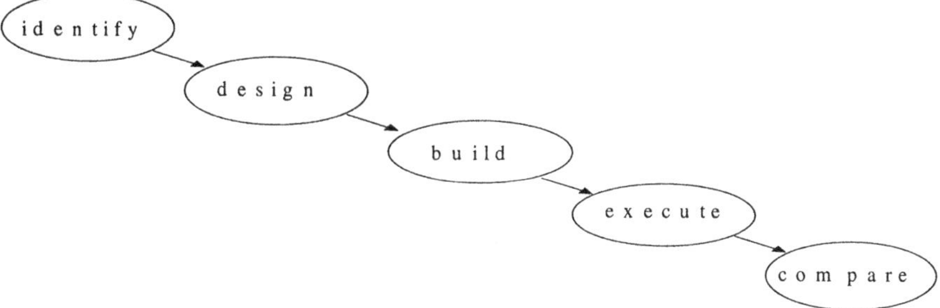

Figure 1. General testing process (adapted from (Fewster and Graham, 1999)).

The testing (also integration and module testing) is composed of different phases (see fig. 1):

identify test conditions (determine, "what" can be tested; which test cases)
design test cases, determine, "how" the "what" is to be tested.
build test cases (implement script, data etc.) by preparing program code for tests as test scripts or special test software (in C/C++, Java, etc) with test inputs and expected outcomes,
execute test cases in the test environment and log the actual outcomes, and
compare test case outcomes to expected outcomes.

We are considering here especially the automatic building of test cases for system testing.

3. SOFTWARE TESTING TECHNIQUES AND TESTING AUTOMATION

There are many tools for software testing, varying from general test management tools to measuring of the dynamic performance of the executed programs. Different testing tools and their location in the V-model is presented in figure 1.

Test identification and design are at their best based on a well defined design methodology or technique. We are considering the three techniques described in further details below.

Equivalence partitioning is a systematic process that identifies, on the basis of whatever information is available, a set of interesting classes of input conditions to be tested, where a class is representative (or covers) a large set of other possible tests. If partitioning is applied to the product under test, the product is going to behave in much the same way for all members of the class (Kit, 1995).

Boundary-value analysis is a variant and refinement of equivalence partitioning with two major differences. First, rather than selecting any element in the equivalence class as being representative, elements are selected such that each edge of the equivalence class is the subject of a test. Second, rather than focusing exclusively on input conditions, output conditions are also explored by defining output equivalence classes (Kit, 1995).

Extended Use Case Test is a test design pattern to develop application-specific tests (Binder, 1999). Extended Use Case Test applies when most, if not all of the essential requirements for the SUT can be expressed as use cases. It is possible to develop test cases by imagining specific ideas for a use case and corresponding expected results.

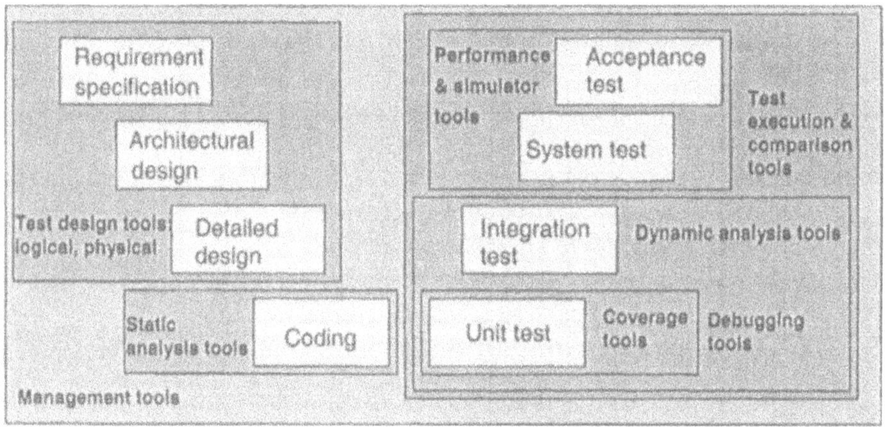

Figure 2. Testing tools vs. software development (revised from Fewster and Graham, 1999).

Component Based Development (CBD) (Carney, 1999) has been leading the way for efficient software development, especially for distributed software systems. Sometimes CBD introduces confusion because of varying interpretations about what is a component and what is not. The definitions given in the following are followed here.

- "A Component is an implementation entity, including source code units, binary code (the output of a translator), and linked, loadable executable files" (Binder, 1999)
- "Components are the packaging construct for the final application. They control, how the application can be delivered and distributed (Kozaczynski and Christerson, 2000)"

Software components are often more or less present in modern software development i.e., within an intra-application composition (e.g., Java beans, Arnold and Gosling, 1999) or inter-application composition using distribution frameworks like Common Object Request Broker Architecture (CORBA, Mowbray and Ruh, 1997), Enterprise Java Beans (EJB; Shannon et. al., 2000), or Distributed Component Object Model (DCOM; Kirtland, 1999). Component based software development offers an additional dimension considering the possibilities for testing automation. Components, or their containers implement a special, common interface, and at the best the tools implement the required testing points (for control or observation) within these interfaces and in application independent points (parts of the component model).

4. COMPUTER AIDED TEST GENERATION (CATG)

Computer Aided Test Generation (CATG) tools are used to automate the "design" and "build" phases of the testing process. CATG tools create abstract or executable test cases based on software requirements or test design. We have developed a test case generator tool prototype, where we create executable test cases based on the requirements and functional specifications of the software under test without needing to explicitly design the test cases. The test case generator takes as inputs a UML Rational Rose® model (Rational, 2001): requirements specifications as system level sequence diagrams, class model of the GUI objects (PCO's) and constraints for the GUI object attributes.

The test case generator parses the UML model and extracts the GUI object data, and creates and shows to the user a table of input attribute values or value constraints acquired from the constraint descriptions in the class model, and a table of output values or value constraints correspondingly. The system can also variate the inputs, i.e., create combinations of input values or constraints for the test cases. The user must create value sets (or rows) of the expected output values by picking combinations of the output value sets. Based on these value sets the system creates final outputs in the form of executable scripts for a GUI test driver environment (WinRunner ® TSL scripts, WinRunner, 2001) and also corresponding script and rows in the constraint tables (input values; expected outcomes).

The strategy for identifying and creating test cases lies in the idea of utilizing the requirements specifications of the software. Either in the requirements specification phase or the analysis phase the components in the user interface are modeled as instances of the available GUI API classes.

Here we consider those GUI components, which have communication with the "operator" actor. In the class model each of the attributes of these objects should get a constraint description, in fact for valid and for invalid values. These constraints are considered here as the sets of equivalence classes for each input and output variable, expressed as algebraic constraints. These can be described e.g., in the Object Constraint Language (Warmer, 1999). During test case generation, an arbitrary value satisfying the constraint (e.g., inside a range) is created and taken into the set of input values of that input variable. Output values are also described as equivalence classes with corresponding constraints. If the output value is a range, then comparison of the actual output value is compared to the range (inside / outside), and if the output value is a single value, then the actual output value is compared to this (equal/unequal). It should be noted, that the constraints could cover both "valid" and "invalid" classes of the input values, or only "valid" ones in which case the "invalid" values could be composed of the complements of the valid value sets. The course of developing the test cases is illustrated within the screenshots in the figure 3.

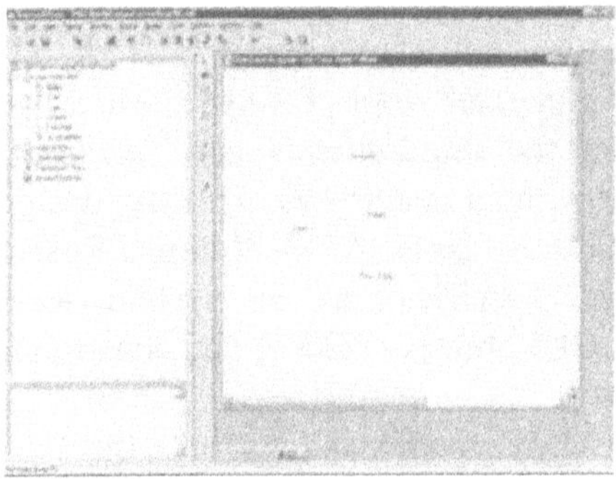

(a) Identify Test Cases:
Req specs in UML (Use Case models)

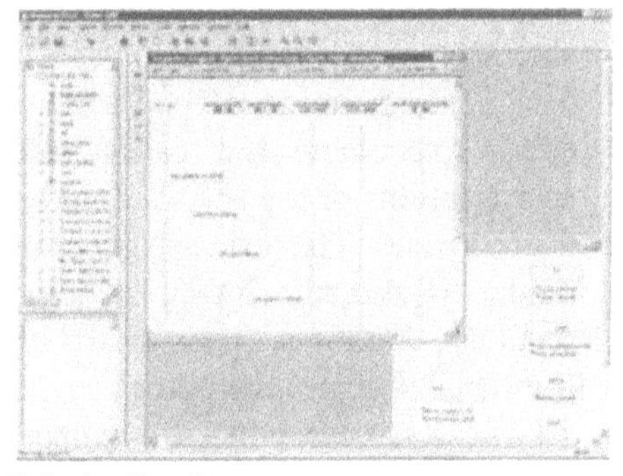

b) Design Test Cases:
Req specs & analysis in UML (interaction models, class/object models)

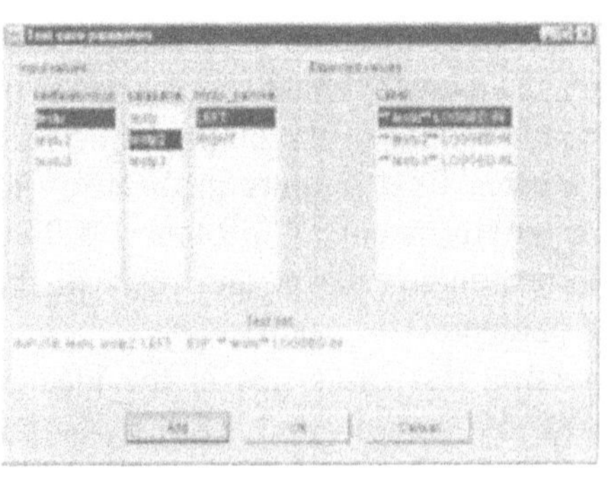

(c) Build Test Cases:

Semiautomatic test case generation

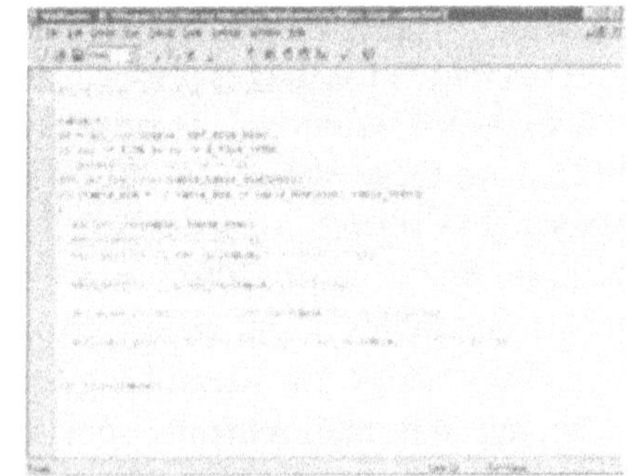

(d) Execute Test Cases:

An executable TSL script

(e) Compare results: WinRunner ® report on a test run

Figure 3. CATG based testing: identify (a), design (b), build (c), execute (d), compare (e).

5. CONCLUSIONS

In this paper techniques and methods concerning software development and software testing automation were discussed. Computer Aided Test Case Generation was considered in more details and a tool prototype was presented. The tool is utilizing UML specifications of the software, developed in a commercial CASE-tool. The tool supports some most general system testing techniques, originating from the equivalence partitioning method.

REFERENCES

Arnold K., Gosling J., The Java Programming Language. Addison Wesley, Massachusetts, UA, 1997. 444p.

Binder R. V., Testing Object-Oriented Systems: Models, Patterns, and Tools. Addison – Wesley, 1999. 1248 p.

Carney D., COTS Product Evaluation and System Design, COTS Spot - Volume 2, issue 1, March 1999. 6 p.

Douglass, B. P., Real-Time UML – Developing Efficient Objects for Embedded Systems. Addison Wesley, Reading, Massachusetts, USA 1998, 400 p.

Dustin E., Rashka J. S., Paul J., Automated Software Testing: Introduction, Management, and Performance. July 1999, Addison-Wesley Pub Co.

Fewster M., Graham D., Software Test Automation – Effective use of test execution tools. Addison Wesley, Oxford, 1999. 574 p.

Grabowski J., Wiles A., Willcock C., Hogrefe D., On the design of the new testing language TTCN-3. 13th IFIP International Workshop on Testing Communicating Systems' (Testcom 2000), Ottawa, 29.8.2000-1.9.2000, Kluwer Academic Publishers, August 2000.

Hodgson R., The X-Model: A Process Model for Object Oriented Software Development. The 4th International Conference on Software Engineering and Its aApplications. Toulouse, France, December 9 – 13, 1991.

Jaaksi A., Aalto J.-M., Aalto A., Vättö K., Tried & True Object development – Industry-proven Approaches with UML. Cambridge University Press, New York, USA, 1999, 315 p.

Kirtland M., Designing Component Based Applications. Microsoft Press, Redmond, Washingotn, USA, 1999. 427 p.

Kit E., Software Testing in the Real World: Improving the Process, ACM Press Books, November 1995, Addison-Wesley, 252 p.

Kozaczynski W., Christerson M., Rose, Rational's Architecture Practice, and Architectureal Reuse. Rose Architect, Winter 2000, pp. 4 – 6.

Kruchten P., The Rational Unified Process, An Introduction, Second edition, Addison Wesley, Cambridge, MA, USA, 2000, 298 p.

McDonnell S., Rapoid Development, Taming Wild Software Schedules. Microsoft Press, Redmond, Washington, 1996. 648 p.

Mowbray T. J., Ruh W. A., Inside CORBA, Distribted Object Standards and Applications. Addison Wesley, Massachusetts, 1997. 376 p.

NetHawk Oy, company info; in "http://www.nethawk.fi"

Newmarch J. D., Testing Java Swing-based Applications. In http://pandonia.canberra.edu.au/java/replayJava/paper.html

Orbiter adds gravity to CORBA. In http://www.nccglobal.com/testing/tmntimes/issue2/tmntimes2_4.htm

Rational Rose, http://www.rational.com

Rosenberg D., Scott K., Use Case Driven Object Modeling with UML – A Practical Approach, Addison Wesley, Reading, Massachusetts, USA, 1999, 172 p.

Schmuller J., Teach Yourself UML in 24 Hours, SAMS Publishing,, Indianapolis, USA, 1999, 422 p.

Segue Launches CORBA products. In http://www.segue.com/html/s_news/press_releases/s_CORBA.htm

Shannon B. et al., Java 2 Platform, Enterprise Edition: Platform and Component Specifications. Addison-Wesley, 2000.

Warmer, The Object Constraint Language . Precise Modeling with UML. Addison Wesley, Reading, Massachisetts, USA, 1999.112 p.

WinRunner GUI Testing SW, in http://www.mercuryinteractive.com

Acknowledgements

This work has been financially supported by the ETX Development Program of the Technology Development Centre of Finland (TEKES), which is greatly acknowledged by the authors.

SESSION VI

TEST AUTOMATION

AUTOMATED TESTING IN PRACTICE: THE HIGHWAY TOLLING SYSTEM *

René G. de Vries, Axel Belinfante and Jan Feenstra
University of Twente – Formal Methods and Tools group
Department of Computer Science
P.O. Box 217, 7500 AE Enschede, The Netherlands
{rdevries, belinfan, feenstra}@cs.utwente.nl

Abstract In this paper we study the application of automated test derivation and execution based on formal specifications. The object of testing is the Payment Box (PB) of the Highway Tolling System, a device which handles electronic payments. Challenges of testing the PB are the transaction speed, parallelism and encryption. We describe a methodology for automated testing and apply this methodology to test the PB. We conclude that automation of the test process is feasible and beneficial, and evaluate our techniques, theory and tools for automated testing.

1. INTRODUCTION

In this paper we study the deployment of methods, techniques and tools which support specification based testing of reactive software systems. Systematic testing of the functionality of reactive systems is crucial in order to check whether they operate correctly. Our research goal is to develop methods and tools to support and, whenever possible, to automate the *conformance testing* process of reactive systems. Conformance testing involves assessing the correctness of a system with respect to its functional specification by means of experimentation. For it we need tools for algorithmic derivation of test suites from specifications and tools for automatic test implementation, execution and analysis. Our challenge is to develop test tools based on a well-defined theory which are well suited for practical applications. Consequently, it is important that the developed tools are applied to realistic case studies from

*This research was partly supported by Interpay Nederland B.V. and by the Dutch Technology Foundation STW under project STW TIF.4111: *Côte de Resyste* – COnformance TEsting of REactive SYSTEms.

industry in order to validate their practical usefulness. In this paper we report on testing a complex industrial device, for which we have not only generated but also executed the tests. We emphasize on the process of setting up and performing automated testing and evaluate how succesful the tools and techniques are.

Automated testing. Test derivation and test execution become increasingly laborious activities, while the complexity of reactive systems grows. Automation of both processes seems to be a solution to reduce the labour. Besides, automated testing is flexible and enables automatic regression testing when a system is modified.

Given the specification of a system, we derive test experiments and execute them on the *Implementation Under Test* (IUT). For automated derivation we need a formal specification of the IUT and formal test theory. Several theories for automated derivation from specifications are known, like [6; 9]. In this paper we adopt the test theory of [9] and use the test tool TorX [1], which exploits this theory.

TorX is also able to execute tests automatically. We use TorX in the *on-the-fly* testing mode. During on-the-fly testing, test derivation and execution occur simultaneously. Instead of deriving a complete test case (one test scenario of a test suite), the test derivation process derives *test primitives* from a specification. These test primitives are actions that are immediately executed in the test run. In this way only the necessary part of a test case is considered, which reduces the amount of computation needed. An important remark is that all computations for one-the-fly testing have to be done at run-time. This can be critical when we need to satisfy an IUT's real-time requirements. An elaborated discussion of test automation based on formal methods and a description of TorX, its architecture, testing modes and configurations can be found in [1].

Highway Tolling System. As case study for the assessment of our approach we will evaluate the testing of the *Payment box* (PB), which is a part of the *Highway Tolling System* (HTS). The Dutch government considers to charge toll on highways as an instrument to reduce the increasing traffic jams. For this purpose, the Highway Tolling System is developed. This system automatically charges fees from vehicle drivers who pass a toll gate on a highway. The fee is paid by an electronic payment which consists of exchanging digital certificates between the PB at the toll gate and an electronic purse on a smart card in the vehicle. When a vehicle passes the toll gate, the system should debit the purse and register a balance increment at the PB.

Interpay B.V., a company owned by the Dutch banks that exploits the electronic purse smart cards, needs to test the system to ensure that the PB processes the money transactions correctly. Because many vehicles can pass a toll gate simultaneously and the vehicles travel at high and different speeds, the number of parallel transactions in progress can be large. Furthermore, for security reasons, the messages exchanged for an electronic payment transaction are encrypted. These issues (speed, parallelism and encryption) contribute to the complexity of the generation, execution and analysis of test experiments to test the PB.

Automated test derivation can make the test generation process faster and more reliable. Test generation is usually done manually by designing and writing test scripts. This is a very laborious and error-prone process, especially in systems with a high level of concurrency. Interpay B.V. tested the PB using traditional test design techniques, although there was automation involved. In order to meet the speed requirements they executed their tests in a dedicated automated execution environment. However, they desire more support for their test process.

Overview. In this paper we report on the testing of the PB using the test tool TorX. We describe the methodology of this approach in Section 2 and report on its application in Section 3. Subsequently, in Section 4 we describe the difficulties and challenges that we encountered and propose some (partial) solutions. In Section 5 we describe the results and observations we made and we finish with some concluding remarks.

2. METHODOLOGY

In this section we describe on an abstract level the process of how to automatically test a system. In the next section we will apply this process to test the PB. Because we test on-the-fly our process does not have the explicit test design phase which is present in batch-oriented testing. Although the process is presented sequentially, in practice it turns out that the process is iterative. We distinguish four phases: preparing the IUT, preparing the test tools, preparing the test environment and performing test execution. We describe them in more detail:

1. *IUT study.* In this phase, firstly we study the system that we are going to test. We investigate all potential interfaces from which we can stimulate and observe the IUT, and study the IUT's observable behaviour. This behaviour may have many features which we do not want to test. So we restrict ourself and identify the behaviour that we are interested in. Secondly, we formalize the behaviour by specifying the system by means of *Formal Description Techniques* (FDTs), e.g. LO-

TOS [5] or PROMELA [4]. Since at this stage (in general), all available system descriptions are informal, we will have to resolve all impreciseness, incompleteness, ambiguities and inconsistencies from which informal specifications suffer. During the development of the formal specification we use automated validation tools to simulate, verify properties of, and model check the formalized behaviour. This gives us insight in obscurities and in anomalous behaviour that was introduced during the functional design phase. Furthermore, these tools support the design of *test purposes*, i.e. means to guide the test derivation.

2. *Tools.* In this phase we determine which tools we are going to use. We investigate what the underlying theory of the tools is, which shall be the basis of interpretation of the test results. Furthermore we investigate the openness of the tools, i.e. the interfaces that the tools have to connect with an IUT.

3. *Test environment.* The test environment is the setup of the test architecture and the application specific test tool components. The *test architecture* describes the relevant aspects of how the IUT is embedded into other systems during the testing process, and how the tester interacts with the IUT. In general we cannot connect the test tool directly with the IUT, but have to use additional devices/components to interface the test tool with the IUT. This phase is decomposed into the following four activities:

Test architecture design. A precise knowledge of the test architecture is required for the test derivation. The tester seldomly communicates directly with the IUT; instead it communicates indirectly via a so called *test context.* The IUT interacts at the *implementation access points* (IAPs) which the tester controls via the test context at the *points of control of observation* (PCOs). Consequently, the test primitives should be derived with respect to the PCOs. The IUT together with its test context is called the *System Under Test* (SUT). The tests are derived from a specification of the SUT, instead of the IUT. The components that are necessary to interface the test tool with the IUT and their functionality have to be identified. These components range from existing generic ones like network services to application specific ones, e.g. for the en- and decoding of messages exchanged between tester and IUT.

Test architecture implementation. In this phase all interfacing components will have to be designed and developed. This is a software engineering task.

System under Test specification. The test context has to be taken into consideration when we derive tests. So, the formal specification of the IUT is extended into a formal specification of the SUT.

Testing the test architecture. We have to check the correctness of our automated test environment. In this phase we debug the text context components and adjust the specification from which we derive tests. This activity is iterative.

4. *Test execution.* In this phase we design *campaigns*, instantiated test environment setups with test goals and strategies. We execute these campaigns and analyse the results.

3. TESTING THE PAYMENT BOX

Here we tell how we tested the PB using the process presented above.

3.1 IUT study

This phase consists of a global IUT study and the construction of a formal specification of the system using an FDT.

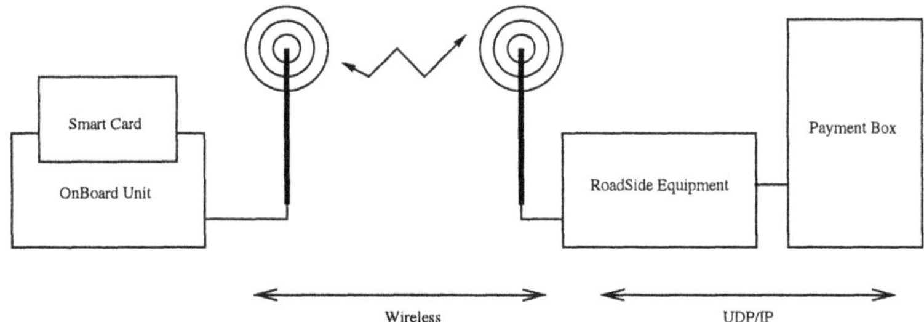

Figure 1. Highway Tolling System

Study IUT. The basic setup of the system is shown in Figure 1. A smartcard containing an electronic purse is inserted into the *OnBoard Unit* device (OBU) in the vehicle. The OBU communicates wirelessly with the *Roadside Equipment.* The Roadside Equipment is the base station in the wireless network that offers a connectionless communication service. The Roadside Equipment itself is connected to the PB by UDP/IP. During a *transaction*, i.e. an electronic payment, several messages are exchanged between the PB and the OBU, following the *PbObu* protocol rules. The protocol is simple. A payment consists of the exchange of a few messages, and there are no message recovery mechanisms. In case of message loss, the message exchange will stop, acknowledged by an error message. The subject of testing is the PB. We want to check the correctness of the electronic transaction processing between multiple smart cards and the PB. So, we will attempt to connect the tester to the PB at the UDP/IP interface and assess the PB for conformance on the PbObu protocol level.

Formal model of IUT. The informal specification of the PB consists of about 50 pages of text. Since the PbObu protocol is simple it was not laborious to make a formal specification of this protocol. The PbObu protocol has been specified in LOTOS and in PROMELA. Every transaction is handled by a separate process instantiation. We used the tools CÆSAR [3] and SPIN [4] to simulate and validate the protocol.

3.2 Test Tools

In this phase we determine the tools that we are going to use, investigate the underlying theory, and identify the facilities offered by the tools to interface with the IUT. In this case study we use TORX.

TorX Theory. TORX is based on the test theory for input output transition systems. In addition to input and output actions, TORX distinguishes the special action δ. The δ action, called *quiescence*, models the absence of output of a system. This absence of output can be explicitly observed by TORX (implemented by a time-out). The notion of correctness between specification and implementation is defined by the *implementation relation* **ioco**. Intuitively, an IUT is considered correct if after a sequence of input, quiescence and output actions, the observed output (including δ) of the IUT is predicted by the specification.

TorX Architecture. The main characteristics of TORX are its flexibility and openness. Flexibility is obtained by using a modular architecture with well-defined interfaces between the components. Openness is achieved by connecting components by pipes over which textual commands and responses are exchanged. The textual interfaces make it simple to debug and test individual components, to experiment using (Unix style) filters to massage the information exchanged, and to distribute the tool over several machines. When needed to link legacy components in the tool environment, we use existing interfaces.

The TORX architecture (in on-the-fly testing configuration) is depicted in Figure 2. The EXPLORER is a specification language-specific component that offers functions (to the PRIMER) to explore the transition-graph of a specification. The PRIMER uses these functions to implement the test derivation algorithm that generates the test primitives from the transition-graph. The optional PARTITIONER is used to steer the on-the-fly derivation process. Normally, when we want to stimulate the SUT, we choose from the set of inputs randomly with a fixed distribution.

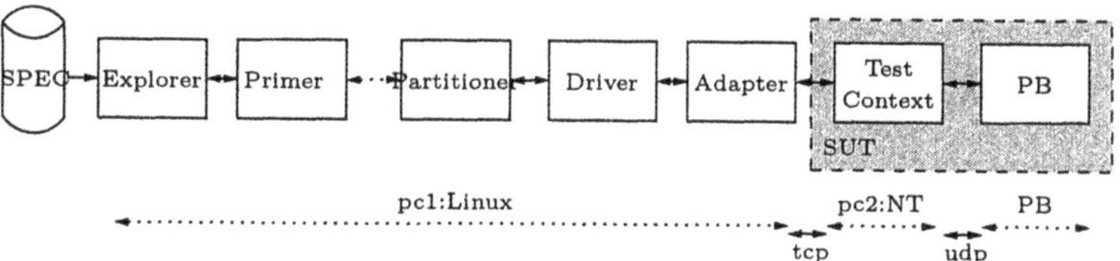

Figure 2. TorX tool architecture

With the PARTITIONER we guide this selection by dividing the possible input test primitives into partitions to which weights (probabilities) are assigned. These weights are taken into account when an input is chosen. PARTITIONERS can be cascaded to partition input actions according to multiple criteria. Similar ideas on probabilities are published in [2]. The DRIVER is the central component of the tool architecture. It controls the testing process, by deciding whether to stimulate or to observe and check the observation. The DRIVER can be run in two modes: a manual mode, in which the user is in full control, and an automatic mode, in which the DRIVER makes all necessary choices randomly. The ADAPTER is the test application specific component that provides the connection with the SUT. It is responsible for sending inputs to and receiving outputs from the SUT on request of the DRIVER, and for encoding and decoding of abstract actions from the DRIVER into the concrete bits and bytes for the SUT, and vice versa, including the mapping of time-outs onto quiescent actions. This clearly makes the ADAPTER dependent on both the specification (version, language), and the SUT.

3.3 Test environment

In this phase we identify the test architecture and implement and test the test environment.

Test architecture design. The PB communicates via UDP/IP, and cannot be approached otherwise. One of the underlying assumptions of testing is that the tester can synthesize every input stimulus for the IUT and can interpret every possible output. This assumption does not hold here. Due to security imposed on electronic transactions, the exchanged messages contain encrypted fields. We can not synthesize nor interpret these fields, since the encryption keys and encryption methods are classified and thus not available. We can indirectly observe and stimulate the PB using the *ObuSim*, a tool running on a Windows NT workstation containing smart cards that host the handling of encryption and decryption. We extend the ObuSim with a (TCP/IP) interface to control the

ObuSim using textual commands. We stimulate and observe the IUT now indirectly. To stimulate, we request the ObuSim to synthesize a message (for which it uses the smart cards) and to send it to the PB. Messages from the PB are received by the ObuSim, decrypted using the smart cards, and the interpretation results are forwarded to the tester.

Exchanged messages and their encryption are mutually related within one transaction, i.e. the format of a message depends on preceding exchanged messages. As a result we can only synthesize, and thus only send, messages for the PB in a particular order. This restriction limits the possibility to exercise the PB behaviour. For example, we can not test for robustness (send arbitrary messages), although it is part of the system's conformance requirements.

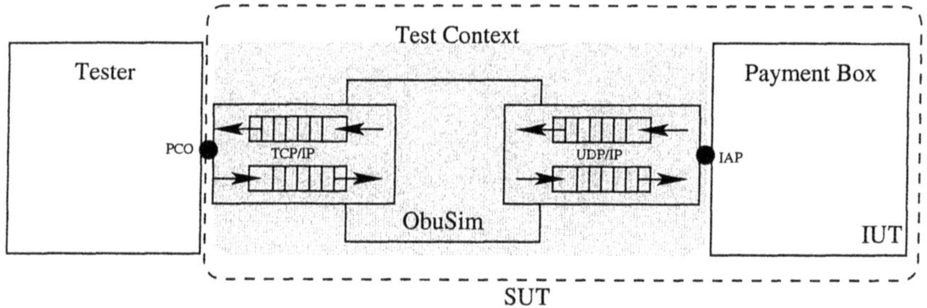

Figure 3. Test architecture

Test architecture implementation. The ObuSim is part of the automated test execution environment developed by Interpay B.V for testing of the PB. The major implementation activity for the test environment was extending this ObuSim with the interface by which TorX can control it. We also developed and parameterized a generic TorX Adapter component that endecodes the abstract specification actions on the message format of this ObuSim control interface.

SUT specification. A UDP/IP service can be modeled as queues, assuming that in our laboratory setting the service is FIFO and reliable. So, a first refinement of the specification is the addition of queues to our model [8]. As previously explained, we should add the behaviour of the ObuSim to the specification from which we derive the tests. The full test architecture is depicted in Figure 3. The tester communicates with PB via the test context (TCP/IP service, ObuSim,UDP/IP service). The PB together with this test context composes the SUT.

Testing the test architecture. Before we can start the "real" test execution, we need confidence in the correctness of both the specification and the test architecture implementation. To gain this confidence we use an iterative debugging process, in which we alternate between running TorX in manual mode and repairing inconsistencies in the specification (where changes made to abstract actions necessitate corresponding changes in the ADAPTER), and bug fixing the test architecture implementation. In this phase we encountered many problems.

3.4 Test execution

Here we report our experiences during the test execution phase.

Introduction to campaigns. In the test environment debugging phase of our process we create multiple versions of specifications and ADAPTERS, and run experiments using multiple configurations. When the test environment is ready and real testing starts, we perform many test executions with varying tool, specification, and possibly also implementation configurations. Previous case studies (e.g. [1]) have shown that it is a laborious task to keep track of the relation between execution results and the tool configuration (including specification and ADAPTER versions).

We set up a semi automatic bookkeeping system to manage the execution phase. In a *test campaign specification language* we specify a *test campaign* which contains all configuration details needed for automatic execution together with archiving information of the execution results. A test campaign tool supports the automatic execution of the specified campaign, i.e. the sequential execution of all experiments specified in the campaign. Related work has been reported in [10].

Campaign design. We designed a test campaign using a single (parameterized) PROMELA specification of the SUT. The configurations in the campaign vary over two parameters: 1) whether or not error stimuli are included, and 2) 78 different values for the random number seed parameter of TorX. So, the campaign describes 2 times 78 executions.

Campaign execution. Due to a minor tool problem (now fixed), and time constraints, of this test campaign only two test executions were performed, consisting of resp. 56167 and 27718 test steps.

Result analysis. During testing we found one conformance violation of the PB. At a certain moment the PB was silent (quiescence), while we expected output. This failure is still under analysis by Interpay B.V. Other conformance violations have not been found.

4. PRACTICAL ISSUES

When we executed the case study, we encountered many difficulties related to the gaps between theory, practice and tool support. We describe some problems in this section.

Model representation. The model of the SUT is decomposed into two main processes: the PB and the ObuSim. Inside both processes we made a decomposition for every transaction, i.e. every possible transaction is modeled by a separate process. This approach is most convenient since it makes the model finite, which is required for both the LOTOS and the PROMELA tools. Additionally, we benefit from the abstraction mechanism of parallelism. Unfortunately, during experimenting with many concurrent transactions, it turned out that for the relatively small model of about 50 processes the LOTOS primer did not perform fast enough to meet the timing constraints of the PB. For the rest of the experiment we used the PROMELA primer, which performed better.

Instantiation of parameters. When we test a system, concrete values have to be given for all data fields of all messages sent to the IUT. However, on specification level, we may abstract from values (free variable) in such input messages, for reasons of generality. Such an abstraction is often applied in writing formal specifications of systems, e.g. for model checking. Here, we have chosen to specify concrete values explicitly in the specification of the PB, to avoid having to instantiate with them elsewhere in the tester (e.g. in the ADAPTER).

Preprocessing specifications. Unfortunately, PROMELA and LOTOS do not support structuring concepts on meta level, e.g. to instantiate a number of processes or to include/exclude a partial behaviour description. As workaround we have used the M4 macro preprocessor [7]. It eases syntactical structuring and consistency keeping of the specification, and offers flexibility when the specification is used for test derivation.

Satisfying time-outs. The PbObu protocol contains time-out scenarios. When an expected message is not received within t_0 seconds, the PB will respond with a timeout message. A typical example of this behaviour is depicted in Figure 4.a. After the reception of the message `SendA` by the PB, the PB expects the message `SendB`. If this message does not arrive within t_0 seconds, the PB responds with the message

TimeOut. The timeout value t_0 (less than 100 milliseconds) is very short compared to the speed with which TORX can deliver test primitives. Especially when we test for many parallel transactions, it can happen that between the delivery of SendA and SendB, many other messages of other transactions are exchanged, so the chance of delivery within the time bound t_0 is very low. To solve this problem, we introduce an "artificial" event SendAB and refine it in the ObuSim. This refinement translates the new SendAB event to a transmission of SendA immediately followed by SendB. However, for various reasons, it can still happen that an error message will be sent after the SendA message. Because we can only observe after we have finished sending a stimulus, and the refinement always sends both SendA and SendB, the observation of this possible error message is delayed, which we have to model explicitly. We do that by adding a queue to the model (Figure 4.b).

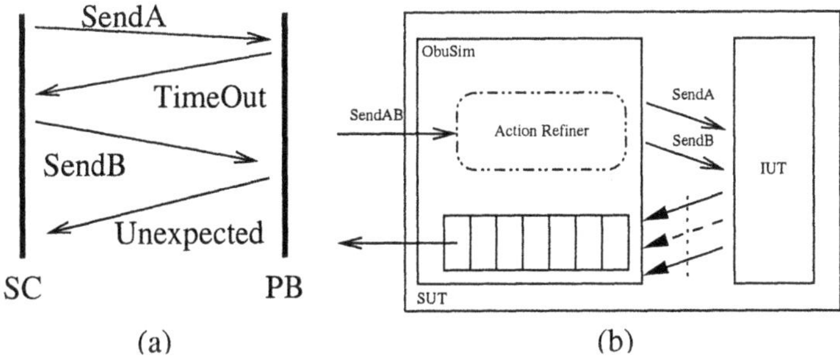

Figure 4. Timing and action refinement

Quiescence and time-outs. The observation of absence of output (quiescence) is implemented by starting a timer when trying to observe any output. If the timer expires after t_q seconds we expect that no output will occur anymore and conclude that we observed quiescence (δ). However, this assumption is too strong for testing the PB. If we choose t_q longer than the timeout t_0 of the PB, we will never make progress in the protocol, i.e. never exercise all behaviour. We prefer to choose t_q shorter than t_0. As a result we might conclude that the PB fails for conformance since after the observation of δ we conclude that we cannot detect any possible output anymore. However, the TimeOut error message may occur after that δ observation. As a pragmatic solution we introduce an additional action Tick. When the IUT is in a state with a time-out scenario, i.e. expects an input, then we generate a Tick output action as long as no other output occurs. The Tick action is explicitly modeled in the specification.

Guarded inputs. Initially we specified parts of the behaviour by a state-oriented machine in PROMELA, i.e. transitions are enabled based on the value of a (global) state variable. However, PROMELA internally translates a predicate into an internal event that blocks based on the evaluation of the predicate, instead of being a blocking condition of an observable action. As a result, the set of actions predicted by the specification is incorrect (this goes wrong with the quiescence predictions), leading to invalid tests. Based on our notion of the semantics of PROMELA and the **ioco** theory, we avoid the use of predicates as internal events. We specified the SUT in a non state-oriented style. Unfortunately this extends the state exploration space.

Probabilistic choice. When running TORX in automatic mode, we noticed that its random input selection strategy (that gives all input actions the same chance of being chosen) did not give us the tests we were interested in. The input actions in our specification fall apart into two categories: one for normal behaviour, and one for error behaviour. In our tests, we do want the main focus on normal behaviour, without completely ignoring error behaviour. The random selection strategy of TORX pays too much attention to error behaviour. To solve this problem, we added the PARTITIONER tool component to TORX, and configured it such that error related actions have a lower chance of being selected. The open architecture of TORX (and the textual interfaces in particular) allowed integration of this new tool component.

Results review. The first execution consisted of 56167 test steps. Of the 17099 transactions which were started, 2200 were successfully completed, 10676 did not meet the timing constraints of the PB, and 4211 did not succeed due to permanent or transitional (21) problems with the smart cards, e.g. insufficient balance. At the end of the execution 12 transactions were still in progress. No error was detected in the PB. Only 61 `Tick` actions occurred, and only once quiescence was observed.

For the second execution, consisting of 27718 test steps, these numbers are respectively 8429 started, 1195 completed, 5237 time constrained, 1992 smart card problems, and 5 still in progress; 24 `Tick` actions, and one quiescence observation. No error was detected in the PB.

The large number of transactions that timed out can be explained by the large number of transactions occurring in parallel, combined with the problems that we had in constructing a specification from which the test events can be derived fast enough.

The low number of `Tick` actions can be explained by the small period of time in which the PB is in a state in which it is waiting for input while all output produced by the PB already has been consumed. The even lower number of quiescent observations is explained in the same way.

5. RESULTS AND OBSERVATIONS

We described automated test derivation and test execution for conformance testing of the PB. We described stepwise the actions that are involved in setting up an automatic on-the-fly test environment and the difficulties and peculiarities that we encountered. We evaluate these:

1. A formal specification for testing differs from a formal specification for validation. This is based on two observations. Firstly, a specification for validation is a model of the IUT. For test derivation we need a model of the SUT. Secondly, a specification for validation can abstract from details which are not of interest for showing a particular property of the system. A specification for conformance testing should describe all possible behaviour at the abstraction level of stimulation and observation.

2. One of the expected benefits of automated derivation, its flexibility, was demonstrated during the engineering phase of the test environment. Since it was hard to identify the SUT in advance , the SUT specification was developed iteratively during the test phase of the test environment and the engineering of the OBUSIM. Adaptations of behaviour, needed to resolve misinterpretation of the informal specification, or to derive specific experiments for validation of the test environment, could easily be solved on specification level, and the proof testing could proceed immediately, since we did not have to rewrite test cases.

3. The flexibility of automated derivation was also shown during testing. By small adaptations of the specification we could easily scale up the experiment (increase the number of concurrent transactions) and direct the tests to a particular test goal. An example of the latter is the disabling of the error generation by the environment, resulting in the increased probability of successful electronic payments transactions. Another issue in the flexibility was shown at the start of the case study. Since we have a formal specification, debugging the specification was easy thanks to the tool support of SPIN and CÆSAR. During the model checking phase, we encountered a functional error in the protocol, which would lead to erroneous money balances. This error has been fixed and new specifications of the HTS have been released.

4. The development of the specification is an iterative process. During the implementation of the ADAPTER more detail of the representation of abstract actions gets known, and our understanding of the SUT increased in the test environment debugging phase.

5. In this case study timing constraints, i.e. handling of time-outs, are dealt with in an ad hoc way. The **ioco** test theory does not offer any theory for handling time-out; neither does TorX. In this application we encountered problems related with the observation of quiescence and specifying time-outs. Since many reactive systems, e.g. protocols, have time-out behaviour, more fundamental theory is needed for testing this real-time class of systems.

6. The assumption that we can synthesize every stimulus and analyze every observation is strong. Because of the encryption involved we delegated the synthesis and analysis to the ObuSim. To resolve timing constraints we used action abstraction and action refinement. More theoretical background on the synthesis of test primitives and action abstraction and refinement in testing is needed to implement generic Adapters for automated test environments.

7. The on-the-fly test approach is challenged when testing systems with real time requirements where the computation of test primitives has to meet certain time bounds to meet an IUT's timing constraints. Although we used an ad hoc solution to cope with the real-time requirements of the PB (stimulate in time), we were not able to generate test primitives fast enough using a Cæsar Primer. A reason could be that the rendez-vous synchronization, where more than 20 processes were involved, slowed down the computation of test primitives. The Promela Primer performed better. Fast computation of test primitives requires efficient handling of the state graph by the Explorer.

8. The automated test derivation from system specifications with a high degree of parallelism is fast and reliable, compared to traditional manual test derivation, which is complex due to the bookkeeping of all interleaving scenarios. By parameterizing the specification we could easily scale up the experiment with respect to the number of concurrent transactions. TorX can handle models of concurrent systems well.

9. The engineering of the automated test execution environment, i.e. the implementation of the Adapter is a laborious task. The hard part was to synthesize the concrete test primitives, i.e. dealing with the smart cards. This conclusion is supported by the conclusions of the traditional test of the PB by Interpay B.V. Also there the whole test execution environment was automated and the implementation of the automated environment was very laborious. Further decomposition into domain specific components of the Adapter can decrease the labour of the development of the application dependent Adapter.

10. The TORX architecture is very flexible. Due to the standardized textual interface between DRIVER and ADAPTER the implementation effort was minimal with respect to this interface. Furthermore, it was easy to cope with multi-platform constraints, i.e. TORX running on a Unix workstation and the ADAPTER on a Windows NT computer. The other TORX components could be reused easily.

11. Due to automation we can execute many tests fast. Since we may use different specifications, TORX tool instantiations (in this case not fully utilized), configurations etc., we will obtain many test executions and test results. Adding the dimension of time, e.g. different releases of the system, specifications etc., even increases the amount of test data. To cope with this complexity we started structuring the test executions and their parameters into test campaigns for which we developed prototype tool support. Initial experiments using campaigns and its tool support demonstrate both the feasibility of such test execution management, and the need for more development on practical and theoretical level.

12. The test campaigns currently only specify (and capture) the elements of the testing process that can be formalized and controlled automatically. Of course, this is not sufficient. Sometimes it is needed to extend the formal experiment description with plain text descriptions of critical test environment parameters that can only be influenced (set up before testing starts) by a human test operator.

13. The results obtained from the execution of a test campaign are large in size and comprehensive to interpret. We need advanced tool support for in-depth analysis of the results, to cope with the complexity.

6. CONCLUDING REMARKS

Summarizing all partial conclusions, we conclude that automated formal test derivation and test execution is beneficial because of the high number of tests that we can execute, and the reliability of these tests (8). Furthermore, automation is feasible due to its flexibility. Adaptations and parameterization of specifications, and test environment configurations are easy (2,3,10). We see the testing of Payment Box as a step ahead in testing realistic industrial applications. However, we need more techniques, theory and tools to support automated testing of real industrial applications. On theory level we need more support for real time behaviour (5,7). On technical and tool level we need more support for system specification (1), result analysis (11,12) and ADAPTER implementation (4,6,9).

Acknowledgments

The authors thank Cornel van Mastrigt and Rommert Jorritsma from Interpay B.V. for their help and support. The anonymous reviewers and Jan Tretmans are acknowledged for their comments.

References

[1] A. Belinfante, J. Feenstra, R.G. de Vries, J. Tretmans, N. Goga, L. Feijs, S. Mauw, and L. Heerink. Formal test automation: A simple experiment. In G. Csopaki, S. Dibuz, and K. Tarnay, editors, 12th *Int. Workshop on Testing of Communicating Systems.* Kluwer Academic Publishers, 1999.

[2] L.M.G Feijs, N. Goga, and S. Mauw. Probabilities in the TorX test derivation algorithm. In Claude Jard Susanne Graf and Yair Lahav, editors, *SAM2000 - 2nd Workshop on SDL and MSC*, pages 173–188, Col de Porte, Grenoble, 6 2000. VERIMAG, IRISA, SDL Forum Society.

[3] H. Garavel. OPEN/CÆSAR: An open software architecture for verification, simulation, and testing. In B. Steffen, editor, *Fourth Int. Workshop on Tools and Algorithms for the Construction and Analysis of Systems (TACAS'98)*, pages 68–84. Lecture Notes in Computer Science 1384, Springer-Verlag, 1998.

[4] G. J. Holzmann. *Design and Validation of Computer Protocols.* Prentice-Hall Inc., 1991.

[5] ISO. *Information Processing Systems, Open Systems Interconnection, LOTOS - A Formal Description Technique Based on the Temporal Ordering of Observational Behaviour.* International Standard IS-8807. ISO, Geneve, 1989.

[6] D. Lee and M. Yannakakis. Principles and methods for testing finite state machines – a survey. *The Proceedings of the IEEE*, 84(8):1090–1123., August 1996.

[7] René Seindal. *GNU m4, version 1.4.* Free Software Foundation, 59 Temple Place – Suite 330, Boston, MA 0211, USA, 1.4 edition, November 1994. Available from URL: http://www.gnu.org.

[8] R. Terpstra, L. Ferreira Pires, L. Heerink, and J. Tretmans. Testing theory in practice: A simple experiment. In T. Kapus and Z. Brezočnik, editors, *COST 247 Int. Workshop on Applied Formal Methods in System Design*, pages 168–183, Maribor, Slovenia, 1996. University of Maribor.

[9] J. Tretmans. Test generation with inputs, outputs and repetitive quiescence. *Software—Concepts and Tools*, 17(3):103–120, 1996. Also: Technical Report No. 96-26, Centre for Telematics and Information Technology, University of Twente, The Netherlands.

[10] T. Vassiliou-Gioles, I. Schieferdecker, M. Born, M. Winkler, and M. Li. Configuration and execution support for distributed tests. In K. Tarnay G. Csopaki, S. Dibuz, editor, 12th *Int. Workshop on Testing of Communicating Systems*, pages 61–76. Kluwer Academic Publishers, 1999.

AD-HOC PROTOCOL MODELLING, VALIDATION AND AUTOMATED TEST SUITE GENERATION

Endre Horváth
Conformance Lab, Ericsson Hungary Ltd. H-1037 Budapest, Laborc u. 1, Hungary
Endre.Horvath@eth.ericsson.se

Abstract This paper describes a trial work connected to research activity in the ad-hoc network protocols area. The goal of this work was to model and validate the Bluetooth baseband protocol layer and to generate test suite in an automated way. This was achieved by using the Telelogic TAU tools: the model was completed in SDL (using SDT), the Validator tool was used to validate it and to generate TTCN test suite.

Key words: SDL, TTCN, Bluetooth, Validation, Test suite generation

1. INTRODUCTION

Real-time aspects in protocol modelling, simulation and validation are very important today. Modern systems in the wireless world, like Bluetooth, have very hard time constraints, so demands on the specification languages, simulation and validation tools used in protocol technology are high. The main goal of my work was to specify a complete system to simulate and validate the Bluetooth baseband protocol layer and to generate TTCN test suite automatically, if it is possible. This paper describes how SDL was deployed in modelling, simulation and validation of Bluetooth, which workarounds were made to prepare the model for automated test suite generation.

Section 2 gives a brief introduction to Bluetooth concentrating on timing aspects. The most important modelling problems and the chosen solutions are described in Section 3, while Section 4 presents the validation procedure.

The test suite generation work is presented in Section 5 and at the end Section 6 summarizes the experiences of my work.

2. BLUETOOTH

Bluetooth is a universal radio interface that enables portable electronic devices to communicate wirelessly via short-range ad-hoc networks [1]. It eliminates the need for wires, cables and connectors between cordless or mobile phones, modems, headsets, personal digital assistants, computers, printers, etc.

Each unit can communicate simultaneously with up to seven other units forming a so-called piconet (Figure 1). One Bluetooth unit acts as the master of the piconet, whereas the other unit(s) act(s) as slave(s). Each piconet can have only one master. However, slaves can participate in different piconets on a time-division multiplex basis. In addition, a master in one piconet can be a slave in other piconet(s) [1].

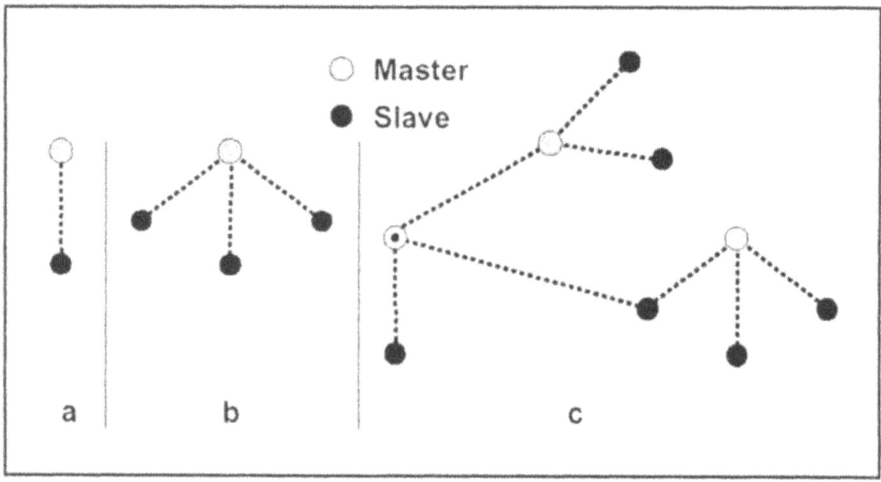

Figure 11. Bluetooth piconets [1]: a) Simple communication; b) Bluetooth piconet; c) Bluetooth scatternet

The Bluetooth radio frequency system is represented as a frequency hopping spread spectrum system in which packets are transmitted in defined time slots on defined frequencies. The channel is represented by a pseudo-random hopping sequence, hopping through the 79 RF channels [1]. The hopping sequence is unique for the piconet and is determined by the master's Bluetooth device-address while the phase in the hopping sequence is determined by the master's clock. The channel is divided into time slots where each slot corresponds to an RF hop frequency. The channel hops to a new frequency in every slot, where the nominal hop rate is 1600 hops/s (slot length is 625 μs) [1]. All Bluetooth units participating in the piconet are time- and hop-synchronized to the channel. To keep this synchronization, a master is required to send packets that synchronize the slaves to the master - even if the master is not sending data. All the slaves in a piconet must be within the radio range of the master, so that every slave can synchronize to the piconet using the master's transmissions.

Every Bluetooth unit has an internal system clock that determines the timing and hopping of the transceiver. The Bluetooth clock is derived from a free running native clock that never needs to be adjusted and is never turned off. For synchronization with other units, only time offsets are used that, when added to the native clock, provide temporary Bluetooth clocks which are mutually synchronized. It should be noted that the Bluetooth clock has no relation to the time of the day; it can therefore be initialized to any value. The Bluetooth clock provides the heartbeat of the Bluetooth transceiver. Its resolution is at least half of the TX or RX slot length (312.5 μs) [1].

For data transmission, a frame is segmented to baseband packets whose length can be 1-5 slots (Figure 2). The data transmission means sending the baseband packets to the destination and listening to the acknowledgement packets in the next slot. The acknowledgement packets are single slot baseband packets by default. A single-bit acknowledgement is used to indicate whether the last packet was received correctly or not.

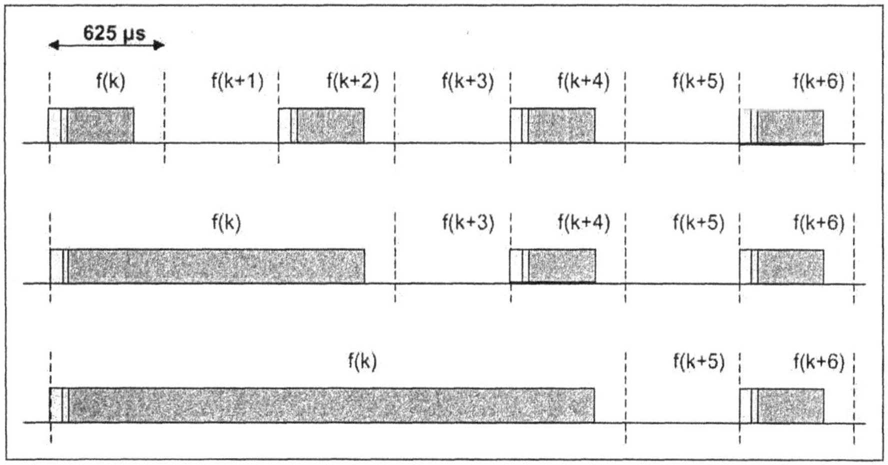

Figure 12. Baseband packets in Bluetooth [1]

3. SDL MODELLING OF BLUETOOTH

Bluetooth was modelled in SDL for validation and testing purposes. The structure of the SDL system is quite simple (Figure 3): the Node block is connected to the environment via two interfaces. The task of the first one is to communicate with the upper layer (User SAP) while the other interface represents the radio channel. This structure also determines the architecture of the generated Test Suite (see Section 5).

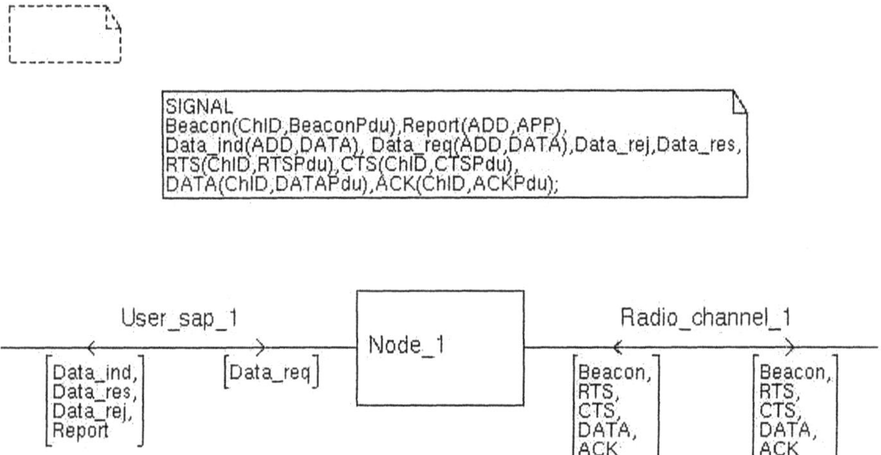

Figure 13. System structure

Unfortunately, real-time features are not fully supported in the current SDL therefore some real-time problems had to be solved by using the available language elements. For example timing in Bluetooth is essential. Every node has an internal clock that determines the timing and hopping of the transceiver. This clock is represented by a 28 bit counter where the least significant bit ticks in units of 312.5 μs (half of the slot length) [1].

An accurate cyclic timer would be nice to model Bluetooth timing in SDL, but it is not supported at the moment. First, there is no cyclic timer in SDL therefore timers have to be restarted immediately after they expired (Figure 4). If a timer expires the timeout signal gets into the input buffer of the process and there is no guarantee that the signal will be processed immediately. A solution for this problem could be to use priority inputs [2] for timeout signals (Figure 4). In this way there is a chance to avoid drifting in the Bluetooth clock.

The 28-bit counter is implemented as a bit-string variable in the SDL model and it is increased after every timeout using a simple procedure (Figure 4). The value of the counter shows the actual status of the Bluetooth clock so it can be included in the Master's advertisement packets sent to the slaves. The actual value of this counter is the input for the frequency hop selection procedure.

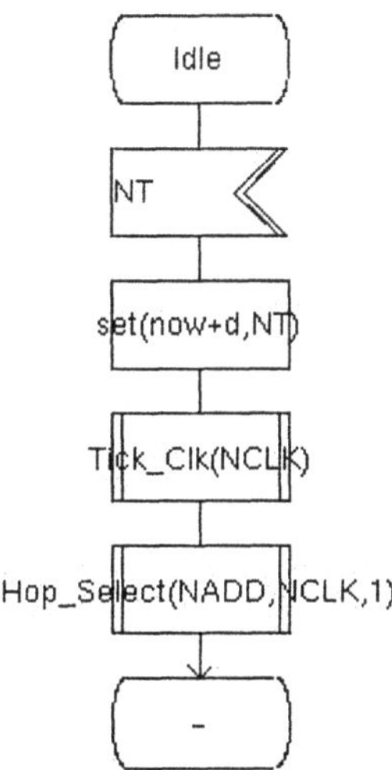

Figure 4. Using priority input for timeout signals

One of the most important tasks of the Bluetooth baseband protocol layer is to control the frequency hopping of the node's transceiver. It is realized in the protocol model by implementing the hop selection algorithm described in the Bluetooth specification [1]. This algorithm generates a pseudorandom number (a channel id) between 0 and 78 according to the MAC address and the clock status of the Master. There is also a third input parameter of the algorithm that controls how often the frequency has to be changed. In the model only two possibilities are distinguished: slow frequency hopping for scanning and fast frequency hopping for other communication. Since there is no physical layer (real transceiver) under the baseband protocol, the channel id is carried in every signal. If a signal is received the model checks whether the node is "hearing" the signal (the channel id in the signal is equal to the node's channel id) or not (Figure 5).

In Bluetooth the data frames are segmented to baseband packets of length 1-5 slots (Figure 2) [1]. There is no frequency change during the transmission of one segment, but the different segments are transmitted on different frequencies (according to the actual clock status of the piconet's master) and every segment has to be acknowledged in the next slot. This simple procedure is not so easy to model by using SDL, because duration cannot be assigned to sending / receiving events. The only solution is to wait until the needed slots are passed which can be achieved by using simple slot counters.

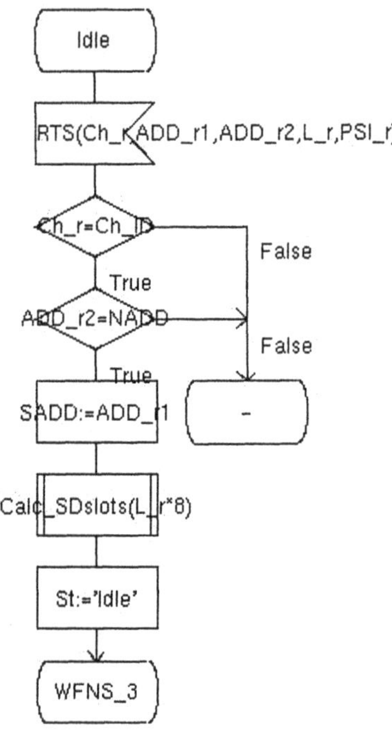

Figure 5. Checking the channel id after a signal reception

4. VALIDATION OF THE MODEL

The protocol model is not simple: there are many states and variables used to specify the baseband protocol of Bluetooth. Therefore the state space to be generated during validation is very large (see Figure 6), so it is not easy (or even impossible) to fully validate this SDL model. That is why the Exhaustive state space exploration algorithm was not applicable on this model and so the Bit-state algorithm was used to validate the SDL system.

Another problem is that the communication with the modelled node is possible only on specified frequencies according to the node's hop sequence. This requires well-constructed test patterns to achieve high coverage in the validation procedure. To solve this problem, the Simulator tool was used to produce some typical test sequences and during simulation some useful test patterns were gained that could be applied in validation, too [3].

Figure 6 shows the result of validation achieved by using simple test signals (produced during simulation) and default Validator settings (Max searching depth = 100). The 72% symbol coverage could be increased up to 80% by defining some erroneous test signals (e.g. negative acknowledgement in data transmission) and by raising the searching depth. The reasons for only 80% symbol coverage are the following:

- The modelled node has a fix MAC address, while the hop selection procedure is executed according to this address. It means that some parts (e.g. permutation according to the input address bits) of this procedure could not be reached at all.
- The length of test data is limited in the Validator, therefore it was not possible to validate all the segmentation functionalities.
- Due to limitations in time and computer resources the searching depth of the Bit-state exploration algorithm was also limited and therewith increasing the searching depth raises the collision risk in application of Bit-state exploration, too.

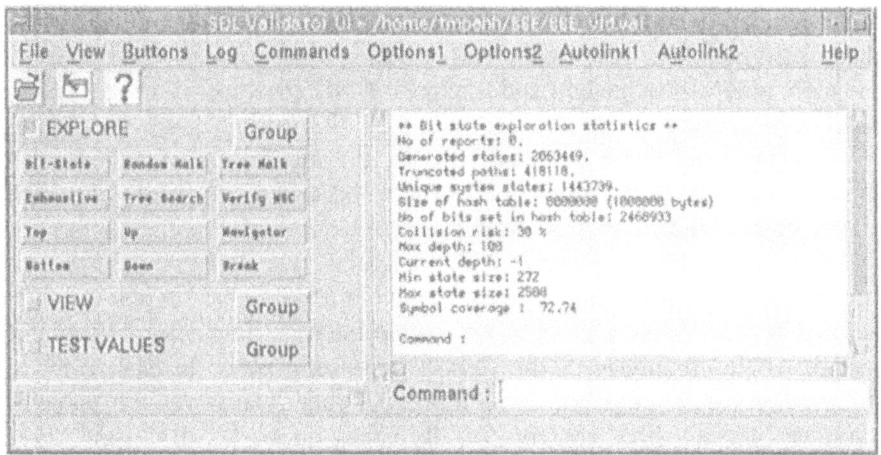

Figure 6. Validation result by using default settings

As a result it can be said that serious problem was not found during validation. The validation procedure was helpful to complete the right SDL model because some design failures were detected and only some model specific problems were occurred like exceeding the maximum transition length (reason: the hop selection algorithm is used very often).

5. AUTOMATED TEST SUITE GENERATION

The Telelogic TAU tools were used for TTCN test suite generation [4]. The starting point of the generation is the SDL specification and the goal is to get a TTCN test suite in an automated way. This procedure has two main parts:

1. Producing MSC diagrams [5] that are the input test purposes for deriving TTCN test cases;
2. Generating a TTCN test suite [6] from the MSC test purposes and the SDL specification.

The second part of the generation procedure is implemented in the TAU Validator in a fully automated way [4] (on demand some translating rules can be defined to personalize the test suite) but the automation of the first part is not so trivial.

To generate MSCs automatically, an appropriate state space exploration algorithm is needed. In case of our Bluetooth model only the Bit-state algorithm could be used, because the Exhaustive algorithm was not applicable at all (see previous section), while other algorithms contain random parts that do not guarantee consistency and applicability with the MSC generation method explained in the following paragraphs. However the most important thing is not which algorithm is used in the MSC generation: the main point is the method and timing of MSC generation during the state space exploration.

A solution for these problems can be the application of an Observer process [2] (Figure 7) to generate Reports according to given rules. The Validator can store how these Reports were reached during the exploration and these paths can be saved as MSC diagrams. The outfit of the MSCs is controlled by the searching depth of the exploration algorithm and the rules defined in the Observer process. Of course the most important part of this method is the definition of the Report–generating rules. In SDL a lot of information can be collected about a process under execution, e.g. value of variables, actual state, contents of the input queue [2]. By using these information the Report generation can be controlled easily.

From a tester's perspective the model is a black box. It means that the tester sends inputs to the IUT (Implementation Under Test) and waits for the reaction. Without any reaction it is not easy to judge whether the system behaves right or not. To produce conventional test cases the outputs of the modelled system have to be observed and a Report should be generated after receiving an output. Unfortunately, observing the outputs of a process under execution is not supported in SDL explicitly, but there is a workaround to solve this problem: by a small modification to the model we can add a counter which value is increased after every sending event and the change of the counter's value can be watched by the observer process.

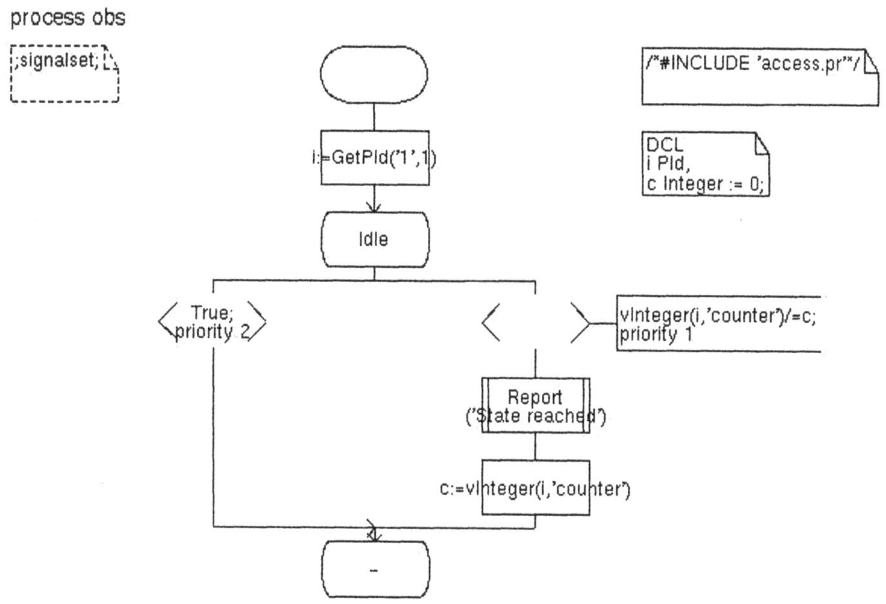

Figure 7. Observer process for MSC generation

By using this method hundreds of MSCs were generated however many of them were not significantly different from one another. The reason is that after a sending event Reports were generated also by reaching a temporal state (e.g. waiting for the next slot) and by getting into the next stable state, too. Therefore another rule was defined to reduce the number of the redundant MSCs by generating a Report only if a stable state is reached. This way 15 different MSCs were generated. An example is shown on Figure 8.

After producing the MSC test purposes the second step of the automated test suite generation was routine work. With some smart scripts and the appropriate configuration the MSCs were translated into TTCN test cases by pressing a button, so the whole test suite was generated very quickly by using the Validator tool. Figure 9 shows the TTCN test case generated from the previously presented MSC.

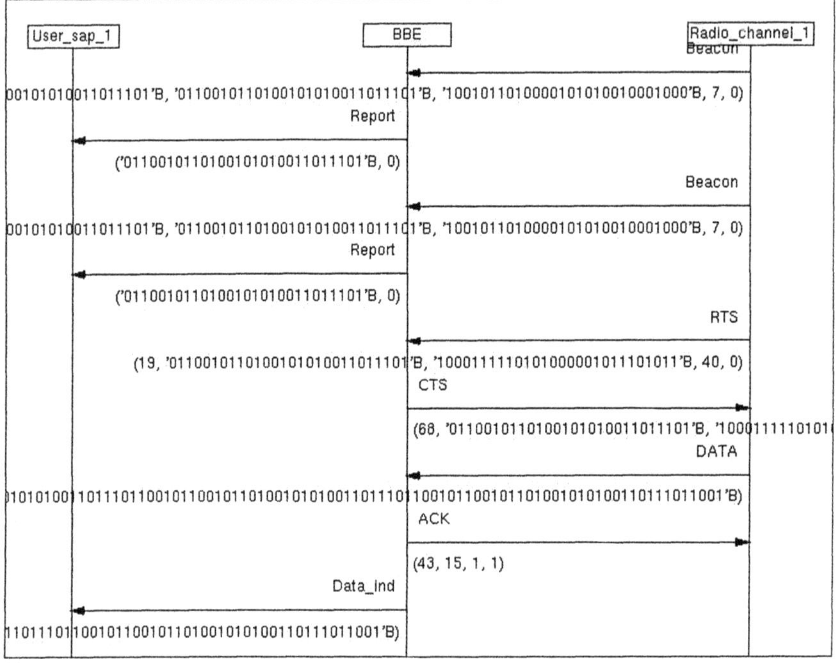

Figure 8. Automatically generated MSC diagram

Test Case Dynamic Behaviour

Test Case Name: BBE_TC_Asse_00007
Group :
Purpose :
Configuration :
Default :
Comments :
Selection Ref :
Description :

Nr	Label	Behaviour Description	Constraints Ref	Verdict	Comments
1		Radio_channel_1 ! Beacon	cBBE_TC_Asse_00001_004		
2		User_sap_1 ? Report	cBBE_TC_Asse_00001_003		
3		Radio_channel_1 ! Beacon	cBBE_TC_Asse_00001_004		
4		User_sap_1 ? Report	cBBE_TC_Asse_00001_003		
5		Radio_channel_1 ! RTS	cBBE_TC_Asse_00001_002		
6		Radio_channel_1 ? CTS	cBBE_TC_Asse_00001_001		
7		Radio_channel_1 ! DATA	cBBE_TC_Asse_00003_003		
8		Radio_channel_1 ? ACK	cBBE_TC_Asse_00003_002		
9		User_sap_1 ? Data_ind	cBBE_TC_Asse_00003_001	PASS	
10		User_sap_1 ? OTHERWISE		FAIL	
11		Radio_channel_1 ? OTHERWISE		FAIL	
12		Radio_channel_1 ? OTHERWISE		FAIL	
13		Radio_channel_1 ? OTHERWISE		FAIL	
14		User_sap_1 ? OTHERWISE		FAIL	
15		User_sap_1 ? OTHERWISE		FAIL	

Detailed Comments:

Figure 9. Automatically generated TTCN test case

The quality of the generated test suite is good but the test cases have to be completed manually since there are no guard timers generated to protect the tester against deadlocks during testing (against waiting for an answer for an indefinite amount of time). However it is very positive that naming of constraints can be controlled with configuration of the generator tool and concurrent TTCN is also supported in the Validator [4].

6. CONCLUSIONS

The completed work described in this paper had three main phases: modelling, validation and test suite generation. The modelled protocol had some specialities that were not too easy to describe in SDL: the problem of accurate timing was solved by using priority inputs, but also the handling of frequency hopping caused some troubles. Frequency hopping was a problem in validation of the model, too. Since the default (automatically generated) test signals were not applicable in validation, the Simulator tool was used to produce the appropriate test patterns (using the right frequency identifiers). In the test suite generation phase frequency hopping was the reason again for many redundant MSCs. Even so the automated MSC generation could be controlled well by using an Observer process, and based on the generated MSCs a TTCN test suite of good quality could be generated easily.

The plan for the future is to continue this work by modelling more (up to 8) Bluetooth nodes communicating with each other. To describe this system an extra process has to be defined for modelling the radio channel. This solution makes it also possible to simulate the losing of data frames and the channel delay. The completed specification is also a very good base for experimenting with real-time extensions to SDL in terms of a European research project called Interval [7].

REFERENCES

[1] Specification of the Bluetooth System (Core), Specification Volume 1, 2001

[2] ITU-T Recommendation Z.100 - Specification and Description Language, 1996

[3] R. L. Probert, A. W. Williams: Fast Functional Test Generation Using an SDL Model, Testing of Communicating Systems, Budapest, Hungary, 1999

[4] M. Schmitt, A. Ek, B. Koch, J. Grabowski, D. Hogrefe: Autolink – Putting SDL-based test generation into practice, Testing of Communicating Systems, Tomsk, Russia, 1998

[5] ITU-T Recommendation Z.120 – Message Sequence Charts, 1996

[6] OSI – Open System Interconnection, Conformance testing methodology and framework – Part 3: Tree and Tabular Combined Notation, ISO/IEC 9646 3, 1997

[7] Preliminary Specification of Timed Extensions; Formal Design, Validation and Testing of Real-Time Telecommunications Systems; Interval project report, 2000

SESSION VII

TEST GENERATION AND SELECTION

GENERATE CERTIFIED TEST CASES BY COMBINING THEOREM PROVING AND REACHABILITY ANALYSIS*

Richard Castanet
Davy Rouillard
LaBRI, Bordeaux I University, 33405 TALENCE Cedex, FRANCE
{castanet,rouillar}@labri.u-bordeaux.fr

Abstract We present a test case generation method which conciliates theorem proving and model checking. Test purposes are expressed by timed regular expressions and then translated into a corresponding automaton using a certified function. This automaton is composed with the system specification and an execution is computed from this sub-specification by an automatic tool. The result is finally re-injected into the theorem prover to be checked.

Keywords: conformance testing, certified test purposes, timed automata, safe computations

1. INTRODUCTION

The life cycle of protocol engineering contains several steps: requirements definition, formal specification, simulation or verification, implementation and finally testing (conformance, interoperability, robustness and performance tests). It is widely recognized that the use of formal model is essential to allow automatic verification as well as automatic test generation. Proof techniques can also be used to validate the critical parts of a system but they are employed still rather rarely in the domain of protocols [14].

The aims of this paper are to show how the test cases generation can be compatible with the proof activity and to exhibit the benefits one may gain in developing a test environment based on a proof assistant. To achieve these goals, we propose to use the general framework *CClair*

*Research partially supported by the French government for the RNRT project Calife.

[8] which supports both verification and testing activities on various kind of automata. For a description of the verification techniques supported by *CClair*, we refer the reader to [7].

The heart of *CClair* is the proof assistant *Isabelle*[17] and its implementation of the *Higher Order Logic.* This logic offers a very rich language in which it is possible to describe complex systems and properties. Thus, it becomes possible to work on systems for which automatic tools fail because of a classical state-explosion problem.

This high expressiveness is also a strong argument for the joint use of proof assistants and automatic procedures because tools such as Isabelle [17], Coq[16] or PVS[20] may work with a great variety of mathematic objects and they have therefore no problems to understand and manipulate the results computed by automatic tools.

Another advantage is that proof assistants deal with theorems i.e. certified objects. This means that all results computed by external procedures have to be checked before been integrated. Furthermore, complex pieces of reasoning may be formalized in order to combine these results. It results in an increased confidence in the validation/testing process since the unavoidable errors due to the merge of several formalisms are immediately detected.

This paper highlights all these concepts by proposing a new approach to generate certified test cases for real-time systems. We are only interested by deriving generic test case without considering a test method. This last aspect will be take account in a next stage of the testing process, following the methodology of the standard ISO9646[13]. To model the specification systems, we use *Parameterized automata* (p-automata) that can be seen as extensions of timed automata or timed I/O automata. The latter have been used in recent works for test generation [12, 4]. The p-automata model has the advantage to allow the use of variables of any type and recent experiments [6] tend to prove it is a convenient formalism to model communication protocols.

The rest of the paper is organized as follows: In section 2, we present the main features of *Isabelle* and *CClair*. In section 3, we describe how *CClair* may be used to formalize the test generation starting from both a specification of a timed system under test and a test purpose that describes a set of behaviors to be tested. In section 4, we introduce a general method to generate test cases by translating test purpose into a p-automaton. This automaton is used as synchronous observer to guide the construction of an execution that satisfies the test purpose. This execution is computed by *Hytech* and then validated in *CClair*. This method is employed in section 5 to generate test cases for the ABR algorithm used in ATM networks. Finally, the section 6 summarizes the results presented in the paper and outlines future works.

2. A GENERAL FRAMEWORK FOR STUDYING AUTOMATA

2.1 *Isabelle*

CClair is developed on top of *Isabelle*, which is a generic proof assistant in the sense that it supports reasoning in various logics : *First Order Logic*, *Zermelo-fraenkel set theory*, *High Order Logic* (HOL in short). In this paper, we are however only concerned by the latter instance of *Isabelle*.

HOL offers a great expressiveness that allows to formalize mathematical principles such as recursion and [co]induction.

Proofs, in *Isabelle*, may be built in a backward-chaining mode : a conjecture is stated and the goal is successively reduced to zero or more new subgoals by applying tactics. When no subgoals remain, the proof is complete and the resulted theorem may be used in further proof. The main tactic is resolution, which mimics the natural deduction: it unifies the conclusion of a proof rule with a selected subgoal and then replaces it by the instantiated premise of the rule. An other important feature is offered by rewriting tactics, which simplify a selected subgoal using possibly conditional directed equalities. Theorems used during rewriting are stored in *simplification sets* that can be extended by any necessary theorems.

Goals may contain *logical variables*, denoted with a question mark $x^?$. Logical variables represent unknown values that can be instantiated by resolution during proofs. Rewriting tactics and logical variables may be combined to perform some computations. For instance,

$$\texttt{filter}\ (\lambda x.\ x = a)\ [a, b, b, c, a] = x^?$$

will instantiate $x^?$ with the list $[a, a]$ using a rewriting tactic.

2.2 *CClair*

The *CClair* project [7] aims to provide the user with an environment for working with transition systems of various kinds. Its kernel is a main theory of plain labeled transition systems, which allows to name states, action labels, transitions, traces and executions, and contains some tools for computing and reasoning. It intends to be *generic* in the same meaning as *Isabelle*: a general framework contains a theory of plain transition systems; various interesting kinds of transition systems, like Büchi, constrained or timed automata are defined in sub-theories.

Executions and traces of a system are formalized using the theory of *lazy* list developed by Paulson[18]. This theory allows us to represent finite as well infinite behaviors in a single representation and provides various usual functions on list such as concatenation and filtering. Executions are therefore naturally declared as lists of transitions.

Properties of executions and/or traces may be expressed via a set of temporal operators ($\bigcirc, \Diamond, \Box$...) (see [9] for example) that define languages of potentially infinite words. Usual operations on languages are also provided, among them `Concat` L_1 L_2 denotes the concatenation of L_1 and L_2, `Star` L is the Kleene-star operation and `Omega` L represents the set of words obtained by infinite concatenations of words in L.

3. TEST GENERATION METHODOLOGY

One of the goal of the *CClair* project is to put in the same framework, verification and testing activities. This section shows that test cases generation may be viewed as a verification task: proving that an unknown execution satisfies a given property. We begin by a description of the p-automata model and its implementation into *CClair*.

3.1 The p-automata model

To model real time systems, we use *Parameterised timed automata* [5]. This model was designed for the formalization and proof of algorithms used in telecommunications and constitutes the heart of the French RNRT scientific project *Calife*.

A p-automaton is a graph associated with a set of variables and a single non resettable clock. Each edge of the graph can be guarded by a condition on the variables (including the clock) and a relation which describes how the values of variables can be modified.

More precisely, a p-automata $P = \langle \mathcal{S}, \mathcal{A}, \mathcal{L}, \mathcal{W}, \mathcal{V}, \mathcal{M}, \mathcal{I} \rangle$ consists of the following components: $\mathcal{S}$ is the *universal clock* that memorizes the elapse of time. $\mathcal{A}$ is a set of *actions*. $\mathcal{L}$ is a set of *locations* that are the vertices of the control graph. $\mathcal{W}$ is a set of *parameters* i.e. variables with values fixed by initial constraints. $\mathcal{V}$ is a set of variables. As usual, we use primed variables to denote the values after a modification and the set of primed of variables is denoted $\mathcal{V}'$. $\mathcal{M}$ is a set of *moves*. Each move $m = \langle l, a, \theta, l' \rangle$ is composed of a source location $l \in \mathcal{L}$, a target location $l' \in \mathcal{L}$ and an action $a \in \mathcal{A}$. The *update relation* $\theta \subseteq (\mathcal{V} \times \{\mathcal{S}\}) \times \mathcal{V}'$ describes the guard condition and modifies the value of variables. Finally, the function $\mathcal{I}$ assigns to each location a constraint on variables called *invariant*.

During an execution, the state of P is given by the triple (s, v, l) that is composed of the value of the clock, a location $l \in \mathcal{L}$ and a vector $v = (v_1, \ldots, v_n)$ that represents a value a_i for each variable $x_i \in \mathcal{V}$. States must be *admissible* i.e. values of variables must satisfy the invariant associated with the location of the state.

P can change its state in two ways: a *discrete* transition associated to a move $\langle l, a, \theta, l' \rangle \in \mathcal{M}$ causes P to change the location from l to l' and the values of variables are updated according the update relation θ. Otherwise, a *delay transition* modifies only the value of the universal clock.

The way in which a p-automaton operates is described by an *execution, i.e.* a sequence of consecutive discrete and delay transitions. However, for reasoning about real-time systems, we are interesting in studying not only the actions that are performed when the system runs, but also the instant at which each action is executed. Therefore, an adequate way to describe the behavior of a p-automaton is given by the notion of *timed trace.* A timed trace is a sequence of pairs $[(a_1, t_1), \ldots, (a_n, t_n)]$ where a_i denotes an action and t_i the instant of execution of a_i. A couple (a_i, t_i) is called a *dated* action.

Behind this general model, a subclass of p-automata called *restricted p-automata* has been identified in [5], where $\mathcal{L}$, $\mathcal{A}$, $\mathcal{M}$ are finite sets, $\mathcal{V}$ is a set of real-valued variables, and update relations and invariants are linear expressions. These constraints allow to translate restricted p-automata into linear hybrid automata [1, 3] on which tools for automatic analysis[11] can be applied.

Example: figure 1 depicts a restricted p-automaton which models a digicode with three keys `A`, `B` and `C`. The correct sequence of keys, i.e. the one which causes the door to open, is `A`, `B`, `A`. Since only three errors are tolerated, the variable *cpt* memorizes the number of errors. Moreover, some delays control the input: `B` must be entered at most 10 seconds after the key `A`. The last key `A` must be entered before 20 seconds. Four successive errors or a too long time between two keys cause the lock of the digicode. A correct timed trace of the digicode is, for instance, the sequence of dated actions $[(\mathtt{A}, 3.2), (\mathtt{B}, 5.4), (\mathtt{A}, 6.1)]$.

3.2 P-automata in *CClair*

The formalization of the model of p-automata in our framework takes the form of an extension of the *CClair* theories on transition systems. It contains the definition of the polymorphic type $(\alpha, l, \nu)\,\mathtt{pa}$ which represents p-automata of actions of type α, locations of type l and variables

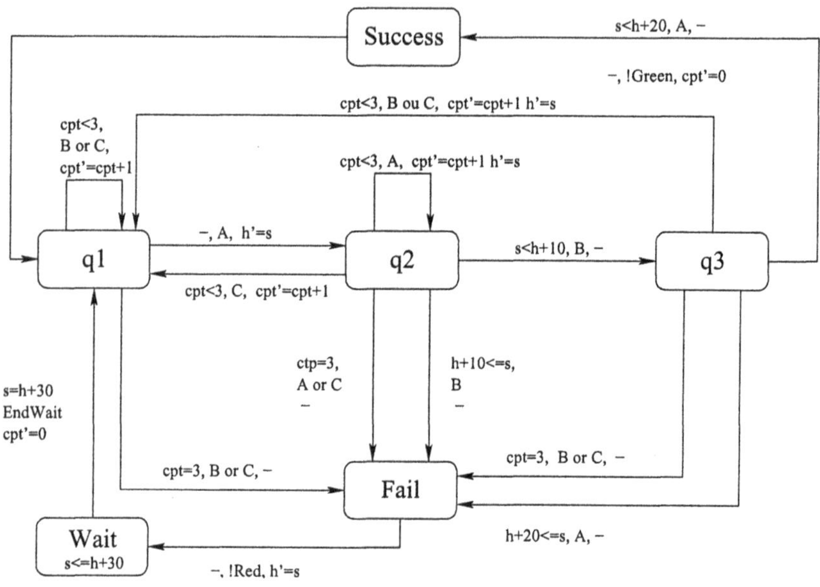

Figure 1. A example of p-automaton

of type ν. Because α, l and ν may be instantiated with any type, it is possible to represent systems with an infinite number of actions or locations. Moreover, variables can contain lists, sets or more complex data structures. A translation of p-automata into plain transition systems is also provided to represent p-automata during execution. Consequently, discrete transition and time delay need not to be defined: it is enough to consider transitions of the translation into the parent theory.

In order to make easier the communication between a finite execution and its associated timed trace, these notions are introduced simultaneous under the form of a predicat defined inductively: given a p-automaton P, $\texttt{F\_TTraces}_P$ contains the objects of the form $s \xrightarrow[P]{\xi, w} s'$ where ξ is an execution of P from the state s to t together with its corresponding timed trace w. $s \xrightarrow[P]{\xi, w} s'$ is called a *run* of P. A run is built with the help of three rules, called *introduction rules*: a run is either empty or obtained by adding a discrete-transition or a delay-transition on the head of an already defined run.

A parallel composition operator, compatible with the *Hytech* composition[11], is provided to modelize complex systems from a collection of automata, each describing a modular component of the system. Consider two p-automata A and B, locations of the parallel composition $A \| B$ are the pairs of location (l_1, l_2) where l_1 is a location of A and l_2 is a location of B. The invariant function of $A \| B$ assigns to (l_1, l_2) the conjunction of l_1 and l_2's invariants.

A move of $A \| B$ is either a move of A or B alone or a combined move if the action is common to A and B. In the latter case, the update relation is the conjunction of the update relation of each component.

Numerous results, about runs of p-automata and their composition, are proven in *CClair*. Among them, the following theorem will be used in section 4.5.

$$\frac{\begin{array}{ll} H1: & \mathtt{acts\_of}\ w \subseteq \mathcal{A}_A \cap \mathcal{A}_B\ \wedge \\ H2: & s \xrightarrow[P\|Q]{x,w} t \end{array}}{\pi 1_{\mathtt{s}}\ s \xrightarrow[A]{\pi 1_{\mathtt{x}}\ x,w} \pi 1_{\mathtt{s}}\ t\ \wedge\ \pi 2_{\mathtt{s}}\ s \xrightarrow[A]{\pi 2_{\mathtt{x}}\ x,w} \pi 2_{\mathtt{s}}\ t} \qquad (1)$$

Given an execution in the composed automaton, this theorem infers an execution with the same timed trace in A and B using the projections $\pi 1_{\mathtt{s}}$, $\pi 2_{\mathtt{s}}$, $\pi 1_{\mathtt{x}}$ and $\pi 2_{\mathtt{x}}$. These are used to project states and executions onto the first and second components. The additional assumption $H1$ requires that all actions mentioned in the trace (collected by the function `acts_of`) are common to A and B.

3.3 A proof approach of the test

Following the definition from standard ISO 9646[13], an implementation conforms to its specification if it satisfies all the conformance requirements which are explicitly mentioned in the protocol standard. Consequently, the process of conformance testing aims at deriving a set of tests cases which will check whether an implementation satisfies all these conformance requirements. In this paper, we focus on the first step of this process which consists in deriving *generic test cases* from the specification i.e. test cases which are independent of any implementation.

Conformance requirements have to be expressed in a formal language and therefore each requirement may involved one or many so-called *test purposes* which are formal descriptions of the constraints to impose on the behavior of the specification in order to decide whether the particular conformance requirements is satisfied. Using terms of theorem proving, we obtain an generic test case if we can prove that it corresponds to an execution of the specification that satisfies a test purpose. Since our aim is also to compute such a test case, we start with an incomplete statement where logical variables replacc the desired execution.

Consequently, deriving a test case amounts to solve a statement of the following form:

$$s \xrightarrow[P]{\xi^?, w^?} s'^? \quad \wedge \quad Q(s, \xi^?, w^?, s'^?) \tag{2}$$

3.4 How to describe Test purposes

Translating conformance requirements into formal language is a non-obvious task: requirements are provided in natural language which often contains many ambiguities. If the formal language used for this translation is too poor, it may lead to errors on the meaning of the requirement. Since the property Q in the goal 2 is a formula of *HOL* logic, one disposes of a large expressive language. Moreover, *CClair* provides many operators, commonly used in verification and testing activities: LTL modalities, language constructors and of course automata. If it is not enough, user may develop his own operators together with a translation into concepts already defined in order to prove the soundness.

Let us emphasize that we are not limited to express test purpose about traces. The reason is that Q takes as argument the execution ξ and an execution contains all information about the successive states of the system. We can therefore formalize constraints on particular value of variables or location. Suppose, for instance, that we seek to obtain a test case where the counter exceeds the allowed value before the system reaches the location $q3$. Using the selectors `cpt` and `loc` to extract the value of the counter and the location from states, the property Q may be: $\xi^? \models \Diamond((\mathtt{cpt} > 3) \wedge \bigcirc\Diamond(\mathtt{loc} = q3))$

3.5 Deriving test cases

Deriving a test case amounts to providing a constructive proof of 2. The basic technique to build an execution is to use of simulation tactics in which introduction rules of the predicat `F_TTraces` are applied. Once a part of the execution is instantiated, the second part of the goal may be simplified through rewriting. If simplifications lead to the formula "False", this means that an error is detected and another execution is searched using backtracking facilities.

This higher degree of interactivity is the price to pay to enable one to work with models known to be undecidable and therefore for which no automatic procedure exists. In this difficult cases, tactics are available to make the task easier. For instance, one may extract the *control graph* of a p-automaton, by ignoring all but action symbols and locations ; if this graph is finite, we can apply certified algorithms on graphs to compute candidates for executions, which are confronted to invariants and update relation of the original automaton.

If automatic procedures may be used, then the generation of certificated test cases is fully automatic as explained in section 4.

4. DERIVING TEST CASES FROM CERTIFIED TEST PURPOSE

This section focuses on the production of test cases for the class of restricted p-automata. Since a restricted p-automaton is a kind of linear hybrid automaton[2], we can invoke the verification tool *Hytech* from *CClair* in order to automatically compute an execution.

Our overall approach is as follows: a temporal test purpose T is expressed using a kind of regular expressions. Then, this expression is translated by means of rewriting rules into a timed-automaton T so that the traces of T satisfy the test purpose. The latter property is established by a pre-proven theorem. Next, T is used as a synchronous observer to guide the construction of an execution which is computed by *Hytech* and finally certified in *CClair*.

4.1 Final location and accepted language

The p-automata model does not permit to declare a final location. For the purpose of defining the language accepted by a p-automaton, we therefore need to extend the model. It is easily done under *CClair* by introducing a new type of automata, called `paf` (p-automata with final location) that adjoins a final location to each p-automata.

$$(\alpha, l, \nu)\,\mathtt{paf} = ((\alpha, l, \nu)\,\mathtt{pa} \times l)$$

A run is accepted by a given automaton (P, f) if there exists a corresponding run in P whose last location is f.

$$(s, w) \in \mathtt{Accepts}_{(P,f)} \equiv \exists\ \xi\ t \mid s \xrightarrow[P]{\xi, w} t\ \wedge\ (\mathtt{loc}\ t = f)$$

4.2 A particular test purpose

Conformance requirements may be formalized by a set of test purposes where each test purpose describes a particular sequence of observable events that the system has to perform in order. As we study timed systems, it is moreover convenient to precise the instant at which each action must be observed. Such test purposes amount to provide a subword of a timed trace of the specification. *CClair* provides a dedicate operator, named `Subword` to express make this class of test purposes. To be more precise, given a sequence of dated actions $l = [(a_1, t_1), \ldots, (a_n, t_n)]$ $(a_i \in \mathcal{A}, t_i \in \mathbb{R})$, $\texttt{Subword}(l)$ specifies the set of timed traces which correspond to the regular expression $(\mathcal{A} \times \mathbb{R})^*.(a_1, t_1).(\mathcal{A} \times \mathbb{R})^* \ldots (a_n, t_n).(\mathcal{A}\times\mathbb{R})^*$ where $*$ denotes the Kleene-star on language and . the concatenation. In other words, Subword allows us to select timed trace whose l is a subword. This means that between two given actions, the system is allowed to perform many other actions.

Using the digicode of the figure 1 as an illustration, $\texttt{Subword}([(\texttt{A}, 3.0), (\texttt{B}, 6.2), (\texttt{A}, 8.3)])$ represents the set of timed traces that contains the two following timed traces.

$$[(\texttt{B}, 1.1), (\texttt{A}, 3.0), (\texttt{A}, 4.6), (\texttt{B}, 6.2), (\texttt{A}, 8.3)]$$
$$[(\texttt{A}, 3.0), (\texttt{C}, 4.9), (\texttt{A}, 5.3), (\texttt{A}, 5.8), (\texttt{B}, 6.2), (\texttt{A}, 8.3)]$$

In order to derive test cases, we are therefore interested in solving the testing statement of the section 3.3 where A is instantiated by Subword:

$$s \xrightarrow[P]{\xi^?, w^?} s'^? \quad \wedge \quad w^? \in \texttt{Subword}(l) \tag{3}$$

4.3 Timed regular expressions

Our purpose is to translate Subword into an automaton so as to use *Hytech* on it. It is a well-known result that regular expressions can be translated into a labeled transition system which accepts the language associated to the expression, and vice-versa. Consequently, it is natural to introduced regular expressions that can be translated into an equivalent automaton and then use these expressions to defined Subword.

A recent paper written by T.Nipkow[15] has explored the ability to formalize the Kleene's theorem into *Isabelle*. However this development cannot directly be reused here for several reasons:

For one, we need expressions that contain time informations and therefore we must translate them into p-automata, not into simple transition systems. For another, Nipkow uses an adhoc representation that differs from our actual formalization of p-automata. A third reason is that the construction presented in [15] is realized in two steps: a automaton with epsilon-transitions is first generated then it is transformed into a deterministic automaton. However, the latter construction involves a non-executable operator on set. Fortunately, to define Subword, we only need a subset of regular expressions, and we can therefore generate, directly from expression, an automaton without epsilon-transitions.

Hence, using the ML syntax, a timed expression on letters of type α is defined by the type α `texp`:

$$\begin{aligned}\texttt{datatype}\ \alpha\ \texttt{texp} = \quad & \mathit{One\_letter}\ \alpha \times \mathbb{R} \\ | \quad & \mathit{Any\_letters} \\ | \quad & \mathit{Conc}\ (\alpha\ \texttt{texp})\ (\alpha\ \texttt{texp})\end{aligned}$$

Following the definition, an timed expression is constructed by concatenation of dated actions. A dated action is either explicitly given using the constructor *One_letter* or taken in the set $\mathcal{A} \times \mathbb{R}$ if the constructor *Any_letters* is used.

Given a regular expression, the primitive recursive function `lang` computes its corresponding set of dated actions word.

$$\begin{aligned}\texttt{lang}\ (\mathit{One\_letter}\ (a,t)) &= \{[(a,t)]\} \\ \texttt{lang}\ (\mathit{Any\_letters}) &= \texttt{Star}\ (\bigcup_{a\in\mathcal{A}} \bigcup_{0\le t} \{[(x,t)]\}) \\ \texttt{lang}\ (\mathit{Conc}\ L_1\ L_2) &= \texttt{Concat}\ (\texttt{lang}\ L_1)\ (\texttt{lang}\ L_2)\end{aligned}$$

Finally, `Subword` is defined as the language of the timed expressions built by the recursive function `sb_exp`.

$$\begin{aligned}\texttt{sb\_exp}([]) &= \mathit{Any\_letters} \\ \texttt{sb\_exp}((a,t).l) &= \mathit{Conc}\ \mathit{Any\_letters} \\ &\qquad (\mathit{Conc}\ (\mathit{One\_letter}\ (a,t))\ (\texttt{sb\_exp}(l))) \\ \texttt{Subword}(l) &= \texttt{lang}\ (\texttt{sb\_exp}(l))\end{aligned}$$

4.4 Deriving a certified automata

The translation of each component of a regular expression into a corresponding p-automaton is depicted on figure 2. The corresponding automata are very simple: locations are natural numbers and no variables, except the universal clock, are required. However, we need a type of variable to declare these automata in our typed framework. One solution is to use the special (ML like) type *unit* which contains the single value υ.

Given an expression E of type `texp`, the result of the translation is the `paf` (T,f) where T is a p-automaton (the timed trace of which are in the language associated to the expression) and f its final location. The desired property is stated by the pre-proven theorem: [1]

$$\forall t_i\ t_f\ (t_i,\upsilon,0) \xrightarrow[T]{\xi,w} (t_f,\upsilon,f) \longrightarrow w \in \texttt{lang}\ E \tag{4}$$

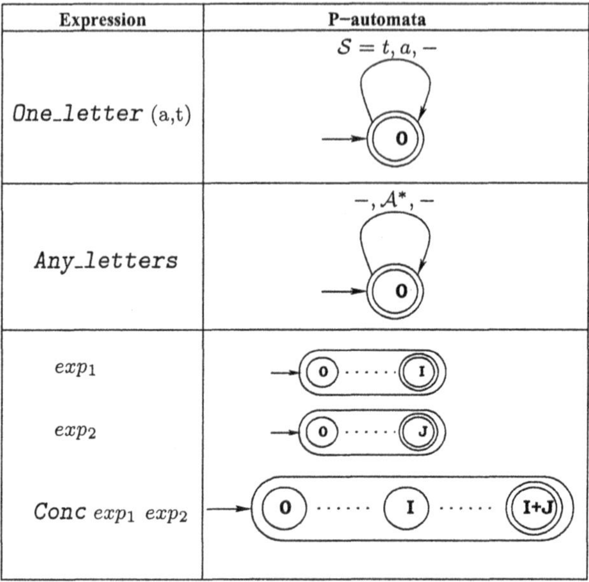

Figure 2. Translation of expressions into p-automata

However, we are only interested in the instance of 4 where E is built using Subword.

$$\forall t_i\ t_f\ (t_i, v, 0) \xrightarrow[T]{\xi, w} (t_f, v, f) \longrightarrow w \in \mathtt{Subword}(l) \tag{5}$$

Let us emphasize that it is an executable translation: definitions use mainly primitive recursions so that a automaton is automatically generated from a regular expression, thanks to the rewriting mechanism of *Isabelle*.

4.5 Validation of the observer technique

Now, if we put 5 on the goal 3, we obtain the following new subgoal:

$$s \xrightarrow[P]{\xi_1{}^?, w^?} s'^? \quad \wedge \quad (t_i{}^?, v, 0) \xrightarrow[T]{\xi_2{}^?, w^?} (t_f{}^?, v, f) \tag{6}$$

The next step consists to validate the well-known technique of observer automata: the basic idea is that the automaton T can be used as a synchronous observer i.e. it can be executed in parallel with the specification automaton in order to find an execution. This step is formalized from to the rule given in 1 proven in section 3.2 and we obtain the following goal :

$$s_c \xrightarrow[P\|T]{\xi^?, w^?} s_c'^? \tag{7}$$

Where s_c (resp. s_c') is the composition of the initial state (resp. final) of the runs in P and T. s_c is completely instantiated but we may take the liberty to let s_c' uninstantiated or to precise a part of the state. It is a means to precisely control the search by constraining the execution to end with particular values of variables. In this case, we have $s_c = (t_i, (v_i, v), (l_i, 0))$ and $s_c' = (t_f{}^?, (v_f, v), (l_f{}^?, f))$.

Notice that *Isabelle* keeps in memory the instantiation made during resolution of the goal 2 with 1 i.e. ξ, ξ_1 and ξ_2 are connected by the equations $\pi 1_{\mathrm{x}}\ \xi = \xi_1$ and $\pi 2_{\mathrm{x}}\ \xi = \xi_2$. When ξ is fully instantiated, it is obvious to compute the value of ξ_1 by rewriting.

4.6 An oracle called *Hytech*

Hytech[11] is a symbolic model checker for linear hybrid systems which may automatically generate a diagnostic trace that explains why a property is (or is not) satisfied by a system description. Therefore the tool *Hytech* can be used to search an execution in the composite specification+observer automaton.

To achieve this task, we need to build an input file that includes descriptions of automata and commands to compute an execution. Because we work with the restricted format of p-automata, the translation into hybrid automata is nearly obvious: all variables are real and declared as *discrete* variables. This ensures that they will not evolve except on explicit update. The universal clock is declared as a variable of type *clock* called *now*. The only difficulty concerns the translation of constraints (update relations and invariants) because *CClair* allows the declaration of any necessary constant to define it. As a consequence, the first step of the translation procedure is to compute a "normal form" which is done through rewriting. The user is responsible for giving all equations needed to expand constants by their definitions.

Two *Hytech* commands are needed to compute an execution in our composed automaton.

```
reached := reach forward from init_reg
print trace to final_reg using reached
```

One must first use forward reachability analysis to compute all states that are reachable from the initial region `init_reg` which contains the single state s_c. The second command causes *Hytech* to generate an execution from `init_reg` to the final region `final_reg` $\{s'_c\}$.

4.7 Validation of the computed execution

Having obtained a desired execution, we then use this result to solve the goal 7. Two choices are offered to us, depending of the level of confidence we have about *Hytech* and our interface with *CClair* : we can admit the computation result as an axiom and directly apply it on 7. A safer alternative is to instantiate the variable $\xi^?$ with the computed execution and then validate it. Let us explain briefly how this latter step can be achieved.

Because all sets involved in the definition of a restricted p-automaton are finite, rewriting mechanism is powerful enough to decide whether a given move is in the set of moves. For instance, $\langle \mathtt{q}_1, C, \mathtt{cpt} = 3, \mathtt{Fail} \rangle \in \mathcal{M}_{digicode}$ is simplified to `True` and therefore is accepted as a move of the digicode.

Concerning the data part of a transition, *Isabelle* provides a decision procedure for linear arithmetic. Therefore the value of variables computed by *Hytech* according to the update relations and invariants are automatically admitted or rejected. As a result, *CClair* provides a tactic which automatically checks the validity of the execution computed by *Hytech*.

5. A CASE STUDY : ABR CONFORMANCE ALGORITHMS

Available Bit Rate[10] is a special kind of connection defined in ATM network architecture : it allows the cell rate to vary during the same session. Therefore, a real-time reactive algorithm is necessary to control that data cells sent by user conform to the negotiated traffic parameters. Two of such algorithms are formalized in [6]. The first one, called $\mathcal{I}$, has the ideal desired behavior but its implementation is impossible in practice because of a too large memory cost. The second one, $\mathcal{B}'$, is therefore an approximation for which a proof of correctness with respect to the ideal algorithm is given. This proof has completely been formalized in our framework[19], including the description of algorithms in terms of p-automata, and proving a set of invariance assertions by induction on execution sequences.

The rate offered to the user depends of the instant at which resource management (RM) cells are received. The crucial point is therefore to test if $\mathcal{B}'$ computes a rate greater or equal to the rate computed by $\mathcal{I}$ for a given sequence of values carried by RM cells and their arrival time. Thus, each sequence corresponds to a test purpose of the form: $\texttt{Subword}([(\texttt{RM}, t_1), \ldots, (\texttt{RM}, t_n), (\texttt{D}, t_{n+1})])$ where the actions RM and D represent respectively the reception of a RM-cell and an user data cell. This allows to apply our *CClair/Hytech* approach for automatically generating certified test cases.

As an illustration, we present an execution obtained from the small test purpose $\texttt{Subword}([(\texttt{RM}, 3), (\texttt{D}, 30)])$.

Actions performed		$\delta(3)$	RM	I1	A7	$\delta(10)$	A9a	$\delta(17)$	D
Value of $\mathcal{S}$	0	3	3	3	3	13	13	30	30
Rate computed by $\mathcal{I}$	0	0	0	1	1	1	1	1	1
Rate computed by $\mathcal{B}'$	0	0	0	0	0	0	1	1	1

The first line presents the trace of the execution : δ denotes time elapse, I1 is an action of $\mathcal{I}$, A7 and A9a are actions of $\mathcal{B}'$. After each step, the value of the clock and the rates computed by $\mathcal{I}$ and $\mathcal{B}'$ are recorded.

We obtain a generic test case by filtering (through rewriting) the actions of the execution. The adaptation of this result according to the test architecture and the available PCO will be done in a further research.

6. CONCLUSION AND FUTURE WORKS

We have presented a general approach for generating generic test cases in the design of real-time systems using an interactive theorem prover. The formal framework is based on HOL specifications and verification environment that includes an expressive specification language and a powerful reasoning system. Furthermore, the use of the model of p-automata, which include truly real-valued variables allows a natural specification of systems.

We have described a technique for automatically deriving certified test cases from formal descriptions of test purposes expressed as a subset of regular timed expressions. This method significantly increases the confidence in the test case generation process since all reasoning steps and computation are checked by the theorem prover.

In future work, one should enrich the language of expressions to provide more refined constraints on the time part of dated actions. We also plan to study a new protocol called PGM[2].

Notes

1. We do not present here the proof of this theorem. All scripts are available online at http://dept-info.labri.u-bordeaux.fr/Davy rouillar/CClair/.

2. see http://www.cisco.com/warp/public/cc/pd/iosw/tech/_fr_xcst_ds.htm

References

[1] R. Alur, C. Courcoubetis, N. Halbwachs, T. A. Henzinger, P.-H. Ho, X. Nicollin, A. Olivero, J. Sifakis, and S. Yovine. The algorithmic analysis of hybrid systems. *Theoretical Computer Science*, 138(1):3–34, 1995.

[2] R. Alur, T. A. Henzinger, and P.-H. Ho. Automatic symbolic verification of embedded systems. In *Proceedings of the 14th Annual Real-time Systems Symposium*, pages 2–11. IEEE Computer Society Press, 1993.

[3] Rajeev Alur, Costas Courcoubetis, Thomas A. Henzinger, and Pei-Hsin Ho. Hybrid automata: An algorithmic approach to the specification and verification of hybrid systems. *Lecture Notes in Computer Science*, 736:209–229, 1993.

[4] B. Baumgarten. Timed systems behaviour and conformance testing - a mathematical framework. In *Proc. 8th PTS*, 1995.

[5] B.Bérard, P.Castéran, E.Fleury, JF.Monin L.Fribourg, C.Paulin, A.Petit, and D.Rouillard. Automates temporisés calife, 2000. http://www.loria.fr/projets/calife/.

[6] B. Bérard, L. Fribourg, F. Klay, and J.-F. Monin. A compared study of two correctness proofs for the standardized algorithm of ABR conformance. Research Report LSV-99-7, LSV, ENS de Cachan, Cachan, France, August 1999. 27 pages.

[7] P. Castéran and Davy Rouillard. Reasoning about parametrized automata. In *Proceedings,* 8th *International Conference on Real-Time System*, volume 8, pages 107–119, 2000.

[8] Pierre Castéran and Davy Rouillard. The cclair project, 1999. `http://dept-info.labri.u-bordeaux.fr/~casteran/CClair/`.

[9] E. Allen Emerson. *Handbook of Theoretical Computer Science (volume B)*, chapter Temporal and Modal Logic, pages 995–1072. Elsevier, 1990.

[10] A. Forum. Atm forum traffic management specification version, 1996.

[11] T. A. Henzinger, P.-H. Ho, and H. Wong-Toi. HYTECH: A model checker for hybrid systems. *Lecture Notes in Computer Science*, 1254:460–463, 1997.

[12] T. Higashino, A. Nakata, K. Taniguchi, and A. Cavalli. Generating test cases for a timed i/o automaton model. In *Proc. IFIP Int'l Work. Test Communicat. Syst. (IWTCS)*, pages 197–214. G. Csopaki, S. Dibuz, and K. Tarnay eds, 1999.

[13] ISO. Information technology, open systems interconnection, conformance testing methodology and framework. *International Standard IS-9646*, CCITT X.290-X.294, 1991.

[14] Jean-François Monin and Francis Klay. Correctness proof of the standardized algorithm for ABR conformance. In *FM'99*, volume 1708 of *Lecture Notes in Computer Science*, pages 662–681. Springer, 1999.

[15] Tobias Nipkow. Verified lexical analysis. In J. Grundy and M. Newey, editors, *Proc. of the 11th International Conference on Theorem Proving in Higher Order Logics*, pages 1–15. Springer-Verlag LNCS 1479, 1998.

[16] Christine Paulin-Mohring. The coq project, 1999. http://coq.inria.fr.

[17] Lawrence C. Paulson. The Isabelle reference manual. Technical Report 283, University of Cambridge, Computer Laboratory, 1993.

[18] Lawrence C. Paulson. Mechanizing coinduction and corecursion in higher-order logic. *J. Logic and Computation*, 7:175–204, 1997.

[19] Davy Rouillard. Le modèle des p-automates dans CClair. Technical Report 1242-00, LaBRI, 2000.

[20] N. Shankar, S. Owre, and J. Rushby. The pvs proof checker: A reference manual. Technical report, CSL, SRI International, Menlo Park CA, 1993.

TEST SELECTION, TRACE DISTANCE AND HEURISTICS

L.M.G. Feijs, N. Goga, S. Mauw*
Eindhoven University of Technology, P.O. Box 513, NL-5600 MB Eindhoven
feijs, goga, sjouke@win.tue.nl

J. Tretmans
University of Twente, P.O. Box 217, NL-7500 AE Enschede, The Netherlands
tretmans@cs.utwente.nl

Abstract

Two heuristic principles for test selection are proposed: *the reduction heuristic* and *the cycling heuristic.* The first assumes that few outgoing transitions of a state show essentially different behaviour. The second assumes that the probability to detect erroneous behaviour in a loop decreases after each correct execution of the loop behaviour. We formalize these heuristic principles and we define a coverage function which serves as a measure for the error-detecting capability of a test suite. For this purpose we introduce the notion of a *marked trace* and a distance function on such marked traces.

Keywords: Test selection, test coverage, trace distance, heuristics, edit distance.

1. INTRODUCTION

The selection of an appropriate set of tests from all possible ones (usually infinitely many test cases), is not a trivial task. We refer to this task as *test selection.* Traditionally, test selection is based on a number of heuristic criteria. Well-known heuristics include equivalence partitioning, boundary value analysis, and use of code-coverage criteria like statement-, decision- and path-coverage [9]. Although these criteria

*This research was supported by the Dutch Technology Foundation STW under project STW TIF.4111: *Côte de Resyste* – COnformance TEsting of REactive SYSTEms; URL: http://fmt.cs.utwente.nl/CdR.

provide some heuristics for selecting test cases, they are rather informal and they do not allow to measure the error-detecting capability of a test suite.

If test cases are derived from a formal specification, in particular if it is done algorithmically using tools for automatic test generation, e.g., AUTOLINK [10], TGV [8] or TORX [3], then the test selection problem is even more apparent. These test tools can generate a large number of test cases, when given a specification in the appropriate formalism, without much user intervention. All these generated test cases can detect potential errors in implementations, and errors detected with these test cases indeed indicate that an implementation is not correct with respect to its specification. However, the number of candidate test cases may be very large, or even infinite. In order to control and get insight in the selection of the tests, and by that get confidence in the correctness of an IUT that passes the tests, it is important that the selection process is formally described and based on a well-defined strategy.

This paper approaches the problem of test selection by making assumptions in an automata-based, or labelled transition system-based formalism. Two different kinds of assumptions are considered in this paper, starting with the ideas of [5]. The first one, called *reduction heuristic*, assumes that few outgoing transitions of a state show essentially different behaviour. The second one, referred to as *cycling heuristic*, assumes that the probability to detect erroneous behaviour in a loop decreases after each correct execution of the loop behaviour.

Section 2 introduces the labeled transition systems and automata. After that we propose a mathematical framework, defining a heuristic as a function on the set of behaviours (traces). This is done in Section 3. When we want to make the two heuristics more precise, defining them as functions according to the definition from Section 3, we observe that an appropriate behaviour representation for them is needed. Therefore in Section 4 we define the *marked trace* representation. After these preparations the definitions of the heuristics as functions on marked traces are easy (Section 5). Subsequently, the notion of isolation and closeness of errors is formalized in Section 6 by defining a *distance* function between behaviours. This idea is taken from [1, 2] and extended to *marked traces*. The trace distance implements the considered heuristics in the sense that the traces which are selected by the heuristics are remote from each other. Every trace which is excluded by the heuristics is close to one of the selected traces. A *coverage function* which may serve as a measure for the error-detecting capability of a test suite is defined based on the maximum distance between selected and non-selected behaviours and a formula for approximating the coverage is given in Section 7.

2. PRELIMINARIES

The basic formalism for our discussion about test selection is the labelled transition system. A labelled transition system provides means to specify, model, analyze and reason about (concurrent) system behaviour.

A *labelled transition system* is a 4-tuple $\langle Q, L, T, q_0 \rangle$, where Q is a non-empty set of *states*, L is a set of *labels*, $T \subseteq Q \times L \times Q$ is the *transition relation*, and $q_0 \in Q$ is the *initial state*. The labels in L represent the actions of a system. An action $a \in L$ is executable in state $q \in Q$ if $(q, a, q') \in T$ for some state $q' \in Q$, which is said to be the *new state* after execution of a; we also write $q \xrightarrow{a} q'$. A finite sequence of pairs $\langle$*state, action*$\rangle$ ending into a state is called a *path*. Similarly, a finite sequence of actions is called a *trace*. The set of all traces over L is denoted by L^*, with ϵ denoting the empty sequence. Abusing notation, we will use p to denote both the labelled transition system and the current (or initial) state of the system.

The traces of a labelled transition system p are all sequences of actions that p can execute from its initial state q_0: $traces(p) =_{\text{def}} \{ \sigma \in L^* \mid q_0 \xrightarrow{\sigma} \}$. Here we use the following additional definitions:

$$q \xrightarrow{a_1 \cdot \ldots \cdot a_n} q' \quad =_{\text{def}} \quad \exists q_0, \ldots, q_n : q = q_0 \xrightarrow{a_1} q_1 \xrightarrow{a_2} \ldots \xrightarrow{a_n} q_n = q'$$

$$q \xrightarrow{\sigma} \quad =_{\text{def}} \quad \exists q' : q \xrightarrow{\sigma} q'$$

For our presentation and formalization we use *minimal*, *deterministic*, *finite-state* transition systems. A finite-state labelled transition system has a finite number of states, i.e., Q is finite. A transition system is deterministic if for any state $q \in Q$ and action $a \in L$ there is at most one successor state, i.e., $T : Q \times L \rightarrow Q$ is a (partial) function. A transition system is minimal if there are no equivalent states, i.e., no two states with exactly the same traces, which means: $\nexists q, q' \in Q : traces(q) = traces(q')$. We (ab)use the word *automaton* for these minimal, deterministic, finite-state transition systems.

Although it may seem a severe limitation to restrict to automata, an important formal test theory, viz. **ioco**-testing [12], can be expressed in terms of so-called *suspension automata*, which are deterministic. So the test selection approach which is presented in this paper can be integrated with **ioco**-testing.

In testing, the traces of the automata are used. A complete (maximal) test suite for an automaton specification s is expressed as $traces(s)$. However, even if s is finite-state, its set of traces will usually be infinite and contain traces of unbounded length. Such a test suite can never be executed within any reasonable limits of time and resources. Consequently, the problem of *test selection* consists of selecting a finite subset $T \subseteq traces(s)$, such that we end up with a reasonably sized set of bounded-length test cases.

The challenge of test selection now is to choose T such that the resulting test suite still has a large error-detecting capability. Moreover, we wish to quantify this capability in order to compare and select test suites. The next sections will present and formalize an approach to selection and quantification.

3. THE TRACE DISTANCE AND THE TEST HEURISTICS

In our test selection method we use heuristics which are applied on traces and distances between traces. This section describes the formal definitions of these notions.

In a formal way a trace heuristic is a function between two sets of traces such that the range is a proper subset of the domain (so the heuristic reduces the size of the initial set).

Definition 1 *Let T be a set of traces.*
i) A trace heuristic h is a function $h : T \longrightarrow T$, where $Ran(h) \subset T$.
ii) A function $d : T \times T \longrightarrow \mathbf{R}_{\geq 0}$ is a trace distance iff: 1) $d(x,x) = 0$; 2) $d(x,y) = d(y,x)$; 3) $d(x,y) \leq d(x,z) + d(z,y)$ for all $x, y, z \in T$.

The pair (T, d) is a metric space. It is customary to express coverages by numbers in the range $[0, 1]$ and therefore we restrict ourselves, without loss of generality, to trace distance functions such that $0 \leq d(x,y) \leq 1$ for all x, y. In order to use a trace distance for test selection the concepts of ε-cover and total boundedness are useful.

Definition 2 *A set T' is an ε-cover of T ($T' \subseteq T, \varepsilon \geq 0$) if for every $t \in T$ there exists $t' \in T'$ such that $d(t,t') \leq \varepsilon$. A metric space (T, d) is totally bounded if for every $\varepsilon > 0$ it is possible to find a finite set $T_\varepsilon \subseteq T$ such that T_ε is an ε-cover of T with respect to distance d.*

Now a link between a heuristic and a trace distance is established: if the subset obtained by the application of that heuristic is an ε-cover of the original set, then the trace distance implements the heuristic.

Definition 3 *Let T be a set of traces and h be a trace heuristic such that $h : T \longrightarrow T$. Let d be a trace distance defined on T. Then d implements the heuristic h iff: $\exists \varepsilon_h \geq 0 : Ran(h)$ is an ε_h-cover of T with respect to the distance d.*

The following definition shows how to obtain the coverage.

Definition 4 *Let T be a set of traces and $T' \subseteq T$ an ε-cover of T with respect to a trace distance d. Let $\varepsilon_m = inf\{\varepsilon \geq 0 \mid T'$ is an ε-cover of $T\}$ be the inferior minimum of the ε values. Then the coverage of T' with respect to T is $cov(T', T) = 1 - \varepsilon_m$.*

4. THE MARKED TRACE REPRESENTATION

When we want to make the two heuristics more precise, defining them as functions according to Definition 1 point i), we observe that an appropriate trace representation is needed. When we apply the *Cycling* heuristic on a trace, we observe that the trace does not have enough information regarding how it was generated, what states it has been going through and how often it went through them. As a result, we will represent the trace in such a way that the information regarding its generation from the automaton will be included. This leads us to a concept called *marked traces.* In the marked trace representation, we associate the cycles with how many times a trace is traversing a state. The name of the state, which is seen as a mark, will serve as the identifier of the cycle. Also we will include the number of cycles through a state.

Definition 5 *Let L be a labelset and Q a set of states. Then a marked trace is inductively defined by: 1) $a \in L$, ϵ and $[\ ]^{0,q}$ $(q \in Q)$ are marked traces; 2) if u $(u \in L$ or $u = [\_]^{-,-})$ and v are marked traces then uv is a marked trace; 3) if u and $[\sigma]^{n,q}$ $(n \in \mathbb{N}, q \in Q)$ are marked traces then $[\sigma\langle u\rangle]^{n+1,q}$ is a marked trace (σ is a sequence of type $\langle\sigma_1\rangle...\langle\sigma_n\rangle$ where σ_i are marked traces, $i = 1, ...n$).*

Example $a_0[\langle bd\rangle]^{1,II}e$, $a_0[\langle bd\rangle\langle bd\rangle]^{2,II}e$ with $II \in Q$ are marked traces.

We will denote the set of all the marked traces over a labelset L and a set of marks Q as L^*_Q. The transformation between the marked representation of a trace and a normal representation of a trace can be made easily by eliminating all the parentheses which occur in the marked representation. For example the marked trace $a_0[\langle bd\rangle\langle bd\rangle]^{2,II}e$ is transformed into the trace a_0bdbde.

In the following example, we will illustrate a way in which a trace of a particular automaton can be transformed into a marked trace. In general, this transformation is not unique.

Example Consider the specification automaton from Figure 1. The labelset is $L = \{b, c, d, e, f\} \cup \{a_i \mid i \in \mathbb{N}\}$ and the initial state is the state *I*. Via a transition a_i from the initial state, one arrives at *II*. This state contains a cycle which goes via *III* using the transitions b and d; the state *III* contains another cycle, via the transition c. From *II* one arrives at *IV* using e or f.

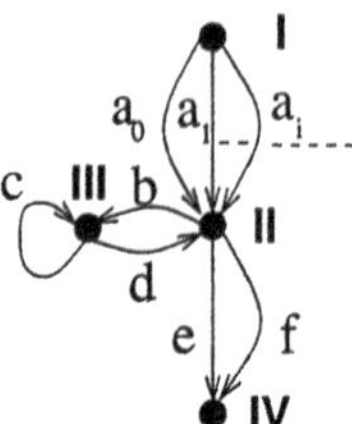

Figure 1. A minimal automaton of a specification

Let us consider the trace $a_0bcdbcde$. Adding boxes to reflect nesting structure, the corresponding path is $Ia_0\boxed{II}b\boxed{\boxed{III}}c\boxed{\boxed{III}}d\boxed{II}b\boxed{\boxed{III}}c\boxed{\boxed{III}}d\boxed{II}eIV$. The state II (surrounded with a box in the path) is repeated three times. Between two occurrences of state II in the path, the state III (surrounded with two boxes) appears twice. If we match every new occurrence of state II in the path with its first occurrence (we will call this way of matching the states *first state matching*), the path will be divided in 4 paths: $\underbrace{{}_Ia_{0\,II}}_{1}[\underbrace{\langle_{II}b_{III}c_{III}d_{II}\rangle}_{2}\underbrace{\langle_{II}b_{III}c_{III}d_{II}\rangle}_{3}]^{2,II}\underbrace{{}_{II}e_{IV}}_{4}$. If we do the same for III in the paths 2) $IIbIII\,cIIIdII$ and 3) $IIbIIIcIIIdII$ and eliminate all the states, we obtain the marked trace $a_0[\langle b[\langle c\rangle]^{1,III}d\rangle\langle b[\langle c\rangle]^{1,III}d\rangle]^{2,II}e$. This marked trace corresponds to the initial trace $a_0bcdbcde$. However, there are also other ways of transforming it into a marked trace. For example, the states of the same trace can be grouped in another way as $Ia_0IIb\boxed{III}c\boxed{III}dIIb\boxed{III}c\boxed{III}dIIeIV$ and this trace has another correspondent marked trace which is $a_0b[\langle c\rangle\langle db\rangle\langle c\rangle]^{3,III}de$.

For this example we see that there is not a unique way of transforming a trace in a marked trace. We leave it as an option to the implementer (the user of our theory) to choose the way by which he transforms a trace into a marked trace. We will give a particular way to implement the transformation of a trace in a marked trace and a way to obtain the set of marked traces. If the implementer chooses another transformation, he can still use the theory presented in this paper if the correspondence between marked traces and traces is unique, and if its set of marked traces respects the property that the widths and the nesting depth are uniformly bounded (we will come to this later).

We obtain a set of marked traces by applying the following function (ALG) on each trace (path) of a finite-state minimal deterministic automaton s. The function builds a marked trace from a trace using a first state match technique like the one we used for the trace $a_0bcdbcde$

at the beginning of the previous example. In ALG we use the following operator, function and procedure: 1) the operator $|_{trace}$ transforms a path to a trace by eliminating all the states which appear in the path and keeping all the labels; 2) the function $NotRepetitivesState(p, Q)$, p a path, Q a set of states, returns true if every state of p which is contained in Q occurs only once in p and 3) the procedure $Divide(p, Q, q, p_1, ..., p_n)$ finds $q \in Q$ and splits p in $p_1, ..., p_n$ ($n \in \mathbb{N}$, $i = 2, ..., n-1$, $p_1 q$, $qp_i q$, qp_n paths) such that: i) $q \in Q$ is the first repetitive state in p, ii) $p = p_1 q p_2 q ... q p_n$ and iii) the set of states of p_j does not contain q ($j = 1, ..., n$).

function ALG (p : *Path*, Q : *SetStates*) : *MarkedTrace;*
var q : *State;*
    $p_1, ..., p_n$: $(\epsilon + Label)(State\ Label)^*(\epsilon + State)$;
begin
  if ($NotRepetitiveState(p, Q)$) **then**
(1)   **return** $p\ |_{trace}$;
  else
(2) $Divide(p, Q, q, p_1, ..., p_n)$;
(3) $Q = Q \setminus \{q\}$;
(4)   **return** $ALG(p_1 q, Q)[\langle ALG(qp_2 q, Q)\rangle ... \langle ALG(qp_{n-1} q, Q)\rangle]^{n-2,q}$ $ALG(qp_n, Q)$;
end

Example Let us consider the path $p = Ia_0IIbIIIdIIeIV$ of the automaton from Figure 1 and the automaton set of states $Q = \{I, II, III, IV\}$. The call of $ALG(Ia_0IIbIIIdIIeIV, \{I, II, III, IV\})$ implies

Apply (2) $Divide(Ia_0IIbIIIdIIeIV, \{I, II, III, IV\}, II, Ia_0, bIIId, eIV)$
where $q = II$ and $p_1 = Ia_0$, $p_2 = bIIId$, $p_3 = eIV$

Apply (3) $Q = \{I, II, III, IV\} \setminus \{II\} = \{I, III, IV\}$

Apply (4) $ALG(Ia_0II, \{I, III, IV\})[\langle ALG(IIbIIIdII, \{I, III, IV\})\rangle]^{1,II}$ $ALG(IIeIV, \{I, III, IV\}) \overset{\text{Apply (1)}}{=} Ia_0II\ |_{trace}\ [\langle IIbIIId$ $II\ |_{trace}\rangle]^{1,II}\ IIeIV\ |_{trace} = a_0[\langle bd\rangle]^{1,II} e$

The set of marked traces is $traces^m(s) = \{ALG(p, Q) \mid p \in path(s)\}$. In the remainder of this paper we will work with marked traces generated with ALG in place of traces.

As one can see, our way of building the set of marked traces is rather complex. One can imagine trivial solutions as for example: every marked trace is the trace itself. But the marked traces built with ALG have nice properties which are required for the application of our test selection theory. For example the width of such marked traces is uniformly bounded (Lemma 7), a property which is used for proving the total boundedness property (a direct consequence of Theorem 13). The marked traces generated with the trivial solution do not have this property.

In conclusion, once we have the set of marked traces, we want to know if it has some specific properties. So for a marked trace of an automaton we want to know if the width of it is uniformly bounded (Lemma 7), and if the nesting depth of it is also bounded (Lemma 9). Here uniformly bounded means that the same upperbound applies at all nesting levels.

Definition 6 *Let s be an automaton. Let L be the labelset and Q the set of states of s. Then the function $width : traces^m(s) \longrightarrow \mathbb{N}$ is : 1) if $a \in L, q \in Q$ then $width(a) = 1$, $width(\epsilon) = 0$, $width([\ ]^{0,q}) = 1$; 2) if u ($u \in L$ or $u = [\_]^{-,-}$) and v are marked traces then $width(uv) = width(u) + width(v)$; 3) if u and $[\sigma]^{n,q}$ ($q \in Q, n \in \mathbb{N}$) are marked traces then $width([\sigma\langle u\rangle]^{n+1,q}) = 1$.*

Lemma 7 *The width of a marked trace generated with ALG from an automaton and the widths of all its component marked traces are less than or equal to $2m - 1$, where m is the number of the states of the automaton. (Without proof)*

Definition 8 *Let s be an automaton. Let L be the labelset and Q the set of states of s. Then the function $nesting : traces^m(s) \longrightarrow \mathbb{N}$ is: 1) if $a \in L, q \in Q$ then $nesting(a) = 0$, $nesting(\epsilon) = 0$, $nesting([\ ]^{0,q}) = 1$; 2) if u ($u \in L$ or $u = [\_]^{-,-}$) and v are marked traces then $nesting(uv) = max(nesting(u), nesting(v))$; 3) if u and $[\sigma]^{n,q}$ ($q \in Q, n \in \mathbb{N}$) are marked traces then $nesting([\sigma\langle u\rangle]^{n+1,q}) = 1 + max(nesting(\sigma), nesting(u))$.*

Lemma 9 *The nesting depth of a marked trace generated with ALG from an automaton is less than or equal to the number of the states of the automaton. (Without proof)*

5. THE HEURISTICS DEFINED FOR MARKED TRACES

As we presented in the introduction, the intuition behind the heuristics *Reduction* and *Cycling* is that they take into account two aspects: the finiteness of 1) the number of outgoing transitions of certain states and of 2) the number of times each cycle can be traversed by every single trace.

When *Reduction* is applied, the labelset L is split in two parts: the selected labels which form a finite set $L' \subseteq L$ and the set of unselected labels which is $L \backslash L'$. This application can be seen as the application of a mapping function *trans*: $L \longrightarrow L'$ which maps every unselected label to a selected label from L' and every selected label to itself. One practical way to make the selection and to obtain L' and *trans* is by defining a distance d_L between labels, such that the metric space (L, d_L) is totally bounded. Let us fix a positive real number $\varepsilon_L \geq 0$. Now L' will be a labelset which is an ε_L-cover of L. The labels which are remote from each other (their distance is greater than ε_L) are selected and the labels from $L \setminus L'$ remain unselected. The function *trans*: $L \longrightarrow L'$ can be defined in this case such that $trans(a) = b$ with $a \in L$ and $b \in L'$ has the minimum label distance to a.

For the *Cycling* heuristic we relate the cycles of the automaton to the marked representation of the trace; limiting the numbers of times of traversing the cycles means limiting the powers of the marked symbols in the marked traces. Now, let us define these heuristics in a formal way.

Definition 10 *Let s be an automaton. Let L be the labelset and Q the set of states of s. Let $L' \subseteq L$ be a finite subset of L and let trans: $L \longrightarrow L'$ be the mapping function. Let l_c be the cycle limit. Then i) The heuristic Reduction: $traces^m(s) \longrightarrow traces^m(s)$ is: 1) if $a \in L, q \in Q$ then $Reduction(a) = trans(a)$, $Reduction(\epsilon) = \epsilon$, $Reduction([\ ]^{0,q}) = [\ ]^{0,q}$; 2) if u ($u \in L$ or $u = [\_]^{-,-}$) and v are marked traces then $Reduction(uv) = Reduction(u)\ Reduction(v)$; 3) if u and $[\sigma]^{n,q}$ ($q \in Q, n \in \mathbb{N}$) are marked traces then $Reduction([\sigma\langle u\rangle]^{n+1,q}) = [Reduction(\sigma), Reduction(u)]^{n+1,q}$.*
ii) The heuristic Cycling: $traces^m(s) \longrightarrow traces^m(s)$ is: 1) if $a \in L, q \in Q$ then $Cycling(a) = a$, $Cycling(\epsilon) = \epsilon$, $Cycling([\ ]^{0,q}) = [\ ]^{0,q}$; 2) if u ($u \in L$ or $u = [\_]^{-,-}$) and v are marked traces then $Cycling(uv) = Cycling(u)\ Cycling(v)$; 3) if u and $[\sigma]^{n,q}$ ($q \in Q, n \in \mathbb{N}$) are marked traces then: a) $Cycling([\sigma\langle u\rangle]^{n+1,q}) = [Cycling(\sigma)\ Cycling(u)]^{n+1,q}$, for $l_c > n$; b) $Cycling([\sigma\langle u\rangle]^{n+1,q}) = [Cycling(\sigma')]^{l_c,q}$, for $l_c \leq n$, where $\sigma = \langle\sigma_1\rangle...\langle\sigma_n\rangle$ and $\sigma' = \langle\sigma_1\rangle...\langle\sigma_{l_c}\rangle$ is obtained by cutting σ after l_c symbols.

Example Let us consider the automaton from Figure 1. For this automaton the set of labels is $L = \{c, b, d, e, f\} \cup \{a_i \mid i = 0, 1, ...\}$. Let $L' = \{a_0, c, b, d, e, f\}$ be a finite subset of L, $l_c = 2$ and *trans*: $L \longrightarrow L'$ $trans(x) = \begin{cases} a_0 & x = a_i, i \in \mathbb{N} \\ x & \text{otherwise} \end{cases}$. Then

i) $Reduction(a_3e) = Reduction(a_3)Reduction(e) = trans(a_3)trans(e) = a_0e$.

ii) $Cycling(a_0[\langle bd\rangle\langle bd\rangle\langle bd\rangle]^{3,II}e) = Cycling(a_0)\,Cycling([\langle bd\rangle\langle bd\rangle\langle bd\rangle]^{3,II})\ Cycling(e) = a_0[\langle bd\rangle\langle bd\rangle]^{2,II}e$.

6. THE TRACE DISTANCE FOR MARKED TRACES

In this section we make the trace distance more precise, defining it as a distance function according to Definition 1 point ii). As explained in the introduction, this gives us an alternative formalization of the ideas behind the heuristics (they will be compared in Section 7). We will combine these ideas with another well-known idea, viz. the edit distance. Section 6.1 introduces the edit distance. After this preparation, the definition of the trace distance function can be given (Section 6.2).

6.1 The edit distance between strings

Because in our trace distance we use the concept of edit distance we shall present this first. Informally the edit distance is defined as the minimum number of insertions, deletions and substitutions required to transform one string into another. Wagner and Fisher ([11]) adopted different costs for the various atomic edit actions. According to Wagner-Fisher transforming a into a b costs $w(a, b)$. Extending this notation, $w(a, \epsilon)$ is the cost of deleting a and $w(\epsilon, b)$ is the cost of inserting b. The cost of editing is the sum of the costs of the atomic edit actions, and $d(x, y)$ is the minimum cost over all possible edit sequences that transform x into y.

Definition 11 *Let $w(a, b)$ be the weighting for the cost of transforming symbol a in symbol b, $w(a, \epsilon)$ be the cost of deleting a and $w(\epsilon, b)$ be the cost of inserting b. Of course $w(a, a) = 0$. Then the edit distance between the strings x and y is denoted as $ED(x, y)$ and it is computed as: 1) $ED(au, bv) = min(w(a, b) + ED(u, v), w(a, \epsilon) + ED(u, bv), w(\epsilon, b) + ED(au, v))$; 2) $ED(au, \epsilon) = w(a, \epsilon) + ED(u, \epsilon)$; 3) $ED(\epsilon, bv) = w(\epsilon, b) + ED(\epsilon, v)$; 4) $ED(\epsilon, \epsilon) = 0$ (where a, b are symbols and u, v are strings).*

6.2 Defining the trace distance

Our test selection technique uses two heuristics. For expressing these heuristics in the trace distance, it is important to remember that in the formalization of the *Reduction* heuristic a label distance was used. The incorporation of this heuristic in the trace distance is achieved in a simple way by using the label distance in the formula of the trace distance. Now a solution should be found for the *Cycling* heuristic.

For the *Cycling* heuristic we simply weight every level k of a cycling symbol (a marked trace of type $[\_]^{n,q}, n \in \mathbb{N}, q \in Q$) with a weight from a series of positive numbers p_k. This series should have the property that $\sum_{k=1}^{\infty} p_k = 1$. The logic behind this weighting is that summing the weights after a given limit (which is the cycle limit) will contribute with a small number reflecting our assumption that the first cycles are more important than the later cycles.

We will define the trace distance for all the possible combinations of the points (1), (2), (3) of Definition 5 (which are generating marked traces). We summarize these combinations below.

Between the marked traces generated with point (1) (such as $[\ ]^{0,q}, q \in Q$ and $a \in L$) we will define a distance function called AtD (atomic distance) because these are the atomic elements which form the marked trace; of course the AtD between two labels will be given by d_L, the distance between these labels; between a label and a marked trace such as $[\ ]^{0,q}$ it will be maximum (one) and between two marked traces such as $[\ ]^{0,q}$,$[\ ]^{0,q'}$ $(q, q' \in Q, q \neq q')$ it will also be one.

Between the marked traces generated with point (2) (such as *af* or *ae*) we will use a distance function called *EdD* (edit distance); we took this option because these traces are generated in a similar style as the strings are formed and it is quite natural to use it because it compares in a good way the terms which form the marked traces (for example in the traces a_0e and $a_0[\langle bd\rangle]^{1,II}e$ the edit distance will recognize that the labels a_0 and e from the first trace are present in the second trace).

Between the marked traces generated with point (3) (such as building $[\langle bd\rangle]^{1,II}$ once we know that $[\ ]^{0,II}$ is a marked trace) we employ the principle that cycles of different marks are very remote and hence have the maximum distance, i.e, 1; when dealing with cycles of the same mark we employ weighting factors p_k with the effect that the later iterations are considered less important than e.g. the first iteration; this can be done by using a function *EdDW* which is an edit distance for which the formula of Definition 11 is modified in such a way to take into account the weights.

The rest of the possible combinations such as (1) with (2), (2) with (3) etc. are defined in a similar style by using one of the techniques mentioned above (*EdD* or *AtD*).

We observe also that this trace distance is to be used in the computation of coverage which should be in the range $[0, 1]$. For simplifying the computation of coverage, we want the trace distance values to be in the range $[0, 1]$. This can be done by dividing all the above mentioned values (generated with an *EdD* or *AtD*) by the maximum width of the marked traces from $traces^m(s)$ (the maximum width is finite, see Section 4). For completing the picture it is necessary to add that the trace distance between a null trace (ϵ) and any other marked trace is maximum (1).

Now we have all the ingredients to define a trace distance on marked traces. We will call it d. In the definition, the distances already mentioned (*EdD* and *AtD*) will be used; also it is implicitly assumed that the definition is symmetric in the sense that $d(x, y) = d(y, x)$, x and y being marked traces and that $d(x, x) = 0$.

As explained above, the function AtD deals with the cases ϵ, $a \in L$ and $[\ ]^{0,-}$. We generalize it to marked traces of the form $[\_]^{-,-}$ as well.

Definition 12 *Let s be an automaton. Let L be the labelset of s, d_L the label distance defined on it and Q the set of states of s. The metric space (L, d_L) is totally bounded and d_L has all its values in the range $[0,1]$. Let l_m be the maximum of the width of the marked traces from $traces^m(s)$. Let p_k $(k = 1, 2, ...)$ be a series of positive numbers such that $\sum_{k=1}^{\infty} p_k = 1$. Then*

1. $d(a,b) = \frac{AtD(a,b)}{l_m}$; $d(a,\epsilon) = d(\epsilon,[\ ]^{0,q}) = 1$; $d(a,[\ ]^{0,q}) = \frac{AtD(a,[\ ]^{0,q})}{l_m}$; $d([\ ]^{0,q},[\ ]^{0,q'}) = \frac{AtD([\ ]^{0,q},[\ ]^{0,q'})}{l_m}$ *with* $a,b \in L, q,q' \in Q$;	*2.* $d(a,uv) = \frac{EdD(a,uv)}{l_m}$; $d(\epsilon,uv) = 1$; $d([\ ]^{0,q},uv) = \frac{EdD([\ ]^{0,q},uv)}{l_m}$ *with* u $(u \in L$ *or* $u = [\_]^{-,-})$, v *marked traces and* $a \in L, q \in Q$;
3. $d(a,[u\langle v\rangle]^{n+1,q}) = \frac{AtD(a,[u\langle v\rangle]^{n+1,q})}{l_m}$; $d(\epsilon,[u\langle v\rangle]^{n+1,q}) = 1$; $d([\ ]^{0,q},[u\langle v\rangle]^{n+1,q}) = \frac{AtD([\ ]^{0,q},[u\langle v\rangle]^{n+1,q'})}{l_m}$ *with* v *and* $[u]^{n,q'}$ *marked traces* $(n \in \mathbb{N}$, $q' \in Q)$ *and* $a \in L, q' \in Q$;	*4.* $d(uv,rt) = \frac{EdD(uv,rt)}{l_m}$ *with* u $(u \in L$ *or* $u = [\_]^{-,-})$, v, r $(r \in L$ *or* $r = [\_]^{-,-})$, t *marked traces;*
5. $d(uv,[r\langle t\rangle]^{n+1,q}) = \frac{EdD(uv,[r\langle t\rangle]^{n+1,q})}{l_m}$ *with* u $(u \in L$ *or* $u = [\_]^{-,-})$ $,v,t,[r]^{n,q}$ *marked traces* $(n \in \mathbb{N}, q \in Q)$;	*6.* $d([u\langle v\rangle]^{n+1,q},[r\langle t\rangle]^{n'+1,q'})$ $= \frac{AtD([u\langle v\rangle]^{n+1,q},[r\langle t\rangle]^{n'+1,q'})}{l_m}$ *with* $v,t,[u]^{n,q},[r]^{n',q'}$ *marked traces* $(n,n' \in \mathbb{N}, q,q' \in Q)$.

where

$$AtD(x,y) = \begin{cases} d_L(x,y) & x,y \in L \\ EdDW(x,y) & x = [\_]^{n,q}, y = [\_]^{n',q}, q \in Q \\ & n,n' \in \mathbb{N}, n \neq 0, n' \neq 0 \\ 1 & \textit{otherwise} \end{cases}$$

$$EdD(uv,rt) = min(AtD(u,r) + EdD(v,t),\ AtD(u,\epsilon) + EdD(v,rt),\ AtD(\epsilon,r) + EdD(uv,t));$$

$EdD(uv,\epsilon) = AtD(u,\epsilon) + EdD(v,\epsilon)$; $EdD(\epsilon,rt) = AtD(\epsilon,r) + EdD\ (\epsilon,t)$;
$EdD(\epsilon,\epsilon) = 0$
with u $(u \in L$ *or* $u = [\_]^{-,-})$, v, r $(r \in L$ *or* $r = [\_]^{-,-})$, t *marked traces;*

$$EdDW([\langle u_1\rangle...\langle u_n\rangle]^{n,q},[\langle v_1\rangle...\langle v_p\rangle]^{p,q}) = EDW^1([\langle u_1\rangle...\langle u_n\rangle]^{n,q},[\langle v_1\rangle...\langle v_p\rangle]^{p,q})$$

$$\begin{aligned} EDW^k([\langle u\rangle\sigma]^{h,q},[\langle v\rangle\sigma']^{g,q}) = min(&p_k \times d(u,v) + EDW^{k+1}([\sigma]^{h-1,q},[\sigma']^{g-1,q}), \\ &p_k \times d(u,\epsilon) + EDW^{k+1}([\sigma]^{h-1,q},[\langle v\rangle\sigma']^{g,q}), \\ &p_k \times d(\epsilon,v) + EDW^{k+1}([\langle u\rangle\sigma]^{h,q},[\sigma']^{g-1,q})); \end{aligned}$$

$EDW^k([\langle u\rangle\sigma]^{h,q},[\ ]^{0,q}) = p_k \times d(u,\epsilon) + EDW^{k+1}([\sigma]^{h-1,q},[\ ]^{0,q})$;
$EDW^k([\ ]^{0,q},[\langle v\rangle\sigma']^{g,q}) = p_k \times d(\epsilon,v) + EDW^{k+1}([\ ]^{0,q},[\sigma']^{g-1,q})$;
$EDW^k([\ ]^{0,q},[\ ]^{0,q}) = 0$
with u_i *and* v_j *marked traces,* $k,h,g \in \mathbb{N}$, $q \in Q$ *and* $u,v,[\sigma]^{h-1,q},[\sigma']^{g-1,q}$ *marked traces.*

We add some explanation. It is easy to check that the definition of *EdD* and *EdDW* are copied from Definition 11 except for the fact that suitable weighting factors p_k have been incorporated. The parameter k in EDW^k indicates the position at which the next edit action takes place. Please note that the recursive definition of EDW^k is well defined because at least one of the right-hand sides of the equation is one symbol shorter than the corresponding left-hand side (therefore, the fact that k is increasing causes no problem). The base case is $EDW^k([\,]^{0,q}, [\,]^{0,q}) = 0$.
Example Let us consider the automaton from Figure 1. For this automaton the maximum width of the marked trace is 3. Let $p_k = \frac{1}{2^k}, k = 1, 2, \ldots$. Let d_L be the following label distance

$$d_L(x, y) = \begin{cases} 0 & x = y \\ \mid \frac{1}{4^{i+1}} - \frac{1}{4^{j+1}} \mid & x = a_i, y = a_j, i, j \in \mathbb{N} \\ 1 & \text{otherwise} \end{cases}$$

1) *The edit distance effect:*
Let us consider the traces $t_1 = a_0e$ and $t_2 = a_0[\langle bd\rangle]^{1,II}e$.
$d(t_1, t_2) = \frac{1}{3} \times EdD(a_0e, a_0[\langle bd\rangle]^{1,II}e) = \frac{1}{3} \times AtD(\epsilon, [\langle bd\rangle]^{1,II}) = \frac{1}{3}$.
The trace distance takes into account that the symbols a_0 and e from the first trace are present in the second trace.

2) *The cycling effect:*
Let us take the traces $t_1 = a_0[\langle bd\rangle]^{1,II}e$, $t_2 = a_0[\langle bd\rangle\langle bd\rangle]^{2,II}e$ and $t_3 = a_0[\langle bd\rangle\langle bd\rangle\langle bd\rangle]^{3,II}e$.
$d(t_1, t_2) = \frac{1}{3} \times EdD(a_0[\langle bd\rangle]^{1,II}e, a_0[\langle bd\rangle\langle bd\rangle]^{2,II}e) = \frac{1}{3} \times EdDW([\langle bd\rangle]^{1,II}, [\langle bd\rangle\langle bd\rangle]^{2,II}) = \frac{p_2}{3} = \frac{1}{12}$;
$d(t_1, t_3) = \frac{1}{3} \times EdD(a_0[\langle bd\rangle\langle bd\rangle]^{2,II}e, a_0[\langle bd\rangle\langle bd\rangle\langle bd\rangle]^{3,II}e) = \frac{1}{3} \times EdDW([\langle bd\rangle\langle bd\rangle]^{2,II}, [\langle bd\rangle\langle bd\rangle\langle bd\rangle]^{3,II}) = \frac{p_3}{3} = \frac{1}{24}$.
When two marked traces are cycling more times through the same cycle, the values of the trace distance start to decrease.

3) *The reduction effect:*
Let us take the traces $t_1 = a_0e$, $t_2 = a_1e$ and $t_3 = a_2e$.
$d(t_1, t_2) = \frac{1}{3} \times EdD(a_0e, a_2e) = \frac{d_L(a_0,a_2)}{3} = \frac{0.23}{3}$;
$d(t_2, t_3) = \frac{1}{3} \times EdD(a_1e, a_2e) = \frac{d_L(a_1,a_2)}{3} = \frac{0.06}{3}$.
When the label distance between the labels (which compose the marked traces) is decreasing, the trace distance is also decreasing.

7. TRANSFORMING THE HEURISTICS INTO A COVERAGE

The trace distance formula depends on the label distance d_L which implements the *Reduction* heuristic and the weights p_k which implement the *Cycling* heuristic. On the other hand, by choosing for each automaton s a finite set $L_\varepsilon \subseteq L$ which is an ε_L-cover of L with respect to d_L

and a cycling limit l_c, a finite set of marked traces $T \subseteq traces^m(s)$ can be obtained. This is done by the application of the *Cycling* and the *Reduction* heuristics on $traces^m(s)$ by taking T =*Ran(Cycling* $\circ$ *Reduction)*. Now for this T and using d we want to approximate its ε-cover of $traces^m(s)$ so that we can compute the coverage $cov(T, traces^m(s))$ – see Definition 4. Intuitively ε should depend on ε_L and l_c. Its formula is given by Theorem 13.

Theorem 13 *Let s be an automaton. Let L be the labelset of s and d_L the label distance defined on it. The metric space (L, d_L) is totally bounded and d_L has all its values in the range $[0,1]$. Let l_c be the cycle limit. Let p_k $(k = 1, 2, ...)$ be a series of positive numbers such that $\sum_{k=1}^{\infty} p_k = 1$. Let l_m be the maximum of the width and z the maximum of the nesting depth of the marked traces from $traces^m(s)$. Let $L_\varepsilon \subseteq L$ be an ε_L-cover of L. Then the finite set T =Ran(Reduction $\circ$ Cycling) of traces obtained by the application of the two heuristics on $traces^m(s)$ is an ε-cover of $traces^m(s)$ with $\varepsilon = \varepsilon^z$ and $\varepsilon^0 = \varepsilon_L$; for $i = 1, ..., z$: $\varepsilon_c^i = \sum_{k=1}^{l_c} p_k \times (max_{j=0,...,i-1}(\varepsilon^j)) + \sum_{k=l_c+1}^{\infty} p_k$; $\varepsilon^i = max_{\text{cycles}=0,...,l_m}(\frac{\text{cycles} \times \varepsilon_c^i + (l_m - \text{cycles}) \times \varepsilon_L}{l_m})$. (Without proof)*

Using the results of Theorem 13 it is easy to prove that the metric space $(traces^m(s), d)$ is a totally bounded metric space and that the trace distance d implements the *Cycling* and the *Reduction* heuristics, in the sense of Definition 3.

For the computation of the coverage we approximate the minimum ε_m from Definition 4 with the ε^z computed in Theorem 13. We will illustrate the computation of the coverage in the following example.

Example Consider the automaton from Figure 1. Let us fix the final state to be *IV*. Let us consider the reduced set $L_\varepsilon = \{a_0, b, c, d, e, f\}$ which is an ε_L-cover of the labelset L with $\varepsilon_L = 0.25$ (ε_L is computed with respect to the d_L defined in the example from Section 6.2). For this automaton the maximum width is $l_m = 3$ and the maximum nesting depth is $z = 2$. Let us fix the series $p_k = \frac{1}{2^k}(k \in \mathbb{N})$ and in the beginning $l_c = 1$. Then the set of traces T which is obtained by the application of the heuristics *Reduction* and *Cycling* is an ε-cover of $traces^m(s)$, with ε computed with the formula from Theorem 13 as:

1) $l_c = 1$, $L_\varepsilon = \{a_0, b, c, d, e, f\}$
$\varepsilon^0 = \varepsilon_L = 0.25$;
$\varepsilon_c^1 = \sum_{k=1}^{1} p_k \times \varepsilon^0 + \sum_{k=l_c+1}^{\infty} p_k = \frac{0.25}{2} + \sum_{k=l_c+1}^{\infty} \frac{1}{2^k} = 0.63$;
$\varepsilon^1 = max_{\text{cycles}=0,...,3}(\frac{\text{cycles} \times \varepsilon_c^1 + (l_m - \text{cycles}) \times \varepsilon_L}{l_m}) = 0.63$; $\varepsilon = \varepsilon^2 = 0.81$;
The coverage is computed via Definition 4 and it is $cov(T, traces^m(s)) = 1 - \varepsilon = 0.19$;

2) $l_c = 2$, $L_\varepsilon = \{a_0, b, c, d, e, f\}$
When we enlarge the set T to T' for $l_c = 2$ we find that $cov(T', traces^m(s)) = 0.51$;

3) $l_c = 1$, $L_{\varepsilon'} = \{a_0, a_1, b, c, d, e, f\}$
When we enlarge the set T to T'' for $L_{\varepsilon''} = \{a_0, a_1, b, c, d, e, f\}$ we find that $\varepsilon''_L = 0.06$ and that $cov(T'', traces^m(s)) = 0.29$.

In this case, one can see that the coverage increases more by adopting a higher value for the cycling limit than by using a larger label subset. But this is not always true, e.g. increasing l_c from 101 to 102 might give lesser increase than taking a larger labelset. Moreover we defined specific values for p_k and d_L.

It can be seen that in this example the monotonicity property required in [4] viz. $T \subseteq T' \Rightarrow cov(T) \leq cov(T')$ is respected. From an intuitive point of view this property is reasonable: if one wants a better coverage, one needs to generate more tests. This property can also be proven to hold in general.

8. CONCLUSIONS

A heuristic is a general guideline for reducing test suites, which must be made more precise to be practically applicable. In this paper we have studied two heuristics for reducing the number of traces in a test suite. Especially for the cycling heuristic we had to introduce additional notation. The reason is that the cycling structure of a trace through a finite-state automaton must be made explicit. We introduced *marked traces* for this purpose, which enabled us to extend the work on cycle reduction by Vuong [1, 2].

In order to introduce a notion of *coverage* for the test suites reduced by means of the above mentioned heuristics, we defined a *trace distance* on marked traces. The results of our studies can be used to effectively calculate the coverage of a test suite reduced with our techniques.

The proposed test selection technique can be compared to the existing theories in this area. In particular, these are the hypothesis theory developed by [6] and the trace distance theory of [1, 2]. The hypothesis theory embodies the trace distance theory (see [6]), but the nice thing about trace distance theory is that it gives a measure for the degree to which a reduced set of traces approximates the original one. So we chose an approach which combines these two theories. In our view, first the heuristics (test hypotheses in the theory of [6]) are to be defined. After that, based on these heuristics a trace distance is built. This gives the possibility to make a test selection with a given ε approximation. The change of the heuristics leads to the change of the trace distance used in test selection.

We have started work on implementing our techniques in the TorX tool environment ([3]). An assumption for implementing our work is that a label distance exists. Because the TorX tools support the input of finite automata defined in LOTOS [7], we could use a label distance on LOTOS labels. This is not trivial because LOTOS labels may be parameterized by arbitrary data types.

References

[1] J. Alilovic-Curgus and S.T. Vuong. A metric based theory of test selection and coverage. In A. Danthine, G. Leduc, and P. Wolper, editors, *Protocol Specification, Testing, and Verification*, pages 289–304. North-Holland XIII, 1993.

[2] J. Alilovic-Curgus and S.T. Vuong. Sensitivity analysis of the metric based test selection. In M. Kim, S. Kang, and K. Hong, editors, *Int. Workshop on Testing of Communicating Systems*, volume X, pages 200–219. Chapman & Hall, 1997.

[3] A. Belinfante, J. Feenstra, R.G. Vries, J. Tretmans, N. Goga, L. Feijs, S. Mauw, and L. Heerink. Formal test automation: A simple experiment. In G. Csopaki, S. Dibuz, and K. Tarnay, editors, *Intenational Workshop on Testing of Comunication Systems*, pages 179–196. Kluwer Academic, 1999.

[4] E. Brinksma, J. Tretmans, and L. Verhaard. A framework for test selection. In B. Jonsson, J. Parrow, and B. Pehrson, editors, *Protocol, Specification, Testing, and Verification*, volume XI, pages 233–248. North-Holland, 1991.

[5] O. Charles and R. Groz. Formalisation d'hypothèses pour l'evaluation de la couverture de test. In *Actes du Colloque Francophone sur l'Ingénierie des Protocoles (CFIP'96)*, Editions Hermes, 1996.

[6] O. Charles and R. Groz. Basing test coverage on a formalization of test hypotheses. In M. Kim, S. Kang, and K. Hong, editors, *Int. Workshop on Testing of Communicating Systems*, volume X, pages 109–124. Chapman & Hall, 1997.

[7] ISO. *Information Processing Systems, Open Systems Interconnection, LOTOS – A Formal Description Technique Based on the Temporal Ordering of Observational Behaviour.* International Standard IS–8807, 1989.

[8] T. Jéron and P. Morel. Test generation derived from model-checking. In N. Halbwachs and D. Peled, editors, *Computer Aided Verification CAV'99*, volume 1633 of *Lecture Notes in Computer Science*, pages 108–121. Springer-Verlag, 1999.

[9] G.J. Myers. The art of software testing. John Wiley & Sons Inc, 1979.

[10] M. Schmitt, B. Koch, J. Grabowski, and D. Hogrefe. Autolink – a tool for the automatic and semi-automatic test generation. In A. Wolisz, I. Schieferdecker, and A. Rennoch, editors, *Formale Beschreibungstechniken für verteilte Systeme*, volume 315. GMD-Studien, St. Augustin, GI/ITG-Fachgespräch, GMD, 1997.

[11] G.A. Stephen. String search. Technical Report TR-92-gas-01, School of Electronic Engineering Science, University College of North Wales, 1992.

[12] J. Tretmans. Test generation with inputs, outputs and repetitive quiescence. *Software–Concepts and Tools*, 17(3):103–120, 1996.

FORMULATION OF THE INTERACTION TEST COVERAGE PROBLEM AS AN INTEGER PROGRAM

Alan W. Williams, Robert L. Probert
School of Information Technology and Engineering,
University of Ottawa, Canada

Abstract A trend in software development is to assemble a system from a number of components. In many cases, the system is expected to function for multiple configurations of interchangeable components, leading to the problem of determining a set of system test configurations to fit a reasonable budget. One approach is to test all configurations that cover, for example, all two-way interactions. We investigate the feasibility of using an integer programming approach to solve the interaction test coverage problem exactly. We also examine the formulation to see if it provides insight into the NP-completeness of the interaction problem.

Key words: Interactions, components, coverage, system testing

1. INTRODUCTION

A common source of system faults is unexpected interactions between system components. The risk is magnified when there are a number of interchangeable components for each element in a system. A manufacturer of a system constructed from heterogeneous components would want to test as many of the potential system configurations as possible, to reduce the risk of interaction problems. However, the number of potential system configurations grows exponentially. The scenario in *Figure 1* has four parameters, each with three values. There are $3^4 = 81$ possible configurations.

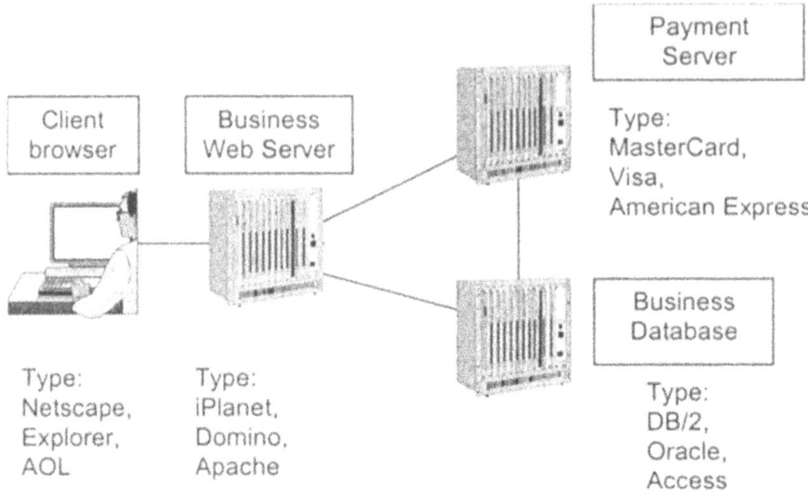

Figure 1. A System Test Scenario.

The system test suite for a single configuration may consist of a large number of tests. Even if there were only 30 tests for the system illustrated in Figure 1, running the entire test suite for every possible configuration would require running 2,430 tests. In practice, systems would have far more parameters and values, and larger test suites for a single configuration.

A system tester faces the constraints of time and money, and all possible configurations cannot be tested within any reasonable allotment. Furthermore, changing between configurations normally requires additional effort, either in physical re-configuration, or in modification of test cases. Therefore, reducing the number of system test configurations will produce significant savings. How, then, can the risk of interaction faults be managed in a realistic test plan?

One approach is to at least test for all two-way interactions among various system components. This leads to a reduced set of test configurations. The assumption is that the risk of an interaction among three or more components is balanced against the ability to complete system testing within a reasonable budget.

Previous work on determining a set of test configurations that covers two way interactions includes 0, 0, 0, 0, 0, and 0. Previous work where this method has been applied to various types of testing includes 0, 0, 0, 0, 0, 0, and 0. In this paper, we extend the work in 0 that formally defines interaction test coverage by investigating an approach that could solve the problem of how to find the smallest set of test configurations to achieve interaction coverage of a specified degree (for example, cover all 2-way interactions). A fast algorithm that finds an approximate solution has been presented in 0; here, we try to solve the problem exactly.

This paper starts with a review of the interaction test coverage problem. We then show that the problem can be formulated as a {0,1} integer programming problem. We show that while the conversion can be done in that direction, a general {0,1} integer programming problem cannot be converted to an interaction test coverage problem. Thus, this relationship cannot be used to show that the interaction test coverage problem is NP-complete. (This is a problem that is still open. 0, 0, 0) Next, we discuss the feasibility of this approach in practice, and conclude with further avenues for investigation.

2. THE INTERACTION TEST COVERAGE PROBLEM

In this section, we set up the problem of selecting test configurations to cover parameter interactions. We subdivide the problem into two parts. The first part is the general problem of selecting from a set of discrete parameter values. In the second part, we look at the problem from the point of view of coverage of sets of interactions. The following is adapted from 0.

2.1 Basic definitions

We start by introducing terminology that will help to define precisely the test interaction coverage problem. The basic inputs to the problem are the number of parameters, and the number of values for each parameter. We begin by presenting notations for these quantities. Let:

p denote the number of independent system parameters.

n_i denote the number of possible values for the parameter with index i. We can assume, without loss of generality, that the parameters are ordered such that $n_1 \geq n_2 \geq \ldots \geq n_p$. In the special case where $n_1 = n_2 = \ldots = n_p$, the common number of values for each parameter will be denoted by n.

v_i denote a **selected indefinite** value in a specific test configuration for the parameter with index i.

1_3 denote a **selected definite** value in a specific test configuration (in this case, parameter 3 takes the value 1).

τ denote a test configuration, where $\tau = \{v_1, \ldots, v_p\}$.

T denote the set of all possible test configurations.

S denote the set of test configurations selected for execution.

d denote the **interaction degree**; the size of the subsets of parameter values for which we wish to detect unwanted interactions.

σ_d denote a subset of the parameter indices of size d; that is, we are choosing d out of p of the parameters.

Φ_d denote the set of all possible parameter subsets σ_d. The size of this set is $|\Phi_d| = \binom{p}{d}$.

The notation for definite and indefinite selected values allows us to keep track, using the subscript, of which parameter has been assigned a value in situations when we shall refer to a partial set of parameter values.

The property of parameter independence means that the selection of a particular value for one parameter affects neither the existence of other parameters, nor the selection of any other parameter values. This may not be the case in general. However, dependencies among parameters can be resolved by substituting a hybrid parameter that enumerates the legal combinations of the dependent parameters 0.

2.2 A general test coverage criterion

In practice, it is not usually possible to test all possible configurations, and therefore we have to select a subset for actual execution. The general test configuration selection problem is to find $S \subseteq T$ such that S satisfies a test coverage criterion.

Normally, an additional objective is to minimize $|S|$, the cardinality of the set of test configurations that satisfy the test coverage criterion. For the moment, we will leave the exact criterion that S satisfies undefined.

We want to find the set of test configurations with minimal size that will satisfy our (currently, undefined) test coverage criterion. Our goal is to define a test coverage criterion using a set of "test units" that need to be covered. We shall investigate what constitutes an interaction testing coverage unit in the next section.

2.3 Applying the criterion to interaction testing

To this point, all of the concepts defined and discussed in this section are generic in nature, in that they do not rely on any particular test selection strategy. In this section, we shall fill in the undefined test coverage criterion from the previous section, by introducing the concept of interaction elements.

The idea behind interaction elements is that they represent a "unit" of test coverage, in terms of system component interaction testing. Other types of test "units" used in other contexts (see, for example, 0) are as follows:

- Control flow testing: statements, branches, flow graph nodes, flow graph edges, conditions
- Data flow testing: definition-use pairs, IO-chains

In the context of system component interaction testing, the approach that we are taking is that there could be unwanted interactions among system components when a particular set of values is assigned to the set of parameters. This would be detected when a test suite is run using the configuration defined by the set of parameter values.

We shall take the view that an unwanted interaction is usually not caused by the particular values of the **entire** set of parameters, but by the values of only a (hopefully, small) **subset** of parameters. The philosophy of test coverage we shall adopt is to try and cover as many subsets of parameters as possible, where we shall limit ourselves to subsets of size $d \leq p$. These subsets will be referred to as interaction elements (or interaction elements of degree *d*, when referring to the cardinality of the subsets).

The aim is to reduce the number of test configurations to the point where the testing can be conducted with a feasible cost in time and money, and still have a good probability of detecting unwanted system interactions.

While it would be ideal to have $d = p$, it is shown in 0 that the number of test configurations to meet this test coverage criterion is be proportional to n^d. In practice, constraints of time and money will usually dictate that a small value of *d*, such as $d = 2$, be used. A study of the effectiveness of various values of *d* is presented in 0.

There is no particular order to the selection of parameters, so we shall use a set of *d* indices as opposed to an ordered *d*-tuple, when selecting a subset of parameters.

2.4 Interaction elements

Suppose that $\tau = \{v_1, \ldots, v_p\}$ is a given test configuration in *T*, and σ_d is a given index subset of $\{1, \ldots, p\}$. An **interaction element of degree *d***, denoted by $\chi(\sigma_d, \tau)$, is defined as $\chi(\sigma_d, \tau) = \{v_j \mid v_j \in \tau \text{ and } j \in \sigma_d\}$.

In other words, we are selecting a subset, of size *d*, of the assigned values for a given test configuration. An interaction element captures a single *d*-way interaction among the parameter values. The notation is chosen to emphasize that there are two parts to constructing an interaction element: selecting a subset of parameters, and that specific values are assigned to those parameters.

Because we have chosen a subset of the parameter indices, there are no repeated elements, and therefore an interaction element will not contain two values for the same parameter. This is a crucial property of a test configuration that we wish to preserve. The set notation is used to indicate that the ordering of the elements is not important. We can recover the parameter associations through the subscripts.

It is time for an example. Suppose that we want to select the values for parameters 1, 3, and 4 from the test configuration $\tau = \{5_1,4_2,3_3,2_4,1_5\}$. For $d = 3$, and $\sigma_3 = \{1,3,4\}$, we have $\chi(\sigma_3, \tau) = \{5_1,3_3,2_4\}$. The subscripts of the interaction element match the index set.

Having defined an interaction element, the next step is to look at the set of all possible interaction elements for specified values of p, n_i, and d. Let us denote this set by X_d, to highlight the dependence on d. The set X_d is:

$$X_d = \{ \{ v_j \mid 1 \leq v_j \leq n_j, j \in \sigma_d, \} \mid \sigma_d \in \Phi_d \}$$

That is, we take all possible index subsets of size d of the parameters. For each index subset, construct a set for every possible combination of d values for the associated parameters. The resulting collection is the set X_d.

Another way to look at the set X_d is consider it to be the set of all interaction elements contained within all possible test configurations. While the definition of interaction elements is dependent on a specific test configuration τ, the set of all possible interaction elements X_d is independent of the choice of test configurations.

For general values of d, the set X_d is the set of all possible interaction elements of degree d. The number of possible interaction elements is $|X_d| = \sum_{i_1=1}^{p-d} \cdots \sum_{i_d=i_{d-1}+1}^{p} (n_{i_1} \ldots n_{i_d})$. In the special case when $n = n_i$ for all i in the range $1 \leq i \leq p$ (that is, all parameters have n values), $|X_d| = \binom{p}{d} n^d$.

2.5 Test configurations as sets of interaction elements

We have previously defined concepts related to system test configuration selection and interaction elements. We can now bring these concepts together to define the interaction test coverage problem.

Suppose that we consider a test configuration in an alternative form: as a set of interaction elements of degree d, where d can be chosen arbitrarily to balance sufficient coverage with a feasible number of test configurations. Within the p parameter values of any test configuration, there are $\binom{p}{d}$ possible subsets of size d of parameter values.

Let $\tau = \{v_1, \ldots, v_p\}$ be a specific test configuration. As an alternative to treating a configuration τ to be a set of p values, a test configuration can be expressed (denoted τ') as a set of $\binom{p}{d}$ interaction elements of degree d:

$\tau' = \{ \chi(\sigma_d, \tau) \mid \sigma_d \in \Phi_d \}$

In other words, τ' is the set of interaction elements produced from all possible index subsets Φ_d for a single test configuration. Each interaction element must be an element of X_d, as X_d contains all possible interaction elements of degree d, over the entire range of values of the parameters.

Alternatively, τ' is the set of all subsets of size d of the assigned values for a specific test configuration. It captures the concept of a test configuration as a set of d-way interactions.

For example, suppose there are three parameters. The test configuration $\{1_1,1_2,1_3\}$ can also be considered as a set of three interaction elements of degree 2, namely $\{\{1_1,1_2\}, \{1_1,1_3\}, \{1_2,1_3\}\}$. In the latter form, we are considering this test configuration to represent the three pairs of 1's produced by selecting parameters, two at a time.

Clearly, each test configuration τ', constructed from an element of T, is a subset of X_d, the set of all interaction elements of degree d. Therefore, the entire set of potential test configurations, T, is a collection of subsets of X_d. This is a significant property that we shall incorporate into our test coverage criterion.

Let T be the set of all possible test configurations. Then, the set of all possible test configurations expressed as interaction elements of degree d, denoted T', is:

$T' = \{ \{ \chi(\sigma_d, \tau) \} \mid \sigma_d \in \Phi_d, \tau \in T \}$.

Each element of T' is a set of cardinality $\binom{p}{d}$, where each of those sets is in turn, a set of cardinality d. There is a one to one correspondence between elements of T', and elements of T, as each element in T' is constructed from an element of T.

Suppose that S is an arbitrary set of test configurations so that $S \subseteq T$. For each test configuration $\tau \in S$, let τ' be the equivalent test configuration expressed as a set of interaction elements of degree d. We can then denote as S' the set of all selected configurations τ' expressed as interaction elements. Since $S \subseteq T$, $S' \subseteq T'$.

2.6 The interaction test coverage problem

We can now define the *interaction test coverage problem*: the goal is to find $S \subseteq T$ (and thus $S' \subseteq T'$), such that every element in X_d belongs to at least one member of S'. In other words, we require that every interaction element be covered by a selected test configuration.

An additional objective is to minimize $|S|$, the cardinality of the set of selected test configurations. We want the minimum number of test configurations that will cover all d-wise combinations among parameter values.

This definition corresponds to other types of test coverage, where the goal is to cover all (or as large a percentage as possible) of some sort of test unit, within the set of selected test configurations. We are using interaction elements as test units for system interaction testing, as one would use control flow branches or definition-use associations in other type of test coverage criteria. Since we are assuming that the parameters are independent, all of our potential test configurations are feasible, and therefore, the test coverage criterion is to cover **all** interaction elements.

If a test coverage criterion based on interaction elements is used, then any interaction problem that is caused by an interaction of up to d specific values can be detected. Interactions of $d + 1$ or more values may not be detected. Thus, the criterion also defines the degree of risk inherent in a set of test configurations.

3. FORMULATION AS A {0,1} INTEGER PROGRAM

In this section, we shall re-formulate the interaction test coverage problem as a constraint-based problem. The result will become a {0, 1} integer programming problem.

Our objective in the interaction test coverage problem is to cover all of the interaction elements using a subset of all possible configurations. That is, given the set X_d of all interaction elements, and the set of all possible test configurations T, select $S \subseteq T$ as the set of selected test configurations. When each element of S is expressed as a set of interaction elements, the set S' is formed as the collection of all covered interaction elements. Then, every element of X_d must be in S'.

3.1 Set up the problem

Suppose that we construct an enumeration of the elements of T. The number of possible test configurations is $|T| = \prod_{i=1}^{p} n_i$. Let $z = |T|$. Furthermore, we will also construct an enumeration of the set of all possible interaction elements. The number of interaction elements is $|X_d| = \sum_{i_0=1}^{p-d+1} \cdots \sum_{i_{d-1}=i_{d-2}+1}^{p} \left(n_{i_0} \ldots n_{i_{d-1}}\right)$. Let $y = |X_d|$. In the special case where all parameters have the same number of values n, $z = n^p$ and $y = \binom{p}{d} n^d$.

Set up variables $\{x_1, \ldots, x_z\}$, where the value of $x_j = 1$ if configuration number j is selected (i.e. contained in S), and 0 if configuration number j is not selected. Since the number of test configurations grows exponentially in the number of parameters, this will be a large set of variables for all but the smallest of test coverage problems.

Now, for each interaction element, determine the set of configurations that cover that interaction element. These will be all configurations where the d parameters in the index set for the interaction element are fixed and the remaining $p - d$ parameters can take any possible value. In the case where there are n values for each parameter, this means that there are n^{p-d} configurations that would cover this interaction element. Define an array of coefficients A such that $a_{ij} = 1$ if interaction element number i is covered by configuration number j, and 0 otherwise. For any i, there will be $p - d$ non-zero values of a_{ij}.

For each of the n^{p-d} configurations, we have a set of n^{p-d} variables representing whether or not the configuration is selected. Therefore, the sum of those variables represents the number of times the particular interaction element is covered. This sum is $\sum_{j=1}^{z} a_{ij} x_j$.

To meet our coverage goal, we require that the sum of those variables is greater than or equal to one, so that the interaction element is covered by at least one test configuration. This represents one constraint on our set of selected test configuration. Therefore, the set of y interaction elements will produce a set of y constraints of the form $\sum_{j=1}^{z} a_{ij} x_j \geq 1$, where $1 \leq i \leq y$.

Additionally, we would like to minimize the total number of configurations that are selected. That is, we would like $\sum_{j=1}^{z} x_j$ to be minimized.

Put together, this forms a {0, 1} integer-programming problem: minimize $\sum_{j=1}^{z} x_j$ subject to the constraints $\sum_{j=1}^{z} a_{ij} x_j \geq 1$, where $1 \leq i \leq y$.

At this point, a comment on the restriction of the values x_j to 0 or 1 is in order. Clearly, the values must be restricted to non-negative integers, as a test configuration cannot be "partially selected" (a fractional value) or "negatively selected". However, suppose that we relax the restriction on the values of x_j to be non-negative integers instead.

Furthermore, suppose that in a minimized sum $\sum_{j=1}^{z} x_j$, there is a value $x_q > 1$. Since all of the constraints are of the form $\sum_{j=1}^{z} a_{ij} x_j \geq 1$, where

$a_{ij} \in \{0, 1\}$, we could replace the value of x_q by 1, and the constraint would still be satisfied. Furthermore, since all of the x_j are non-negative integers, the sum $\sum_{j=0}^{z-1} x_j$ would be reduced by the amount $x_q - 1$, which contradicts the assumption that the sum was minimized. Therefore, in the minimized sum, all of the $x_j \in \{0, 1\}$.

The result is that the restriction $x_j \in \{0, 1\}$ does not exclude any potential minimal solutions. The restriction may be useful in practice, as we can provide an integer-programming solver with the information that the variables are binary in nature. This allows the integer-programming solver to discard potential solutions more quickly. (Note that either of these are still much more difficult to solve as compared with a linear programming problem.)

Here is an example. Suppose that there are three parameters, and there are two possible values for each parameter. There are $2^3 = 8$ possible test configurations, and $\binom{3}{2} 2^2 = 12$ interaction elements to be covered. We define a set of variables $\{x_1, \ldots, x_8\}$ such that $x_j \in \{0, 1\}$. We will have $x_j = 1$ if configuration j is selected, and 0 otherwise. *Figure 2* illustrates the resulting $\{0,1\}$ integer programming problem.

In *Figure 2*, the sets of test configurations are listed in the column headings, and the sets of interaction elements are listed in the row headings.

	Configurations								
Interaction Elements	{1,1,1}	{1,1,2}	{1,2,1}	{1,2,2}	{2,1,1}	{2,1,2}	{2,2,1}	{2,2,2}	
$\{1_1,1_2\}$	x_1	$+x_2$							≥ 1
$\{1_1,1_3\}$	x_1		$+x_3$						≥ 1
$\{1_2,1_3\}$	x_1				$+x_5$				≥ 1
$\{1_1,2_2\}$			x_3	$+x_4$					≥ 1
$\{1_1,2_3\}$		x_2		$+x_4$					≥ 1
$\{1_2,2_3\}$		x_2				$+x_6$			≥ 1
$\{2_1,1_2\}$					x_5	$+x_6$			≥ 1
$\{2_1,1_3\}$					x_5		$+x_7$		≥ 1
$\{2_2,1_3\}$			x_3				$+x_7$		≥ 1
$\{2_1,2_2\}$							x_7	$+x_8$	≥ 1
$\{2_1,2_3\}$						x_6		$+x_8$	≥ 1
$\{2_2,2_3\}$				x_4				$+x_8$	≥ 1

Figure 2. Formulation of a test coverage problem as an integer program.

If we minimize $x_1+x_2+x_3+x_4+x_5+x_6+x_7+x_8$, subject to $x_1+x_2 \geq 1$, $x_1+x_3 \geq 1$, $x_1+x_5 \geq 1$, $x_3+x_4 \geq 1$, $x_2+x_4 \geq 1$, $x_2+x_6 \geq 1$, $x_5+x_6 \geq 1$, $x_5+x_7 \geq 1$, $x_3+x_7 \geq 1$, $x_7+x_8 \geq 1$, $x_6+x_8 \geq 1$, $x_4+x_8 \geq 1$, we will have obtained the set of test configurations of minimal cardinality that covers all interaction elements.

3.2 Solving the integer program

For experimental purposes, a linear programming solver called "lp_solve" 0 written by Michel Berkelaar was used. Lp_solve is available as free-ware from Eindhoven University. The input file format is straightforward, given the above discussion:

```
min: x0 + x1 + x2 + x3 + x4 + x5 + x6 + x7;
x0 + x1 >= 1;
x1 + x2 >= 1;
x1 + x3 >= 1;
x1 + x5 >= 1;
x3 + x4 >= 1;
```

```
x2 + x4 >= 1;
x5 + x6 >= 1;
x5 + x7 >= 1;
x3 + x7 >= 1;
x7 + x8 >= 1;
x6 + x8 >= 1;
x4 + x8 >= 1;
int x1, x2, x3, x4, x5, x6, x7, x8;
```

The first line represents the objective function, and indicates that it should be minimized. The constraints are listed, and the final line indicates that variables `x1` through `x8` should be restricted to integers. An implied constraint is that all variables are greater than or equal to zero.

The output produced by lp_solve for the above input file is:

```
CPU Time for parsing input: 0.01s (0.01s total since program start)
CPU Time for solving: 0s (0.01s total since program start)
Value of objective function: 4
x1                    1
x2                    0
x3                    0
x4                    1
x5                    0
x6                    1
x7                    1
x8                    0
```

The value of the objective function is 4, which is the sum of `x1` through `x8`. This indicates that four test configurations are sufficient to provide coverage of all interaction elements. The specific values of the solution variables indicate that the test configurations {1, 1, 1}, {1, 2, 2}, {2, 1, 2}, and {2, 2, 1} should be selected. The configurations can be determined quickly by representing the variable number (plus 1, to allow for indexing from 1 instead of 0) in binary, and increasing each value by 1: for example, `x4` is binary 101, which indicates {2, 1, 2}.

By formulating the interaction test coverage problem as a {0, 1} integer programming problem, solving the resulting integer program exactly will produce the best possible solution.

3.3 Difficulties with the approach

We run into problems because the number of variables required grows exponentially. If there is the same number of values, n, for each parameter, we have the following results:

The row dimension will be $\binom{p}{d} n^d$, which is the number of interaction elements. This is somewhat manageable, since the power in the exponent is only d.

The column dimension will be n^p, which is the number of configurations. This will be extremely large in most cases.

The number of non-zero a_{ij} per row will be n^{p-d}

The number of non-zero a_{ij} will be $\binom{p}{d} n^p$

To get an idea of how quickly this becomes infeasible to calculate in practice, here are some experimental results using the lp_solve tool:

Table 1. Results of running lp_solve on test configuration problems.

# parms	# values per parm	# constraints	# variables	Result: # configs	Run time (s)
3	2	12	8	4	<0.01
4	2	24	16	5	0.01
5	2	40	32	6	0.70
6	2	60	64	6	16.57
7	2	84	128	6	441.21
4	3	54	81	9	0.08
5	3	90	243	13*	*

The * in *Table 1* indicates the best possible solution found at the point when the process was killed after running for about 6.5 hours. Some results provided by other users of lp_solve, (included as documentation in the distribution) indicate lp_solve will have difficulties for problems that have more than about 100 **integer** variables. The above results support this statement.

3.4 Is the interaction test coverage problem NP-complete?

We have reformulated the interaction test coverage problem as a {0, 1} integer programming problem, which is NP-complete 0. We now present an argument why a general {0, 1} integer programming problem does not reduce directly by this mapping to a test configuration problem.

In a general {0, 1} integer programming problem, we could have, for example, the following set of constraints:

Constraint 1: $x_1 + x_2 + x_3 \geq 1$
Constraint 2: $x_4 + x_5 \geq 1$
Constraint 3: $x_6 + x_7 \geq 1$
Constraint 4: $x_1 + x_4 + x_7 \geq 1$
Constraint 5: $x_2 + x_5 + x_1 \geq 1$

We have seven variables and five constraints and the key point that seven is a prime number. Now, the number of variables represents the number of configurations, which is $\prod_{i=1}^{p} n_i$. However, if we have a prime number as the number of configurations, then there can be only one parameter with more than one value. This parameter must have seven possible values.

Now, the number of interaction elements is $|X_d| = \sum_{i_1=1}^{p-d} \ldots \sum_{i_d=i_{d-1}+1}^{p} (n_{i_1} \ldots n_{i_d})$, and this is the number of constraints in an interaction test coverage problem. However, we know of the existence of at least one parameter with seven values, and therefore this sum is at least seven. We cannot have any terms of this sum less than zero, since this would represent a parameter with a negative number of values, and that is definitely not an interaction test coverage problem. However, our integer program has only five constraints, and therefore cannot represent the number of interaction elements for any problem with seven variables.

Thus, we have found a counter-example to the hypothesis that a general {0,1} integer programming problem can be represented directly as an interaction test coverage problem.

Therefore, we cannot reduce a general {0, 1} integer programming problem to a test configuration problem, and therefore we cannot obtain a result as to whether the interaction test coverage problem is NP-complete using this approach.

There is regularity to how the 0 and 1 coefficients appear in the constraint grid, of which the integer programming formulation does not take advantage. That regularity is also enough to guarantee that there is a feasible minimum solution to the integer-programming problem constructed out of a test configuration problem. There has to be at least one feasible solution since we are guaranteed to cover every interaction element by selecting every possible test configuration. Of course, the minimum ought to be much less than that, but we have shown the existence of at least one solution, and therefore a minimum has to exist.

4. CONCLUSIONS AND FURTHER WORK

We have shown that the interaction test coverage problem can be solved exactly by formulating the problem as a {0,1} integer program. Unfortunately, this leads to difficulties in practice because the latter is NP-complete. The experiments we have run show that only the very smallest of interaction test coverage problems can be solved with this approach.

We have also shown the reverse mapping is not possible; a general {0,1} integer programming problem cannot always be converted to an interaction test coverage problem. Therefore, we cannot establish that the interaction test coverage problem is NP-complete by this route.

For further work, one avenue of investigation is whether a linear programming approximation will produce useful results. Our initial experiments indicate that such an approximation is possible, but the results do not appear to be as good as the recursive covering array construction of 0.

Other work is needed in extending the results of 0 to cover interactions of degree higher than 2, and to investigate recursive covering array construction for parameters with varying numbers of values.

REFERENCES

Beizer, B. *Software Testing Techniques*, Second Edition, Van Nostrand Reinhold, New York NY USA, 1990.

Berkelaar, M., "lp_solve," version 3.0. Linear programming solver developed at Eindhoven University, available at ftp://ftp.ics.ele.tue.nl/pub/lp_solve

Brownlie, R., Prowse, J., and Phadke, M.S. Robust Testing of AT&T PMX/StarMail using OATS. *AT&T Technical Journal 71*, 3 (May/June 1992), 41-47.

Burroughs, K., Jain, A., and Erickson, R.L. Improved Quality of Protocol Testing Through Techniques of Experimental Design. In *Proceedings of Supercomm/ICC '94*, (1994), 745-752.

Cohen, D.M., Dalal, S.R., Fredman, M.L., and Patton, G.C. The AETG System: An Approach to Testing Based on Combinatorial Design. *IEEE Transactions on Software Engineering, 23*, 7 (July 1997), 437-444.

Cohen, D.M., Dalal, S.R., Parelius, J., and Patton, G.C. The Combinatorial Approach to Automatic Test Generation. *IEEE Software 13*, 5 (Sept. 1996), 83-88.

Crescenzi, P., Kann, V., editors. A compendium of NP-complete problems. On-line at http://www.f.kth.se/~viggo/problemlist/compendium.html

Dunietz, I.S., Ehrlich, W.K., Szablak, B.D., Mallows, C.L., and Iannino, A. Applying Design of Experiments to Software Testing. In *Proceedings of the 19th International Conference on Software Engineering (ICSE '97)*, (Boston MA USA, 1997), 205-215.

Karpinski, M. Polynomial Time Approximation Schemes for Some Dense Instances of NP-Hard Optimization Problems. In Proceedings of the 1st Symposium on Randomization and Approximation Techniques in Computer Science, Lecture Notes in Computer Science 1269, Springer-Verlag, 1997, 1-14.

Karpinski, M. and Zelikovsky, A. Approximating Dense Cases of Covering Problems. ECCC Technical Report TR97-004. On-line at ftp://eccc.uni-trier.de/pub/eccc/reports/1997/TR97-004/index.html.

Perkinson, W.B. A Methodology for Designing and Executing ISDN Feature Tests Using Automated Test Systems. In *Proc. of IEEE GLOBECOMM '92*, (1992).

Ryu, J., Kim, M., Kang S., and Seol, S. Interoperability Test Suite Generation for the TCP Data Part Using Experimental Design Techniques. In *Proceedings of the 13th International Conference on the Testing of Communicating Systems (Testcom 2000)*, (Ottawa ON Canada, 2000), 127-142.

Stevens, B. and Mendelsohn, E. Efficient Software Testing Protocols. In *Proceedings of the 8th IBM Centre for Advanced Studies Conference (CASCON '98)*, (Toronto ON, 1998), 279-293.

Williams, A.W., and Probert, R.L. A Practical Strategy for Testing pair-wise Coverage of Network Interfaces. In *Proceedings of the 7th International Conference on Software Reliability Engineering (ISSRE '96)*, (White Plains NY USA, 1996), 246-254.

Williams, A.W. Determination of Test Configurations for Pair-Wise Interaction Coverage. In *Proceedings of the 13th International Conference on the Testing of Communicating Systems (Testcom 2000)*, (Ottawa ON Canada, 2000), 59-74.

Williams, A.W., and Probert, R.L. A Measure of Component Interaction Test Coverage. In *Proceedings of the ACS/IEEE International Conference on Computer Systems and Applications (AICCSA 2001)*, (Beirut Lebanon, 2001), 304-311.

SESSION VIII

TESTING DISTRIBUTED SYSTEMS

PRINCIPLES OF DISTRIBUTED TEST SYNTHESIS BASED ON TRUE-CONCURRENCY MODELS

Claude Jard
IRISA/CNRS
Campus de Beaulieu
F-35042 RENNES Cedex
France
Claude.Jard@irisa.fr

Abstract Automatic synthesis of test cases for conformance testing has been principally developed with the objective of generating sequential test cases. In the distributed system context, it is worth extending the synthesis techniques to the generation of multiple testers. We base our work on our experience in using model-checking techniques, as successfully implemented in the TGV tool. Continuing the works of A. Ulrich and H. König, we propose to use a true-concurrency model based on graph unfolding. The article presents the principles of a complete chain of synthesis, starting from the definition of test purposes and ending with a projection onto a set of testers.

Key words: Test, Distributed systems, Synthesis, True-concurrency models, Inter-operability

1. INTRODUCTION

Algorithms for automatic test synthesis have been proposed both in the academic world, and in industry. However, the use of these tools reaches a limit when testing distributed systems. This is because they are dedicated to the synthesis of sequential test cases (represented by event sequences or finite automata). Such synthesis is not always well-suited to test systems containing parallel activities. It is also known that a state representation of a specification with parallelism often suffers from a combinatorial explosion.

The interest in generating distributed test cases was recognised a few years ago, as demonstrated by the inclusion of concurrent constructs in the TTCN standard. We retain three main motivations to synthesise distributed test cases:

- It can be naturally imposed by the test architecture under consideration. Let us consider a system geographically scattered on a network. The idea is to design a set of testers, each tester being located at the communicating entity to be checked, and communicating with the other testers to co-ordinate the test activity and the production of diagnosis.
- It allows more compact and clear test cases to be obtained. This is the case when the system under test produces concurrent observable events: a sequential representation would require all possible interleavings to be computed. This rapidly suffers from a combinatorial explosion as the concurrency increases.
- In certain cases parallel testing is needed to check particular behaviours. For example, one often considers for controllability reasons that the testers must wait for the system stabilisation before injecting new interactions. Under this assumption, it was shown by [2] that a distributed test case can position the system under test into states which are not reachable by a sequential test. More generally, the situation will also occur in the context of real-time testing.

One can distinguish two main approaches to synthesising distributed test cases:

- The generation of sequential test cases, followed by their automated distribution. The idea is to produce a set of communicating testers which behave like the sequential test (i.e. in the sense of trace equivalence). The advantage of this approach is that it requires no more than the current state of the art; it can even be used on hand-written test cases. The major drawback is that it does not take into account the intrinsic parallelism of the system under test. In general, one does not know how to distinguish between parallelism and interleaving; in practice this leads to useless synchronisation between the local testers.
- The re-examination of the synthesis, retaining the parallelism information contained in the formal specification during the construction of the test cases. We discuss this extreme approach in the paper. The main difficulty is the use of a true-concurrency model in which causality and concurrency are explicitly represented, in place of the usual automata or transition system models. This kind of model has been mainly developed by theoreticians and has not yet been fully exploited. The synthesis of distributed test cases appears to be an interesting context to use the explicit parallelism included in the model.

The question of the automatic synthesis of distributed testers is relatively recent. It has appeared gradually from the notion of multiple, then distributed interfaces. For example, in [18], the system under test is modelled by a single finite state machine with several distributed interfaces. A test generation method is sketched, based on the idea of synchronisable test suites. In [19], multiple testers are generated by considering only particular synchronous behaviours of the parallel specification. Co-ordination of the testers makes the assumption that the communications between entities of the system under test are observable. The idea of using true-concurrency models in the case of asynchronous systems came from two research groups separately (one in Korea, driven by M. Kim, the other in Germany, driven by A. Ulrich and H. König). In Kim's approach [20,21], they adopt a specific model, which consists in computing particular concurrent paths from a communicating finite state machines view. The introduction of event duration makes the computation easier. It is not clear however to know the algorithmic complexity of the method and how it scales up in a real testing methodology (abstraction, selection, ...). We chose to follow the Ulrich and König's approach [22], mathematically based on theoretical and algorithmic results on Petri nets. The partial order semantics of Petri nets and its implementation in the "unfolding" algorithmic has been developed for many years, but rather confined in the theoretical computer science community. We think it is enough sound and advanced to be applied in several domains... like distributed testing. In [22], the unfolding of "behaviour machines" is used to propose a "partial order transition cover" as a general heuristics to select partial order test cases, which could be later projected on parallel testers. In the same vein, [23] has tempted to avoid the use of Petri nets and to directly generate the partial orders (event structures) in the context of asynchronous communication.

The rest of the paper is organised as follows: First, we give an overview of a test synthesis method based on model-checking and sequential transition systems, as implemented in the TGV tool. We then propose to revisit the whole test-production chain using partial-order representations of the behaviours. This is presented in Section three, following the different steps of the methodology: the partial order view of a specification (the notion of "tile") and of a test purpose, the construction of an unfolding (the "puzzle game"), its partial order abstraction, and its final projection onto several testers. Particular attention is paid to the algorithmic complexity and its potential to scale up, in the perspective of developing a real prototype. Some indications of possible future developments are given in the conclusion.

2. SYNTHESIS BASED ON TRANSITION SYSTEMS

We mainly rely on our experience in conformance testing. The TGV tool (Test Generation using the Verification technology) [3,4], jointly developed by our group at Irisa and a group at Vérimag, is a real-size implementation of synthesis techniques based on transition systems. We thus begin by recalling the main principles.

2.1 Our example

Let us consider the small example depicted in Figure 1. This is a simple connection-disconnection protocol, modelled with two interacting finite automata communicating through one-bounded channels. The users can use the protocol by asking for a new connection (event **a**), or asking for the disconnection of a previously opened connection (event **b** from one side, event **c** from the other side). Each request is acknowledged by the local process after having performed the corresponding action (events **a**, **b** and **c**). The protocol manages a possible collision of disconnect messages by exchanging a disconnect confirmation, named d. The scenario presented in Figure 1 illustrates the three possible repeatable behaviours (connection is closed by the initiator, connection is closed by the other side, and collision). The message exchanges between processes are neither controllable, nor observable.

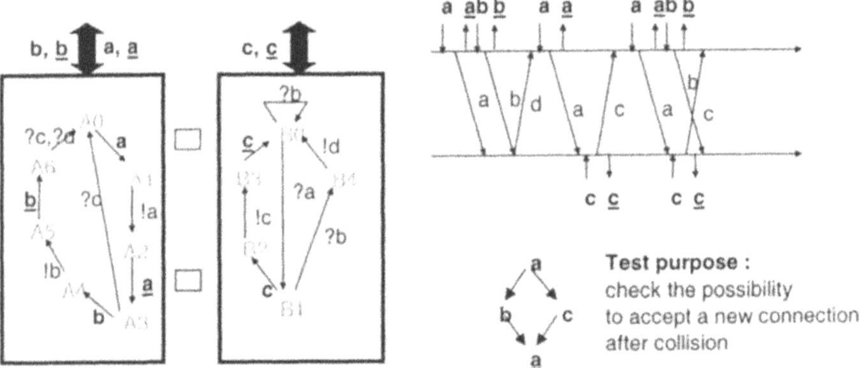

Figure 1. A small example of connection-disconnection protocol and a possible test purpose.

The test objective here is to check the possibility to accept a new connection after collision (collision management is known to be a fragile aspect of this kind of protocol). This can be naturally described by the partial order given in Figure 1: **a** must precede **b** and **c**, which precede **a̲**. The description by communicating finite automata is just for illustration purpose. In the real use of TGV, models are described in higher-level languages like SDL, Lotos or UML [5,6,7], the associated compiler providing the state representation.

2.2 The state-graph representation

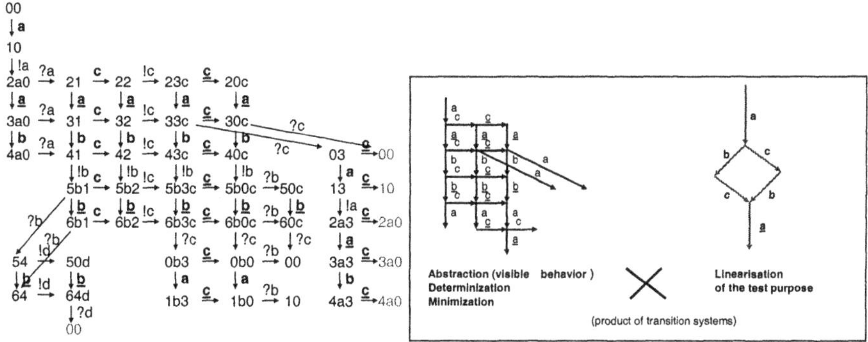

Figure 2. Finite automata, trace-equivalent to the communicating automata of Figure 1; its visible abstraction, guided by the automaton of the test purpose. Each state of the test purpose accepts all the events (the single loops are not represented). The sink state is labelled by *accept.*

The exhaustive simulation of the protocol, starting in the initial state A0B0 with empty channels, and keeping track of the global states reached by the simulator gives the graph depicted in Figure 2. Notice that cycles are built when reaching a previously generated state. This state graph captures all the possible traces of the protocol (the interleaving is computed in the case of concurrent events). From this graph, one can compute a trace-equivalent automaton restricted to the alphabet of visible events. A part of this graph can be selected using the test purpose in order to keep only the traces it accepts (leading to the sink state PASS).

2.3 Test synthesis

The resulting graph representing all the visible traces of the specification, consistent with the test purpose, defines a set of possible test cases (up to the inversion of interactions). In general, to reduce the complexity, one extracts only one test case using some heuristics. For example, we consider that a test case must be (globally) controllable, which means that there is no choice between an emission from the tester and another interaction. In our example, the resulting test case is given in Figure 3. To be complete, we must mention that the test case is augmented with verdicts (PASS in the final state, FAIL for possible receptions that are not in the graph, INCONCLUSIVE when the reception is not on a path selected by the test purpose) and timers (to prevent the test from dead-, live- and output-locks). The generated test cases are guaranteed to be safe (they cannot reject a conformant implementation in the sense of *ioco* conformance [8]). The method is also complete in the sense that it is able to reject any non-conformant implementation (assuming the provision of a corresponding test purpose, and some fairness assumptions about the implementation).

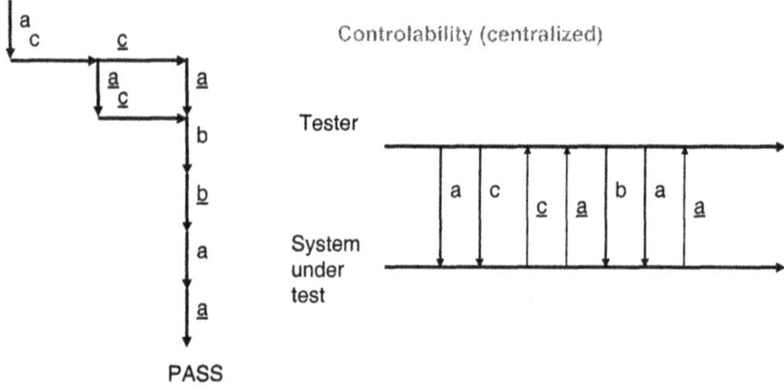

Figure 3. Resulting test case under controllability assumption.

In the complete version of TGV, these different graphs are not built in sequence. Their construction is performed on-the-fly during the synthesis of the test case through the use of APIs at different levels [10], as depicted in Figure 4. The algorithms are mainly based on adaptations of Tarjan's algorithm [9], computing the strongly connected components of a graph via a depth-first search. The complexity is linear in the size of the state graph (though the graph itself may be exponential in the size of the model, notably when the concurrency is significant). Determinisation remains exponential, but is applied to the graph of visible behaviours, which is much smaller than the state graph.

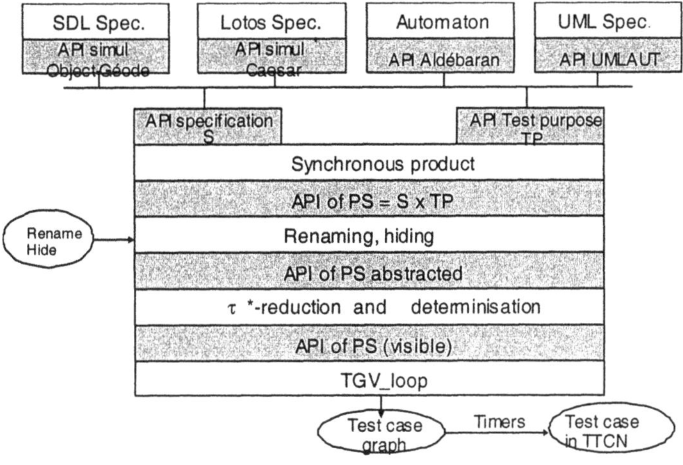

Figure 4. The on-the-fly organisation of TGV.

3. PARTIAL ORDER VIEW OF THE SYSTEM

3.1 Tile systems

In this section we introduce our mathematical framework. Tiles correspond to partial transitions and a system is defined as a collection of tiles.

Let **V** be a finite set of variables. Each variable $v \subset \mathbf{V}$ takes its values in some finite domain D_v. For $V \subseteq \mathbf{V}$, we set $X_V = \prod_{v \in V} D_v$. Elements of X_V are denoted by x_V and are called *V-states*, or local states. For $v \in \mathbf{V}$, we denote by $v(x_V)$ the value of the variable v in state x_V. We shall consider local transitions relating local states, very much in the same way as transitions relate states in standard automata. These local transitions will be referred to as tiles in the sequel. Formally, a *tile* is a 4-tuple $\tau = < V, \bar{x}_V, \alpha, x_V >$, where $V \subseteq \mathbf{V}$ is a subset of variables, and $(\bar{x}_V, \alpha, x_V)$ is a local transition, relating the previous V-state $\bar{x}_V \in D_V$, and performing event α where α ranges over some set A of possible event labels. For τ a tile, we shall sometimes denote by V_τ its set of variables. A system is a triple

$\Sigma = < V, X_0, \mathrm{T} >$, where $V \subseteq \mathbf{V}$ is a finite set of variables, X_0 is a set of initial states, and T is a finite set of tiles and $V = \bigcup_{\tau \in \mathrm{T}} V_\tau$.

Figure 5 shows the tile system of our example, as it is entered in our prototype.

```
% Variables
var A : 0..6 init 0;
    B : 0..4 init 0;
    M : (O,a,b) init O;
    N : (O,c,d) init O;

% Tiles
?A  pre A(0) label ?A post A(1);
?b  pre B(0) M(b) label ?b post B(0) M(0);
!a  pre A(1) M(0) label !a post A(2) M(a);
?a  pre B(0) M(a) label ?a post B(1) M(0);
!A  pre A(2) label !A post A(3);
?C  pre B(1) label ?C post B(2);
?B  pre A(3) label ?B post A(4);
!c  pre B(2) N(0) label !c post B(3) N(c);
?c  pre A(3) N(c) label ?c post A(0) N(0);
```

Figure 5. The tile system of the example of Figure 1 in textual form.

The interleaved sequence of states and events $x_0, \alpha_1, x_1, \alpha_2, x_2, \ldots, \alpha_k, x_k, \ldots$ is a *run* of system Σ if $x_0 \in X_0$ and,

1. for each $k > 0$, there exists $\tau = < V_\tau, \bar{x}_{V\tau}, \alpha, x_{V\tau} > \in \mathrm{T}$ such that, $\forall v \in V_\tau : v(x_{k-1}) = v(\bar{x}_{V\tau}), \alpha_k = \alpha, v(x_k) = v(x_{V\tau})$, and,

2. $\forall v \notin V_\tau : v(x_{k-1}) = v(x_k)$.

Since tiles define local transitions, it may be the case that two successive tiles of a given run involve disjoint sets of variables, i.e. modify different local states. In this case, exchanging the order of the tiles yields to an equivalent run. This is why we will adopt a partial ordering of tiles instead of considering the different runs.

3.2 Construction of the unfolding

Given a run, the sequence of successive tiles forms a graph, by superimposing the pre-condition of a tile $v(\overline{x}_{v\tau})$ onto an equivalent condition in the existing graph (like a puzzle game). This graph contains two types of nodes: the conditions (the different values of the variables used in pre and post conditions of the tiles), and the events of the tiles. Given two nodes *n* and *n'* (condition or event), we say that *n causes n'*, written $n \leq n'$, if either $n = n'$ or there is a path of arrows from *n* to *n'*. We say that *n* and *n'* are in *conflict*, written $n \# n'$, if there is a condition *m*, different from *n* and *n'*, from which one can reach *n* and *n'*, exiting *m* by different arrows. Finally we say that *n* and *n'* are *concurrent* if neither $n \leq n'$, nor $n' \leq n$, nor $n \# n'$ hold. A *co-set* is a set of concurrent nodes. From a tile system $\Sigma = < V, X_0, \mathrm{T} >$, the basic algorithm for the construction of the graph is the following:

Puzzle := X_0;
repeat
if there exists a tile $\tau \in \mathrm{T}$ *such that* $\overline{x}_{v\tau}$ *is a co-set of Puzzle then append* τ *to Puzzle*
forever

Figure 6 shows the graph obtained after 8 steps of the above algorithm.

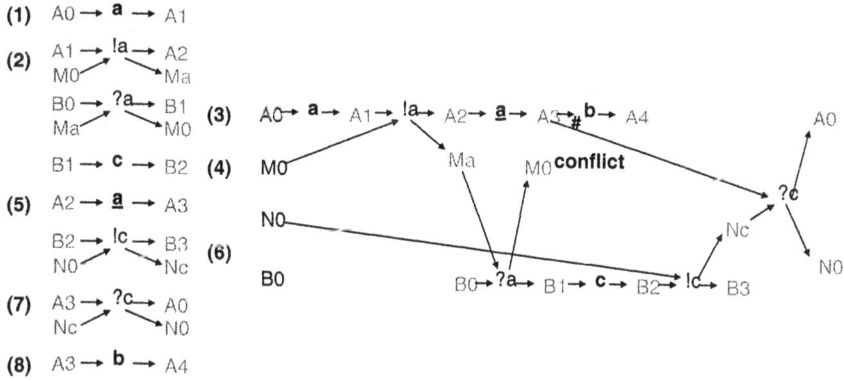

Figure 6. Result of the application of these 8 tiles in sequence. Conflict between tiles 7 and 8 is pointed out by the branching from condition A3.

This graph is generally infinite (in the case of infinite behaviour), it has no circuits, every condition has at most one input node, every node has a finite number of predecessors in the graph, and no node is in self-conflict. It is in fact an occurrence net in the framework of Petri nets. We can use the corresponding terminology. A *cut* is a set of conditions c satisfying the following two properties: c is a co-set, and c is maximal (it is not properly included in any other co-set). A *configuration* is a set of nodes κ satisfying the two following properties: κ is causally closed (if $n \in \kappa$ and $n' < n$, then $n' \in \kappa$) and conflict-free (no two nodes of κ are in conflict). Furthermore, we require for convenience that all maximal nodes (if any) of configurations shall be conditions. Finite configurations and cuts are closely related. In particular, given a finite configuration κ the set of conditions *Cut(κ)* is a reachable global state, which we denote *GS(κ)*. The basic algorithm will eventually produce any reachable global state under only the fairness assumption that every tile candidate to be added is eventually chosen to extend the puzzle (the correctness proof follows from the definitions and from the results of [11]).

It appears that the unfolding is of fractal nature, and can be reduced to a finite generator part, called a finite complete prefix. A prefix *U* of the unfolding is complete if for every reachable global state *S* there exists a configuration *C* in *U* such that $GS(C) = S$ and for every tile τ enabled by *S* there exists a configuration $C \cup \{e\}$ such that $e \notin C$ and *e* is the event of τ. A complete prefix contains as much information as the unfolding, in the sense that we can construct the unfolding from it as the least fix-point of a concatenation operation on patterns defined by maximal configurations of the prefix . In order to construct such a prefix, the question is to locate the events (called the *cut-off events*) from which the extension in the unfolding can be stopped. We will denote *[e]* the set of predecessors of *e* (the set of events *e'* such that $e' \leq e$). An event *e* of the prefix is a *cut-off event* (with respect to a particular order $\prec$) if the prefix contains an event *e'* such that $GS([e]) = GS([e'])$, and $[e'] \prec [e]$. The algorithm to construct a finite complete prefix is the following:

Finite_Puzzle := X_0;
cut_off := {};
<u>*repeat*</u>
  Select a tile τ *such that* $\overline{X}_{V\tau}$ *is a co-set of Finite_Puzzle;*
  live := τ *exists* <u>*and*</u> $\overline{X}_{V\tau} \cap$ *cut_off*={};
  <u>*if*</u> *live* <u>*then*</u> *append* τ *to Finite_Puzzle;*
    <u>*if*</u> $\exists\, u \prec t : GS(u)=GS(t)$ <u>*then*</u> *cut_off* := *cut_off* $\cup\, X_{V\tau}$
<u>*until*</u> *not live*

The correctness of the algorithm requires that the partial order $\prec$ be correctly chosen. In [12], it is proved that $\prec$ must be *adequate*, that is defined as an order that is well-founded, which refines the set inclusion and which is preserved by finite extensions. The size of the prefix also depends on this order, but it is possible to guarantee that the prefix is never larger than the global reachability graph (states + transitions).

> The running time of the algorithm is $O\left(\left(\frac{|C|}{\varphi}\right)^{\varphi}\right)$, where C is the set of conditions of the prefix, and φ denotes the maximal size of the pre-conditions of the tiles in the original system.

Figure 7 shows the complete prefix of our example as computed by the Esparza-Römer-Vogler's unfolding algorithm (available through the "Model-Checking Kit" of the Technical University of Münich [26]). The slowest part of the algorithm is locating the possible conditions that can be covered by a new tile. This is implemented by coding the concurrency relation and providing a method of maintaining it. This deteriorates as the size of the prefix increases, since the amount of memory needed to store the concurrency relation may be quadratic in the number of conditions in the already built part of the prefix. A recent improvement proposed in [13] structures the set of events in order to speed up the search in practice, not by trying the events one by one, but several at once, merging the common parts of the work.

The unfolding can be generated from this prefix by considering three maximal configurations ended by the sets {A0,M0,N0,B0}, {A4,M0,N0,B1} and {A2,Ma,N0,B0} respectively, shown as dashed lines in Figure 7. From these maximal nodes in the prefix, the unfolding can be continued by gluing the pattern starting from a similar cut in the prefix.

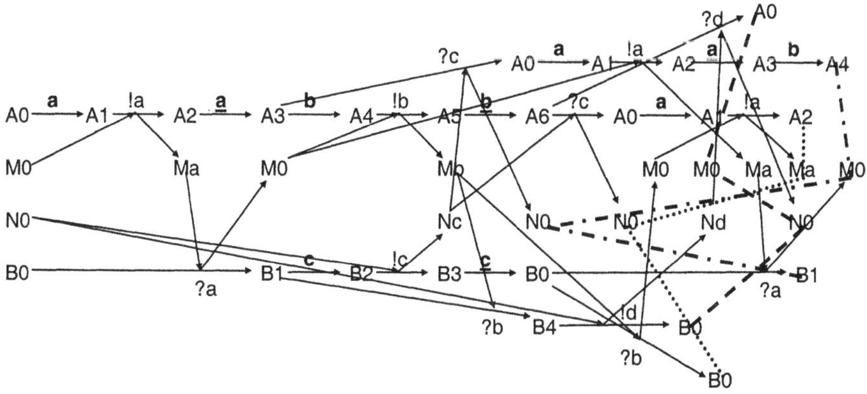

Figure 7. Complete finite prefix of our example.

3.3 Guiding by test purposes

Test purposes are a very interesting feature when dealing with large specifications. Their role is to mark out a relevant part of the specification in which a test must be found. This concept, present since the beginning in the ISO methodology, is rich enough to continue to arouse discussions in a broader community [14,15]. In TGV, a test purpose is given by a finite automaton with sink states labelled by *accept* or *refuse*. A transition of the specification is triggered if there exists a similar transition in the test purpose. It thus allows some transitions to be cut in the state graph representation. The accept state will become the PASS state in the final test case.

This point of view can be easily ported to partial order models, by considering that test purposes are particular tile systems, with two terminal specific tiles having accept or refuse as post-conditions. From the two tile systems (the specification and the test purpose), one can derive a new tile system, coding the product. The principle is as follows: for each tile of the test purpose, let us consider a tile of the specification with a similar event label and build a new tile by making the conjunction of pre-conditions and the conjunction of post-conditions. This can increase the number of tiles. The unfolding is then carried out on this new tile system. An alternative could be to perform the product on-the-fly during the construction of the unfolding, instead of pre-computing the new tiles. This would imply to keep the maximal configurations in the prefix in order to be able to continue the unfolding if required by the test purpose. Placing a tile containing an accept or refuse condition is considered as a cut event in the algorithm. Figure 8 shows the tile system of the test purpose chosen in our example.

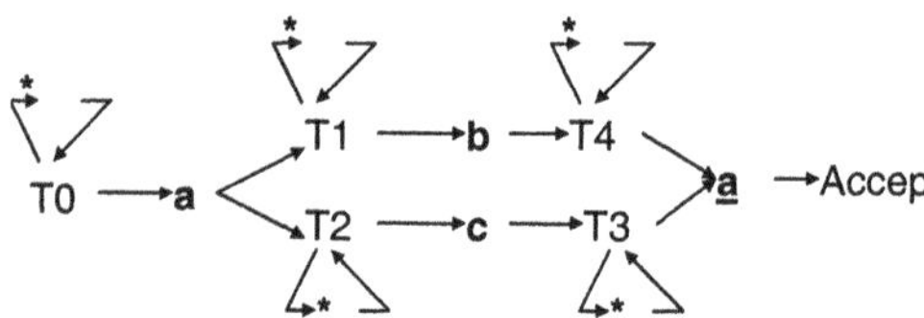

Figure 8. A partial ordered test purpose. "*" means any event label of the specification, except the outgoing events.

3.4 Abstraction

At this step, the complete prefix contains all the information needed to generate a test case (no further unfolding is needed, since all the realisation of the test purpose has been considered in the new tile system, resulting from the product of the specification with the test purpose). We consider that the relevant semantics for a test case is the partial order of its events. It can be extracted from the prefix by considering the observable events only and the paths in the graph linking them. The graph of the test case is the partial order defined as follows: the nodes are the events of the observable tiles, and a node *n* precedes a node *n'* if and only if there exists a path of arrows from *n* to *n'*. This operation is linear in the size of the prefix (computation of a sub-order). To be rigorous, we must distinguish the situation in which two nodes labelled with concurrent events have a common predecessor, from the case where the events are in conflict. The latter situation will be resolved in the projection phase, while the first will generate a local choice.

Some more pruning can be done on the graph. First, the only interesting paths are those leading to *Accept*. The others can be deleted, while keeping the branching information on the relevant paths in order to be able to set possible INCONCLUSIVE verdicts. Second, we generally require that test cases are controllable. In our framework, we consider *local controllability* only, which means that a reception in the tile system, occurring on a local process cannot have the same direct predecessor as another event of this process. Figure 9 shows the partial order of the abstraction in our example and the extracted sub-graph.

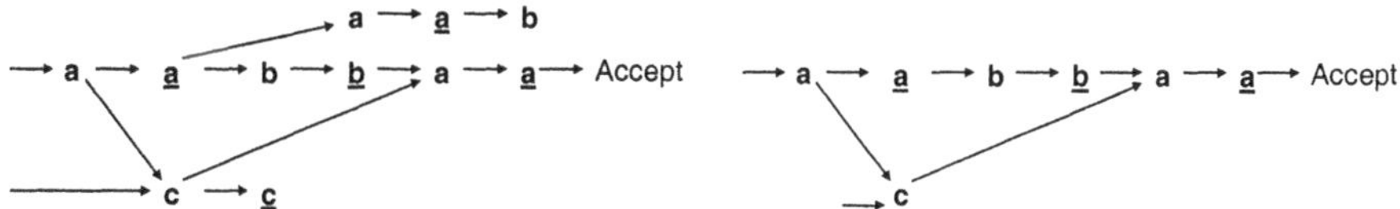

Figure 9. Abstraction and selection of a test graph.

3.5 Projection

The last step is the projection of the test graph onto the different testers. The principle is the following:

- the events of the testers are the mirror images of the events of the test graph (receptions from the point of view of the specification are the emissions of the testers, and vice versa),
- the graph of events of a tester is the projection of the test graph, keeping only the local events (another sub-order construction). At this step, it is advisable to build the transitive reduction of the local graph, in order to avoid redundant synchronisation (this is of cubic complexity, but the algorithm is applied generally on small graphs),

- a direct link between two events located on different testers is implemented by exchanging a synchronisation message (this particular message is emitted after the occurrence of the first event, and received by the other tester before performing the second event).

This is standard way to distribute the behaviour of an automaton. By construction, the partial order defined by the test graph is preserved by projection. Thus, all the traces are preserved too [16,17]. The result of the projection for our example is shown on Figure 10.

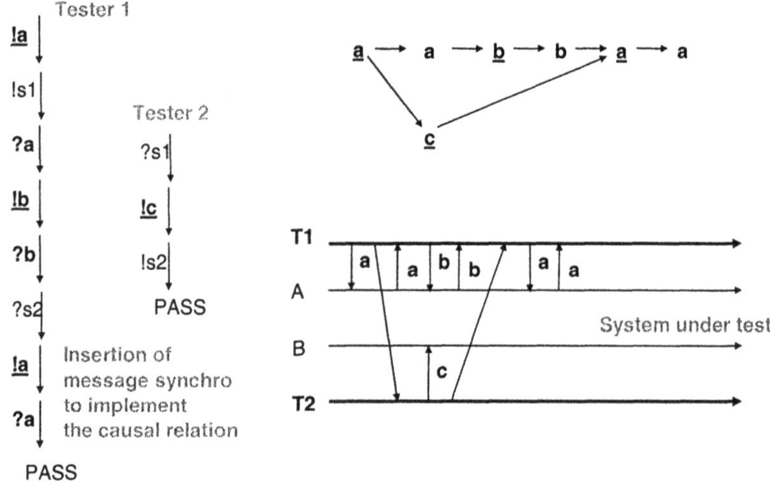

Figure 10. The resulting testers in our example.

It is interesting to compare this distributed test case with the sequential one of Figure 3. The automatic distribution of the test case of Figure 3 would produce much more synchronisation. Of course, the diamond (a,c) in the centralised test case is represented by real parallelism in the distributed test case. Furthermore, we can see that interaction !b (and ?b) is concurrent with !c in the distributed case. This situation seems impossible to infer from the sequential test case.

4. CONCLUSIONS AND PERSPECTIVES

Pursuing the approach initiated by Ulrich and König, we propose a complete chain of test synthesis based on a true-concurrency model. This is done by revisiting the TGV methodology based on test purposes and of graph manipulation (product, abstraction, projection, controllability). The theoretical basis of our proposal relies on sound and scalable algorithmic, based on the construction of prefixes of unfoldings. The main perspective is to continue the implementation of these ideas. We have also several research directions to explore:

- The use of UML as modelling language. Beyond its popularity, there is a real challenge to deal with the partial order semantics of UML, as given in the action semantics currently specified.
- The required algorithms seem to be implementable on-the-fly, like in TGV. But the situation is much more complex on unfoldings than in simple transition systems.
- There are specific questions of controllability in a distributed context [24], which deserve further study.
- Finally, it is tempting to refine the standard conformance relation based on sequential traces to a kind of partial order inclusion. This could be achieved by considering a distributed observation of the communication between the entities under test [25], i.e. by instrumenting the implementation by a vector clock mechanism.

5. BIBLIOGRAPHY

[1] ISO/IEC 9646 IT-OSI, OSI Conformance Testing Methodology and Framework

[2] M. Törö. Decision on Tester Configuration for Multiparty Testing. Proc. of the 12th int. Workshop on Testing of Communicating Systems. Budapest, Hungary, 1999.

[3] JC. Fernandez, C. Jard, T. Jéron and C. Viho. Using on-the-fly verification techniques for the generation of test suites, Conference on Computer-Aided Verification (CAV '96), New Brunswick, New Jersey, USA, Alur, A. and Henzinger, T. editors, Springer, LNCS 1102, july 1996.

[4] JC. Fernandez, C. Jard, T. Jéron and C. Viho. An Experiment in Automatic Generation of Test Suites for Protocols with Verification Technology, Science of Computer Programming, Groote, J.-F. and Rem, M. editors}, Elsevier Science, number 29, pages 123-146, 1997

[5] L. Doldi, V. Encontre, JC. Fernandez, T. Jéron, S. Le Bricquir, N. Texier and M. Phalippou. Assessment of Automatic Generation Methods of Conformance Test Suites in an Industrial Context, IFIP TC6 9th International Workshop on Testing of Communicating Systems, Baumgarten, B. and Burkhardt, H.-J. and Giessler, A., Chapman & Hall, september 1996.

[6] A. Kerbrat, C. Rodriguez, and Y. Lejeune. Interconnecting the ObjectGéode and CADP toolsets. In Proceedings of SDL forum'97. Elsevier Science (North Holland), 1997.

[7] T. Jéron, JM. Jézéquel and A. Le Guennec *Validation and Test Generation for Object-Oriented Distributed Software*. International Symposium on Software Engineering for Parallel and Distributed Systems (PDSE'98), Tokyo, Japan, April 1998.

[8] J. Tretmans, *Test Generation with Inputs, Outputs and Repetitive Quiescence*. Software, Concepts and Tools (1996) 17: 103-120.

[9] R. Tarjan. *Depth-first Search and Linear Graph Algorithms*. SIAM Journal Computing, 1(2):146-160. June 1972.

[10] T. Jéron and P. Morel. *Test Generation Derived from Model-Checking*. 11th intern. Conf. On Computer Aided Verification (CAV'99), Trento, Italy, July 1999. LNCS 1633, pp. 108-122.

[11] J. Engelfriet. *Branching Processes of Petri Nets*. Acta Informatica 28, pp. 575-591 (1991).

[12] J. Esparza, S. Römer. *An Unfolding Algorithm for Synchronous Products of Transition Systems*. Proc. Concur'99, Springer, LNCS 1664 (1999) 2-20.

[13] V. Khomenko and M. Koutny. *Towards an Efficient Algorithm for Unfolding Petri Nets*. Proc. Concur'2001. Springer, LNCS 2154 (2001): 366-380.

[14] Y. Ledru, L. Du Bousquet, P. Bontron, O. Maury, C. Oriat, and ML. Potet. Test Purposes: Adapting the Notion of Specification to Testing. To appear in the proc. of the IEEE Automated Software Engineering Conference (ASE'2001). San Diego, November 2001.

[15] RG. De Vries and J. Tretmans. *Towards Formal Test Purposes*. In Formal Approaches to Testing of Software (FATES), Aalbord, Denmark, August 2001.

[16] B. Caillaud, P. Caspi, A. Girault and C. Jard. *Distributing Automata for Asynchronous Network of Processors*. European Journal on Automated Systems (JESA), 31(3): 503-504. May 1997.

[17] C. Jard, T. Jéron, H. Khalouche and C. Viho. *Towards Automatic Distribution of Testers for Distributed Conformance Testing*. . Formal Description Techniques and Protocol Specification, Testing and Verification, 18, pp. 353-368. IFIP, Kluwer, November 1998.

[18] G. Luo, R. Dssouli, Gv. Bochmann, P. Venkaratan and A. Ghedamsi. *Test Generation with respect to Distributed Interfaces*. Computer Standards and Interfaces 16 (1994): 119-132.

[19] R. Castanet and O. Koné. *Deriving Co-ordinated Testers for Interoperability*. Protocol Test Systems, VI (C-19), O. Rafiq (Ed). Elsevier Science B.V. (North-Holland). 1994 IFIP.

[20] M. Kim, S.T. Chanson, S. Kang and J. Shin. *An Approach for Testing Asynchronous Communicating Systems*. Proc. of the 9th int. Workshop on Testing of Communicating Systems. Darmstadt, 1996, pp. 141-155.

[21] M. Kim, J. Shin, S.T. Chanson and S. Kang. *An Enhanced Model for Testing Asynchronous Communicating Systems*. Formal Description Techniques and Protocol Specification, Testing and Verification, 19, pp. 337-355. IFIP 1999. Beijing, China.

[22] A. Ulrich and H. König. *Specification-based Testing of Concurrent Systems*. Formal Description Techniques and Protocol Specification, Testing and Verification, 17. T. Mizuno, N. Shiratori, T. Higashino & A. Togashi (Eds.), 1997 IFIP. Published by Chapman & Hall.

[23] O. Henniger. On Test Case Generation from Asynchronously Communicating State Machines. Testing of Communicating Systems. Vol. 10. M. Kim, S. Kang & Al. (Eds). Chapman & Hall, pp. 255-271, September 1997.

[24] A. Ulrich and H. König. *Architectures for Testing Distributed Systems*. Proc. of the 12th int. Workshop on Testing of Communicating Systems. Budapest, Hungary, 1999, pp. 93-108.

[25] L. Cacciari and O. Rafiq. *Controllability and Observability in Distributed Testing*. Information and Software Technology 41 (1999): 767-780. Elsevier.

[26] http://wwwbrauer.informatik.tu-muenchen.de/gruppen/theorie/KIT/)

FAULT DETECTION WITHIN A COMPONENT OF A SYSTEM OF COMMUNICATING FSMS

Ana Cavalli[1], Svetlana Prokopenko[1], Nina Yevtushenko[2]
1 Institut National des Telecommunications, 9 rue Charles Fourier 91011 Evry France
Email: Ana.Cavalli@int-evry.fr, Svetlana.Prokopenko@int-evry.fr
2 Tomsk State University, 36 Lenin av. 634050 Tomsk Russia
Email: Yevtushenko@elefot.tsu.ru

Abstract In this paper, we consider the problem of detecting faults within a component of a system of communicating FSMs. These faults are detected by a given set of external test cases, which satisfy appropriate test purposes. Given a component FSM and an external test case, we propose a procedure for deriving the set of all output faults of the component machine, which can be detected with this test case. Applications range from test suite minimization to derivation of diagnostic tests for a component FSM. In this paper, we use the above technique for augmenting a given test suite in order to detect all output faults within a component under test. The same approach can be used with respect to any other finite set of faults within the implementation of a component FSM.

Key words: Finite State Machine (FSM), communicating FSMs, test suit

1. INTRODUCTION

There are a number of methods for test suite derivation based on an FSM model. Some methods return a test suite, which satisfies appropriate test purposes [1, 2]; other return a complete test suite w.r.t. an appropriate fault domain [3-10]. Traditional test purpose approaches are based on the following idea: to traverse an appropriate set of transitions. If each transition is traversed then the obtained test suite is known to detect any output fault of an implementation system and to have a rather good quality. However, usually traversing all the transitions is impossible for a large system and a test engineer selects a subset of them. There are a number of papers [see, for example, 1, 2] with recommendations how to select such a subset in the best way. When coming to communicating FSMs the test purpose often is to traverse each possible transition of each component FSM [2, 11]. In the case of communicating FSMs, each transition of the overall system comes from a combination of transitions of some modules. By this reason, a proper subset of all the global transitions that usually is much less than the set of all global transitions satisfies such a test purpose. The fault coverage of the obtained test suite remains unknown. In the paper [10], the authors show that under the assumption that we can observe internal outputs of each component FSM a test suite traversing each possible transition of each component FSM detects any single output fault of each component FSM.

In this paper, we continue to study a fault coverage of the above test suite. A method is proposed for determining which output faults of an implementation component FSM are detected with a given test suite when no access is granted to the internal outputs of an appropriate component machine. We also show how these faults influence a behavior of the overall implementation. In particular, we show how to relate to each test case of a given external test suite a finite set of output faults of a possible implementation of a component under test that can be detected with this test case and how the approach can be used for test minimization without a loss of completeness.

The novelty of the work presented in this paper is that we consider all output faults of the component FSM, not only single output faults. We illustrate that when no access to internal outputs is granted it is not enough to traverse an appropriate transition of the component even for detecting a single output fault. Additional test cases are necessary to guarantee complete fault coverage and we propose a technique how to derive them.

2. PRELIMINARIES

2.1 I/O Finite State Machines

An I/O finite state machine (often simply called a FSM or a machine throughout this paper) is an initialized, possibly partially specified, deterministic machine denoted by a 6-tuple $A = (S,X,Y,\delta,\lambda,D_A,s_0)$ where S is a finite set of states with $s_0 \in S$ as the initial state, X is a finite nonempty set of inputs, Y is a finite nonempty set of outputs, while δ and λ are next state function δ: $D_A \rightarrow S$ and output function λ: $D_A \rightarrow Y$, where $D_A \subseteq S \times X$ is the specification domain. The machine A is *complete* if $D_A = S \times X$; otherwise, the machine is *partial*. In the usual way, the function λ is extended to input sequences with results in the set of output sequences. The set I_A is the set of all input sequences where a behavior of the FSM A is defined. The $\lambda(\alpha)$ denotes the output sequence that is produced by the FSM when an acceptable sequence α of the set I_A is submitted. As usual, given input sequence $x_1...x_k$ and output sequence $y_1...y_k$, the sequence $x_1/y_1, ..., x_k/y_k$ is called *a trace* of the A if $\lambda(x_1...x_k)= y_1...y_k$.

Given two FSMs $A =(S,X,Y,\delta,\lambda,D_A,s_0)$ and $B=(T,X,Y,\Delta,\Lambda,D_B,t_0)$, FSM A is said to be a *reduction* of FSM B, denoted $A\leq B$, if the set of traces of A is a subset of that of the FSM B. For partial deterministic FSMs the reduction relation coincides with a so-called quasi-equivalence relation [12]. Deterministic FSM A is a reduction of deterministic FSM B if and only if B is quasi-equivalent to A.

2.2 Composition of FSMs

We consider a system composed by several FSMs C_i, $i=1, ..., k$, as shown in Figure 1. We refer to symbols of alphabets X_i as to *external inputs*, to symbols of alphabets Y_i as to *external outputs* while referring to symbols of alphabets Z_{ij}, $i\neq j$, as to *internal actions*. In fact, some alphabets can be empty but the union of X_i (Y_i) over all $i\in I$ is not empty. We refer to the component FSM as to an *embedded FSM* if the component FSM has no external inputs and outputs. The system always has a single message in transit, i.e. the alphabets are pairwise disjoint and the environment submits the next input only when the system has produced an output to the previous input. Under this assumption, a component machine accepting an input may produce either an external or a single internal output. If the component machines fall into infinite internal dialog when an appropriate external input sequence is submitted we say the system falls into live-lock under the input sequence and its behavior is said to be not specified. If the behavior of one of component FSMs is not specified under a submitted input we also assume the system behavior is not specified. Under the above assumptions we can simulate a behavior of the composition under an external input sequence.

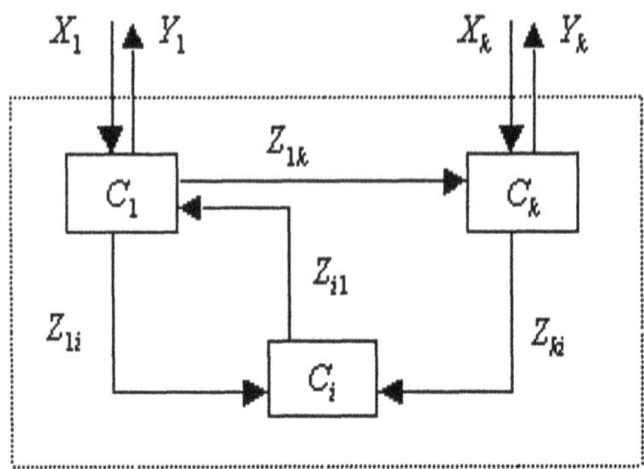

Figure 1. System of communicating FSMs.

Let a component FSM C_i have the set Q_i of states. Then the composite FSM is a FSM over the union of alphabets X_i and Y_i with the state space that is a subset of the Cartesian product of Q_i, $i \in I$. States of the Cartesian product are divided into stable and transient states. By definition, the initial state q_{10} ... q_{k0} is stable. Otherwise, the state is stable if it has been reached immediately after the system has produced an external output. We start from the initial state q_{10} ... q_{k0}. The algorithm for simulating a behavior of the system w.r.t. an external input sequence is based on the derivation of a partial reachability graph induced by the input sequence [5, 10] that then is projected onto external alphabets. The composite reference FSM $RM = \Diamond C_i$, $i=1,\ldots, k$, can be derived using the above procedure. In this case, we derive the global reachability graph [4].

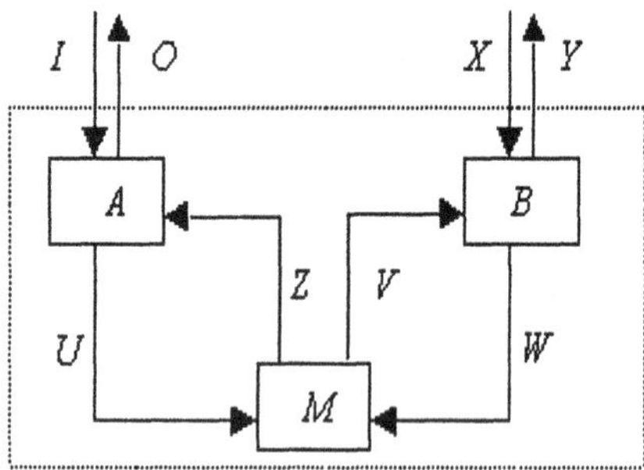

Figure 2. System under test.

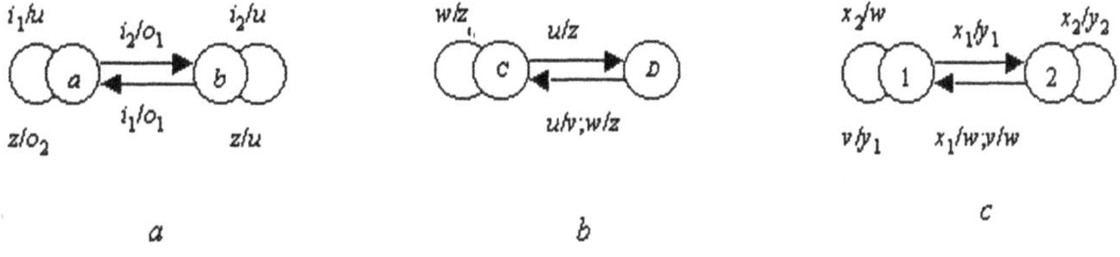

Figure 3. Component FSMs *A* (*a*), *M* (*b*) and *B* (*c*).

We illustrate the procedure by a simple working example that has communicating FSMs *A*, *B* and media *M* through which component machines *A* and *B* communicate (Figures 2 and 3). Media *M* has no external inputs and outputs and can be considered as an embedded component FSM. Consider external input sequence x_1x_1. When x_1 is applied at the initial state $aC1$ of the system the component *B* produces external output y_1 and enters state 2. Thus, the system produces the output y_1 and enters a stable state $aC2$ when the input x_1 is submitted. When the next input x_1 is applied to the reference system at stable state $aC2$ the component *B* produces internal output *w* and came back to state 1, i.e. the system enters a transient state $aC1$. The media *M* at state *C* replies with output *z* to input *w* and remains at state *C*, i.e. the system remains at the transient state $aC1$. Input *z* is then applied to *A* at state *a*; the *A* produces external output o_2, i.e. the system reaches the stable state $aC1$. The composite FSM is shown in Figure 4. However, we do not need to construct the composite FSM; the reference external output response to an external input sequence is derived by simulating a system behavior under the input sequence.

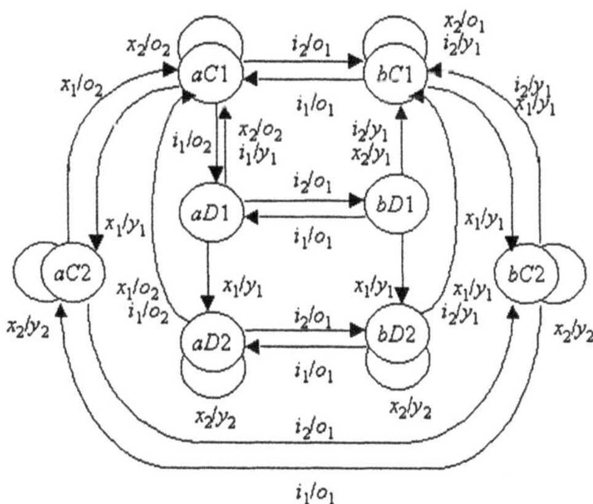

Figure 4. The composite FSM.

2.3 Fault domain

One important aspect of test generation is to specify an appropriate fault model. As mentioned above, it is natural to assume that the structure of the reference system is preserved in all potential implementations and at most one component FSM can be faulty [see, for example, 5, 13, 14, 15]. We refer to a FSM modeling the reference system as to the *reference* FSM while calling the *fault domain* the set $\Re$ of FSMs modeling all possible systems under test. As usual, we assume an implementation is completely specified, i.e. any input sequence can be applied to the implementation. Moreover, each component FSM can produce an error signal to the environment if an applied input is unexpected for the specification component FSM at a current state. The implementation FSM $IM \in \Re$ is called a *faulty* or a *nonconforming* implementation if the reference FSM is not a reduction of *IM*; otherwise it is a *conforming* implementation.

A *test suite* is a finite set of finite input sequences of the reference machine *RM*. A test suite, which detects any nonconforming implementation, is called a *complete* test suite w.r.t. the fault domain $\Re$. Thus, if a system under test is modeled by an FSM $IM \in \Re$ and is not detected by a complete test suite w.r.t. $\Re$ then one concludes that the reference system is a reduction of the system under test, i.e. a behavior of the system under test coincides with that of the reference system under any input sequence where the behavior of the reference system is specified.

In this paper, we are concerned about detecting output faults in implementations of component FSMs. A test suite is complete if it detects all output faults in the implementation of each component FSM. As a guide, we use a widely used test purpose for a system of communicating FSMs [16]. A test suite satisfying the test purpose must traverse each possible transition of each component FSM in the reference system. Test selection is performed in order to obtain a test suite satisfying the above test purpose such that the result test suite detects the maximum of output faults within implementations of component FSMs.

Our first step is to evaluate which output faults in the implementation of a component FSM can be detected by a test suite traversing each transition of the component that is involved in interaction with other component FSMs. To describe these faults we use an approach originally proposed in [8] for test minimization for an embedded component and developed in [10] for single output faults.

3. DETECTING OUTPUT FAULTS IN A COMPONENT MACHINE WITH AN EXTERNAL TEST CASE

We consider a reference system composed by k deterministic FSMs, as shown in Figure 1. Let α be an external test sequence, i.e. a sequence over external input alphabet. If we are concerned only about faults within a component FSM C_i we need to describe which output faults of the component FSM can be detected with the sequence α. We further assume that live-locks in the implementation system can be detected by a timer and show below that all the faults of the component FSM C_i detected by α can be described by a collection of finite subsets of output faults.

3.1 Detectable output faults

Our first step is to illustrate a relation between an external test case and output faults in a component machine, which can be detected with the test case. Consider the composition of FSMs A, B and M shown in Figure 2 and input sequence x_1x_2. Suppose that implementations of machines A and M are faulty-free while an implementation Imp_B of FSM B can have output faults. The reference composition has an external output response y_1y_2 to x_1x_2. We are interested which faults in the implementation Imp_B of the component FSM B can be detected with the external test case x_1x_2.

Let x_1 be applied when component FSMs A, M and B are at their initial states a, C and 1. The implementation FSM Imp_B produces y_1, y_2 or w to the input x_1 and enters state 2. If the implementation machine Imp_B at the initial state produces the output y_2 to x_1 then the overall implementation system produces an unexpected external output response y_2 to the test case x_1. Therefore, if the Imp_B has the output fault $(1, x_1, y_2)$ then the implementation system is detected with the test case x_1 independently of its other output faults. Let the implementation machine Imp_B at the initial state produce the output w to x_1 that then is applied to the machine M at the initial state C. The machine M produces the output z to w and remains at the state C. The output z is applied to the machine A at the state a and A produces an unexpected output response o_2 to x_1. Thus, if the Imp_B has the output fault $(1, x_1, w)$ then an implementation system is detected with the test case x_1 independently of other output faults.

Let the implementation machine Imp_B at the initial state produce the reference output y_1 to x_1 and enter state 2. We then apply the next input x_2 to the implementation system. The implementation machine Imp_B at the state 2 produces y_1, y_2 or w to x_2. If the Imp_B produces y_1 the overall system produces unexpected output y_1 to x_2. Thus, if the Imp_B has output fault $(2, x_2, y_1)$ it is detected with the test case x_1x_2. If the Imp_B at the state 2 produces the output w to x_2, it remains at the state 2, and then after some transitions where Imp_B is not involved the implementation system produces o_2 to x_2. Thus, when the Imp_B has the output fault $(2, x_2, w)$ it is detectable with the test case x_1x_2. The construction is illustrated in Figure 5 where wrong external outputs are shown in bold.

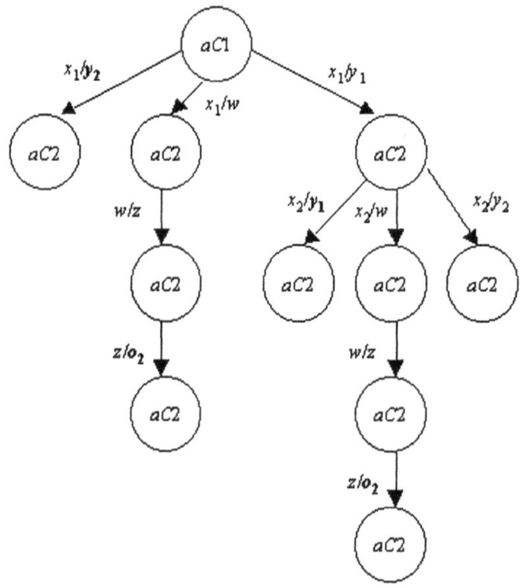

Figure 5. An example of the detection of output faults of the component FSM with an external test case.

The above example clearly shows that given an external test case and a component under test, we can construct the set of all output faults detected within the component machine with the given test case. However, the number of these sets may be exponential. We obtain most interesting case when an external test case *completely tests* an appropriate transition. These faults are detected by a test case independently of other faults within the implementation of the component FSM. In fact, such a test case detects $|Y|^{|Q\times X|-1}$ output faults where Q is the state set while X and Y being the component's input and output alphabets. Here we notice that to completely check a transition usually it is not enough to traverse this transition.

Given an external input sequence α and a set Out_i of output faults of the component FSM C_i, the set Out_i is *detectable* with α if any implementation system where the set of output faults of an implementation of the C_i contains Out_i, has an unexpected output response to α at Points of Observation (POs).

If a test case completely checks a component transition then for short, we include the only transition into the set Out_i.

3.2 Constructing the set of detectable output faults

Given a component FSM C_i that can be faulty, and an external input sequence $x_1 \ldots x_m$, we first derive an acceptor $F(C_i, x_1 \ldots x_m)$ that represents all possible composition traces when an implementation of each component machine different from C_i is faulty-free. By a designated state *Fail* the acceptor recognizes those traces that imply an unexpected behavior of the composition. The acceptor is derived based on the component FSMs and is then projected onto Input/Output (I/O) pairs of the component C_i in usual way [10]. I/O pairs of the components different from C_i are replaced with the empty word. To determinize the obtained acceptor we use a subset construction and replace each subset having the state *Fail* by a designated state *Fail* without outgoing transitions. Moreover, each state, for which there exists an input that takes the projection only to the *Fail* state, is replaced with the *Fail* state. The expected external output response $y_1 \ldots y_m$ to input sequence $x_1 \ldots x_m$ is obtained by simulating a behavior of the reference system applying the input sequence.

Formally, the state set of the acceptor $F(C_i, x_1 \ldots x_m)$ is a subset P of $Q_1 \times \ldots \times Q_{i-1} \times Q_i \times Q_{i+1} \times \ldots \times Q_k \times \{0, \ldots, m\}$. The acceptor is constructed for inputs $x_1, \ldots, x_m$ in succession. States of the set P are divided into stable and transient states. By definition, the initial state $q_{10} \ldots q_{k0}0$ is stable. Otherwise, the state is stable if it has an incoming transition with an external output. The stable states cannot be merged with transient states. Two transient states with the same names in the segment for the same external input are merged if they have an incoming transition labeled with a pair with the same output part. We start from the initial state $(q_{10} \ldots q_{k0})0$.

Given a state $(q_{1t} \ldots q_{kt})j$ and I/O pair a/b of the component C_p, the a/b takes the acceptor from state $(q_{1t} \ldots q_{pt} \ldots q_{kt})j$ to a stable state $(q_{1t} \ldots q'_{pt} \ldots q_{kt})(j+1)$ if b is the expected external output of the system to input x_{j+1}. Here q'_{pj} is the state where the input a takes the component FSM C_p from the state q_{pi}. If b is an unexpected external output of the system to input x_{j+1} or a is an unexpected input at state q_{pi} then the a/b takes the acceptor from state $(q_{1t} \ldots q_{kt})j$ to the designated state *Fail*. If b is an internal output of the component machine C_j then the a/b takes the acceptor from state $(q_{1t} \ldots q_{jt} \ldots q_{kt})j$ to a transient state $(q_{1t} \ldots q'_{jt} \ldots q_{kt})j$. The a/b also takes the acceptor to the state *Fail* if there appears a cycle labeled only with internal actions in the acceptor. The only difference between the component FSM C_i of our interest and other component FSMs is that we consider all possible outputs to the input a when a is applied to the C_j which keep the deterministic implementation of C_i, while considering only the reference output for all other component FSMs. We denote $D(C_i,x_1\ldots x_m)$ the deterministic projection of $F(C_i,x_1\ldots x_m)$ onto I/O pairs of the component FSM C_i. To reduce the projection we replace with the *Fail* state each state for which there exists an input that takes the projection only to the *Fail* state.

By construction, the acceptor $D(C_i,x_1\ldots x_m)$ is an acyclic graph and comprises complete information about all sets of detectable output faults of the component FSM of our interest.

We say a state p of the acceptor $D(C_i,x_1\ldots x_m)$ different from the *Fail* state is *deterministically reachable* from the initial state if for each prefix α of the input sequence taking the acceptor from the initial state to state p there is the only output sequence β such that α/β does not take the acceptor from the initial state to the *Fail* state.

For each state p deterministically reachable from the initial state in the acceptor $D(C_i,x_1\ldots x_m)$ and every branch from the state p to the *Fail* state, we derive the set Out_i including into the set all transitions of the branch. To reduce the obtained collection we remove each item that comprises another item and denote $Out(C_i,x_1\ldots x_m)$ the obtained set system.

Theorem 3.1. Given an external input sequence α, a nonconforming implementation Imp_i of C_i is detectable with α if and only if it has a set of output faults that contains an item of the set system $Out(C_i,\alpha)$.

In fact, an implementation system with component FSMs C_1, ..., C_{i-1}, Imp_i, C_{i+1}, ..., C_k is detected by α if and only if it has a trace that takes the acceptor $F(C_i,\alpha)$ from the initial state to the designated state *Fail*. The latter is possible if and only if the component machine Imp_i has the set of output faults that contains I/O pairs of the component FSM which occur through the corresponding projection of the path, i.e. has the set of output faults that contains an item of the set system $Out(C_i,\alpha)$.

The set system $Out(C_i,\alpha)$ can be reduced if some test cases are already included in the test suite. In this case, constructing the acceptor we do not have to consider at least all wrong I/O pairs of the component C_i of the transitions completely tested with other test cases. We denote $Out(C_i,\alpha/T)$ such a system where T is the part of a test suite that is already derived. For example, in our working example, $Out(A, i_2i_2i_2/\{i_2x_1x_1i_2\})$ is empty.

4. APPLICATION TO TESTING COMMUNICATING FSMS

Theorem 3.1 provides a guide of what part of the behavior of a component FSM can be tested with a given test suite. The above result can be used in various applications, which range from test selection, test suite minimization to derivation of diagnostic tests for a component FSM. Test minimization w.r.t. arbitrary faults in the implementation of a component FSM has been considered in [8, 17]. In this paper, we consider how the above construction can be used for test minimization w.r.t. output faults and for selecting test cases.

4.1 Test selection for a system of communicating FSMs based on a composite FSM

When a test suite is derived for a system of communicating FSMs the test purpose usually is to traverse every possible transition of each specification component FSM at least once. Test selection is performed based on the test purpose. We here propose how to reach the test purpose while having a test suite with a higher fault coverage. The technique is based on the composite FSM; however, it can easily be modified in order to use only parts of the composite machine with a predefined length of input sequence.

In the paper [16] the method of test derivation based on the composite FSM is presented. The idea of the method is as follows.

Every transition of a component FSM is involved in a number of global transitions. We assign a distinguished color for every transition of each component FSM and use this color for each global transition where the component transition is involved. To reach the test purpose we need to find a minimum set of input sequences of the composite FSM, which cover all the colors.

Using the results of the previous section we can associate with each test case the set of output faults within a component under test which are detected with the test sequence. For example, given an input sequence, we can consider the number of completely tested transitions as scope of the sequence. In this case, we are required to derive a minimum set of input sequences with maximum scope, which cover all the colors. Using the above technique we will reach the test purpose and simultaneously the obtained test suite will have the good fault coverage, in particular, w.r.t. output faults in implementations of component FSMs.

Consider the composition of three FSMs Imp_A, M and B and a test case i_2. By direct inspection (Figure 6), one can assure the test case traversing the transition (a, i_2) within the component FSM A does not completely check this transition.

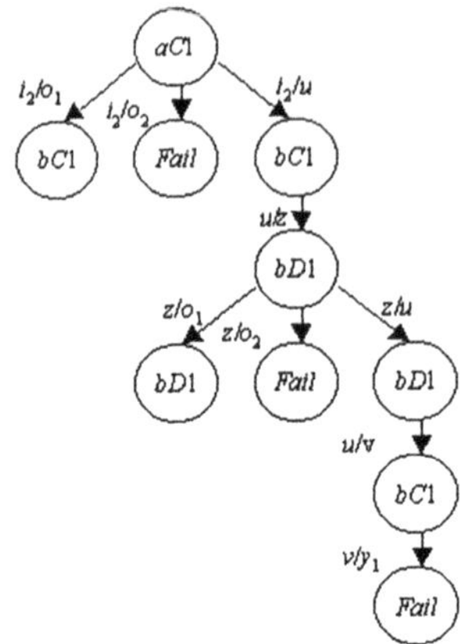

Figure 6. The test case traversing the transition (a, i_2).

If the implementation Imp_A of the component FSM A has two output faults (a, i_2, u) and (b, z, o_1), i.e. Imp_A is a submachine of the FSM shown in Figure 7, then the composition of Imp_A, B and M has the reference output o_1 to i_2. However, this composition reaches the state $bD1$ that is different from the state $bC1$ of the reference composition. Therefore, to detect this fault we can combine a non-deterministic FSM presented in Figure 7 with component FSMs B and M and to derive an input sequence distinguishing reference state $bC1$ from the state $bD1$ of the obtained composition.

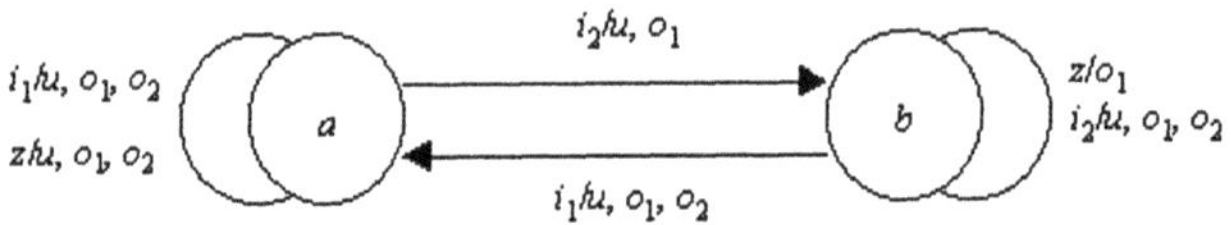

Figure 7. The implementation Imp_A.

As it is shown in Figure 8, in our case, such a sequence exists and is equal to i_2i_2. The reference system at the state $bC1$ has the output y_1y_1 to i_2i_2 while for the composition where the output fault (a, i_2, u) occurs, we have at the state $bD1$ outputs o_1, o_2 or y_1 to i_2. If the faulty implementation produces the reference output y_1 to i_2 then it produces the unexpected output o_1 to the next i_2, since at state b the implementation component FSM Imp_A produces o_1 to z (Figure 7). Therefore, the transition (a, i_2) is completely tested by the test case $i_2i_2i_2$.

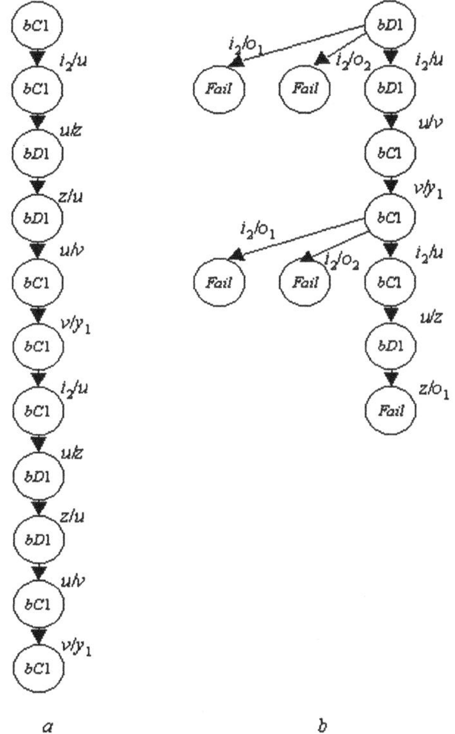

Figure 8. An input sequence distinguishing the reference state $bC1$ (a) from the state $bD1$ (b) of the composition where an implementation of component FSM A has output faults (a, i_2, u) and (b, z, o_1).

The method for deriving input sequences distinguishing states of two non-deterministic FSMs is proposed in [18]. However, if the reference state cannot be distinguished from the given state of the obtained composition we do not guarantee that it cannot be distinguished at all. Possibly, the cause is the compact representation of all possible implementations as a unique non-deterministic FSM. In this case, one can try to add to a given test case all input sequences of length up to an appropriate integer, say two, and check if the transition can be completely tested. If no then we give up to completely test the transition and add nothing to the given test case. The latter approach can also be applied in the case when the reference composite FSM is not derived.

The procedure can be shortened when some of test cases are already included into the test suite. In this case, we are not to check transitions, which are completely tested by included test sequences.

For our working example, a test suite completely checking all transitions of the component FSM A is $TS = \{x_2i_1x_1x_1;\ i_2i_1x_1x_2i_2;\ i_2x_1x_1i_2i_2;\ i_2x_1x_2i_1;\ i_2i_2i_2\}$.

By direct inspection, one can assure the same test suite checks each transition of FSM M and FSM B.

4.2 Test suite minimization w.r.t. output faults of component FSMs

When a test suite has been derived from the reference composite FSM [see, for example, 19, 20] it can be expected to be redundant when only one component FSM can be faulty. In this section, we propose a procedure for test suite minimization without a loss of its fault coverage w.r.t. output faults of the component FSMs. In particular, the procedure can be used for minimization of interoperability tests [21, 22].

Given a complete test suite w.r.t. an appropriate fault model, we can minimize it without loss of its fault coverage based of Theorem 3.1 under an assumption that at most component FSM C_i can be faulty.

Theorem 4.1. Given a complete test suite TS for the reference FSM $RM=\Diamond C_j$ w.r.t. the fault domain $\mathfrak{I}$ and proper subset $T\subset TS$, let $\mathfrak{R}$ be the set containing each FSM of the fault domain $\mathfrak{I}$ that is a composition of the component FSMs C_1, ..., C_{i-1}, Imp_i, C_{i+1}, ..., C_k where Imp_i is an implementation of C_i, possibly with output faults. If each set of output faults detected by test cases of the test suite TS also is detected with an appropriate test case of the set T then the set T is a complete test suite w.r.t. the fault domain $\mathfrak{R}$.

In other words, if a proper subset T of a given test suite TS satisfies the conditions of Theorem 4.1 then T and TS detect the same set of output faults within the component FSM C_i. Here we notice that conditions of Theorem 4.1 are sufficient but not necessary. The reason is the sets of detectable output faults may be changed if some sequences are already included into the test suite.

We now propose a straightforward procedure for test minimization for a system of communicating FSMs under an assumption that at most one component FSM can be faulty. Given a test suite TS for a system of communicating FSMs and the sets $Out_\alpha(C_i)$, $\alpha\in TS$, where $Out_\alpha(C_i)$ is a set of output faults of C_i detected with α, the procedure returns subset T of TS that detects the same set of faulty implementations of each component FSM C_i as the initial test suite TS. We enumerate test cases in $TS = \{\alpha_1, ..., \alpha_k\}$ and iteratively for each test case α_j, consider $T = TS\backslash\{\alpha_j\}$. If $Out(C_i,\alpha_j/T)$ is empty then we can delete α_j from the current test suite TS without a loss of its completeness.

Here we notice that in the proposed approach we do not enumerate all the output faults, a number of which is exponential. We try to treat output faults in parallel. However, the result returned by the above procedure usually depends on the order of the test cases in the set *TS*. Just now we can only recommend to try first the test case that completely tests a maximum number of transitions. Another procedure based on a Boolean matrix [8] can be proposed for a test suite minimization. In this case, the problem of determining a minimum subset of a given test with the same fault coverage reduces to the problem of deriving a minimum cost cover of a Boolean matrix.

Given test suite $TS = \{x_2i_1x_1x_1;\ i_2i_1x_1x_2i_2;\ i_2x_1x_1i_2i_2;\ i_2x_1x_2i_1;\ i_2i_2i_2\}$ for our working example, by direct inspection one can assure that its subset $\{x_2i_1x_1x_1;\ i_2x_1x_1i_2;\ i_2x_1x_2i_1\}$ detects the same set of output faults in implementations of the component FSMs. Moreover, the test case $i_2x_1x_2i_1$ cannot be replaced with $i_2i_1x_1x_2i_2$ without a loss of its fault coverage, because the latter does not check a transition (a, i_2) completely, despite of the fact that both subsets of the initial test suite traverse the same set of transitions in each component FSM.

5. CONCLUSION

In this paper, given a system of communicating FSMs, we establish a relation between an external test case and output faults of a component machine, which can be detected with this test case. We also demonstrate an application of the established relation for test selection and minimization for communicating FSMs. The relation can also be useful when calculating fault coverage of a given external test suite w.r.t. faults within the implementation of a component FSM [23] as well as when deriving diagnostic tests for output and transfer faults of a component FSM.

REFERENCES

[1] J.-C. Fernandez, C. Jard, T. Jeron, and C. Viho, *Using on-the-fly verification techniques for the generation of test suites.* In CAV, LINCS 1102, USA, July, 1996.

[2] Cavalli, A., Lee, D., Rinderknecht, C., and Zaidi, F., *Hit-or-Jump: An algorithm for embedded testing with applications to IN services.* Proceedings of Joint Inter. Conf. FORTE/PSTV99, pp: 41-58.

[3] Petrenko, A., Yevtushenko, N. and v.Bochmann, G. (1996), *Testing deterministic implementations from their nondeterministic specifications.* Proceedings of 9th IWTCS, pp: 125-140.

[4] Petrenko A., Yevtushenko, N., and v. Bochmann, G. (1996), *Fault models for testing in context.* Proceedings of Joint Inter. Conf. FORTE/PSTV96.

[5] Lima, L.P., and Cavalli, A.R. (1997), *A pragmatic approach to generating test sequences for embedded systems.* Proceedings of 10th IWTCS, pp: 288-307.

[6] Lima, L.P., and Cavalli, A.R. (1997), *Application of embedded testing methods to service validation.* Second IEEE Intern. Conf. on Formal Engineering methods.

[7] A. Petrenko, N. Yevtushenko, *Testing faults in embedded components.* Proceedings of 10th IWTCS, pp: 272-287.

[8] Yevtushenko, N., Cavalli, A.R., and Lima, L.P. (1998), *Test minimization for testing in context.* Proceedings of 11th IWTCS, pp: 127-145.

[9] Lima, L.P. (1998), *A pragmatic method to generate test sequences for embedded systems.* Ph.D.Thesis. Insitut National des Telecommunications, Evry, France.

[10] Cavalli, A.R., Prokopenko, S., Yevtushenko, N. (2000), *Fault detection power of a wide test suite for a system of communicating FSMs.* Proceedings of 13th IWTCS, pp: 35-56.

[11] Lee, D., Sabnani, K.K., Kristol, D.M., and Paul, S. (1996), *Conformance testing of protocols specified as communicating finite state machines - a guided random walk based approach.* IEEE Transactions on Communications, 44(5): 631-640.

[12] Gill, A., *Introduction to automata theory.* Mc Graww-Hill, NY, 1962.

[13] Petrenko, A., Yevtushenko, N., v. Bochmann, G., and Dssouli, R. (1996), *Testing in context: Framework and test derivation.* Computer Communications Journal, Special issue on protocol engineering, pp: 1236-1249.

[14] Information technology (1991), *Open systems interaction. Conformance testing methodology and framework.* International standard IS-9646.

[15] Petrenko, A., Yevtushenko, N., and Dssouli, R. (1994), *FSM based strategies for testing communicating FSMs.* Proceedings of 7th IWTCS.

[16] C. Besse, A. Cavalli, and D. Lee, *Optimization Techniques and Automatic Test Generation for TCP Protocols.* IEEE Automated Software Engineering, Conference ASE'99, Cocoa Beach, Florida (USA), 12-15 October 1999.

[17] Yevtushenko, N., Cavalli, A.R., and Anido, R. (1999), *Test suite minimization for embedded nondeterministic finite state machines.* Proceedings of 12th IWTCS, pp: 237-250.

[18] I. Koufareva, *Using non-deterministic FSMs for test suite derivation.* Ph.D.Thesis, Tomsk State University, Russia, 2000 (In Russian).

[19] Chow, T.S. (1978), *Test software design modeled by finite state machines.* IEEE Transactions on Software Engineering, 4(3): 178-187.

[20] Fujiwara, S., v.Bochmann,G., Khendek, F., Amalou, M., and Ghendamsi, A. (1991), *Test selection based on finite state models.* IEEE Transactions on Software Engineering, 17(6): 591-603.

[21] C.Besse, A. Cavalli, M. Kim, F. Zaidi, *Two methods for interoperability tests generation. An application to the TCP/IP protocol.* Research report N01002-LOR, INT, June 2001.

[22] C. Viho, S. Barbin and L. Tanguy, *Towards a formal framework for interoperability testing.* Proceedings of Joint Inter. Conf. FORTE2001, pp: 53-68.

[23] J.Zhu, S.T.Vuong, and S.T.Chanson, *Evaluation of test coverage for embedded system testing.* Proceedings of 11th IWTCS, pp: 111-126.

INVITED TALK II

HARDWARE/SOFTWARE INTEGRATION TESTING FOR THE NEW AIRBUS AIRCRAFT FAMILIES

Jan Peleska
Center for Computing Technologies TZI
University of Bremen, Germany
jp@tzi.de

Abstract In this presentation, we describe the methods and techniques currently applied in the test of the cabin management controllers for the Airbus families A318, A340-500/600 and A380. The hardware-in-the-loop testing environment is described and we explain, how an integrated approach for software testing, hardware/software integration and system testing allows to re-use test specifications on these different levels. Moreover, the concepts for automatic test data generation and test evaluation, as well as the utilisation of generic test specifications are introduced. Our approach has been elaborated by research and development teams at Airbus Deutschland, KID-Systeme, Verified Systems International and the Author's research group at the University of Bremen. Tool support is provided by the RT-Tester real-time test tool developed by Verified Systems and the University of Bremen.

Keywords: Airbus Cabin Communication System, Software Integration Testing, Hardware/Software Integration Testing, Test Automation

1. INTRODUCTION

Motivation. In this article, we describe state-of-the-art concepts and novel approaches to embedded systems testing for avionics control systems. These are currently applied by Verified Systems International GmbH in collaboration with the author's research group at Bremen University for the test of the Cabin Management System CIDS, designed for the Airbus aircraft families A340-500/600 and A318. CIDS has been developed by KID-Systeme in Buxtehude, a subsidiary of Airbus Deutschland.

In the eighties and early nineties of the last century, the test of computerised avionics control systems still required a high degree of manual interaction: On system integration level, the inputs to the system under test (SUT), the checking and recording of SUT reactions, as well as the evaluation of test results were performed interactively by testing personnel, and a large portion of the test documentation consisted of paper listings filled in and maintained in a manual way. Only some external systems which interacted with the SUT in the real operational environment but were not available for SUT testing were replaced by automatic computer simulations. However, the variation possibilities for the behaviour modelled by these simulations were still limited and required a considerable amount of manual interaction. On HW/SW integration level, several manufacturers of aircraft controllers already applied *hardware-in-the-loop testing*: The stimulation of inputs to the SUT as well as the simulation of external systems were performed by computers acting as test drivers, and the SUT reactions were recorded automatically. A joint time base for stimulated inputs and recorded outputs allowed to analyse the causal relationships between the test events observed. However, the generation of inputs was mostly based on sequential test scripting languages: Each input to the SUT had to be "programmed" into the test script in a manual way, and the scripts processed these inputs on a one-at-a-time basis, which did not allow to generate complex scenarios of simultaneous inputs on several SUT interfaces. Moreover, the recorded SUT reactions had to be checked manually against the applicable requirements specifications.

Like KID-Systeme, some manufacturers changed their testing approach within the last decade towards hardware-in-the-loop testing enhanced by new techniques in order to achieve a higher degree of automation. These – often very ambitious – campaigns were motivated by the following problems:

- The growing complexity of applications increased the amount of test cases needed to achieve sufficient test coverage in a considerable way.
- The growing demand for customer-specific modifications and extensions increased the frequency of new system releases which have to be accompanied by regression testing.

An analysis of these problems performed by KID-Systeme, Verified Systems and the author's research group at the University of Bremen resulted in the integrated SW- and HW/SW-integration testing environment described in this article.

Overview. In Section 2, we give a more detailed analysis of the problems listed above and describe the testing approach and tool concept resulting from these considerations. This is the main part of this article and illustrates the main ideas which according to our understanding have been crucial for the success of our approach. The full hardware-in-the-loop test configuration is sketched in section 3. Section 4 contains the conclusion.

Background and Related Work. From the application-oriented point of view, the work presented in this article is based on the author's experience with the development of test systems for avionics controllers in the early nineties:

- Software integration test system for an earlier version of CIDS developed for the Airbus A330/340,

- Hardware-in-the-loop testing environment for a BMW-Rolls Royce aircraft engine controller.

The experiences gained from these systems resulted in the development of the RT-Tester system [18] which is used for the testing approach described in this article and for other testing projects in the fields of railway, space and automotive control systems. Reports about other industrial applications can be found in [12] (test of tramway crossing control system) and [16] (test of fault-tolerant computer for the International Space Station).

From the theoretical point of view, the problems of automatic test generation, test execution in hard real-time and test evaluation have been investigated by the author and his research team at Bremen University in collaboration with several other scientists. In [11, 13, 14] the theory for automated testing of reactive systems without timing requirements are described. The foundations of the theory are based on Hennessy's testing equivalence elaborated for process algebras with acceptance tree semantics [3]. For real-time testing, our formalisms are based on the semantics of Timed CSP (Communicating Sequential Processes) as given by Schneider [20]. Comprehensive introductions to CSP are given in [5, 17]. For the associated algorithms implemented in the RT-Tester tool we made use of a theorem about the executability of CSP specifications in hard real-time, which has been formulated by the author [15] and established in complete form by Oliver Meyer [9].

The field of test automation based on formal methods is currently investigated world-wide by several research groups. We name [1, 10, 19, 21] as a set of representative publications which also give an extensive overview of existing publications in this research area.

The examples from CIDS presented in this article have been simplified in order to focus on the underlying concepts. See [7] for a more detailed description of CIDS.

2. TESTING APPROACH AND TOOL ENVIRONMENT

To overcome the two main problems about growing testing complexity and regression testing workload described in the introduction, five main goals were defined and implemented in the testing environment. These will be described in the subsequent paragraphs. Throughout this section, we will refer to the organisational structure of the testing environment, as represented in Figure 1.

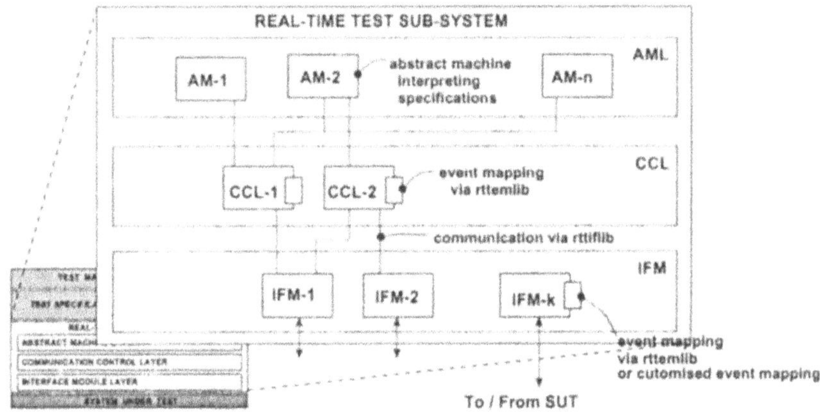

Figure 1. Organisational Structure of the Test System.

2.1 Re-use of specifications on different integration levels

Deficiencies of the conventional approach. The classical approach to embedded systems testing used different testing environments and different test specification techniques on module test, SW integration test, HW/SW integration test and system integration test level. Typically, the specifications used for module and SW integration testing referred to SW functions and data structures, while the higher integration test levels referred to events observable at various system interfaces. As a consequence, the test results achieved on these different integration levels were very difficult to compare, since the terms used in software tests had to be translated to associated terms about data passed along system interfaces. Moreover, it was impossible to re-use test specification parts on different levels without translating them into other representations.

Re-use by Interface Abstraction. The testing efficiency can be considerably increased if a single set of *interface abstractions* is used from software integration (or even module) testing level to system integration. This allows specification parts referring to system interfaces only to be re-used on all test levels. (Of course, internal software interfaces manipulated or monitored during software integration testing cannot be accessed by system integration testing.) For the RT-Tester system we choose CSP-style channel specifications for interface definition syntax on all integration levels. The abstract channel specification is mapped onto concrete interfaces that depend on the test integration level. To facilitate the setup of different test configurations, the test system is structured into three conceptual layers (see Figure 1): The *abstract machine layer AML* contains the mechanisms to create test data and check SUT responses (see the more detailed description below). This is done on the abstract level of CSP events, and each abstract machine is equipped with a CSP channel interface specification. The *interface modules (IFM)* are used to map abstract CSP events onto concrete SUT interfaces and vice versa. The *communication control layer (CCL)* relays events between abstract machines and interface modules. Whenever an interface is accessed on different test integration levels, the same CSP channel description is used: we only need to exchange the associated IFM according to each level's interface semantics.

Example: Interface from Flight Attendant Panel to CIDS Reading Lights Application. The CIDS Reading Lights application controls the switching of reading lights throughout the Airbus cabin: External systems, e. g., control panels installed for the cabin crew, will send reading lights control commands to the CIDS controller which reacts by switching the lights associated with the respective command. The interfaces involved in the operational environment have been sketched on the left-hand side of Figure 2. For the *"Reading Lights Off"* command, the CSP channel representation for these inputs to the SUT is given as

```
fap_id_t = { 1..10 }
channel FAP_key_cil_rl_off : fap_id_t
```

A test event `FAP_key_cil_rl_off.1` represents the situation where at flight attendant panel (FAP) 1, the "Reading Lights Off" key has been pressed.

For software integration testing, we observe that the Reading Lights Control software component accesses key events using a driver function call `keyEvent = getKey()`. This function is exchanged for testing purposes by a stub with identical interface, which reads the `keyEvent` data object to be returned to the caller from a shared memory buffer (see right-hand side of Figure 2). An interface module accepts abstract CSP channel events like `FAP_key_cil_rl_off.1` which have been generated by abstract machines simulating user interactions at various FAPs, transforms them into new `keyEvent` data objects which are placed into the shared memory buffer.

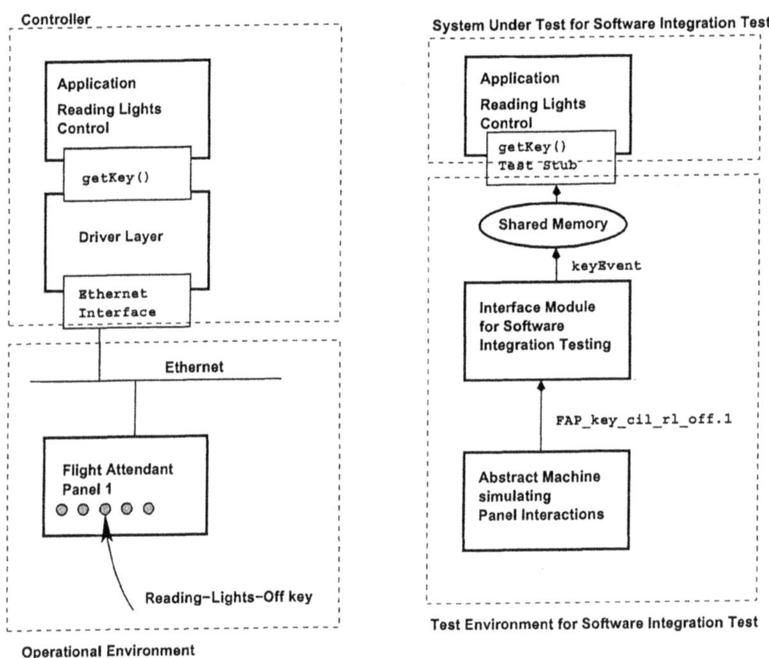

Figure 2. Interfaces in the operational system versus software integration test interfaces.

For HW/SW integration testing, we would like to utilise the same abstract machines, but have to take into account that the interfaces to be accessed on this integration level is given by an Ethernet-based protocol (see left-hand side of Figure 3). A new IFM accepts the same CSP events from abstract machines. Now the CSP events are transformed into telegrams encoding the key event, and the telegrams are transmitted using TCP/IP.

For system integration testing (see right-hand side of Figure 3), the CSP interface and the generating abstract machines still remain the same, but now another IFM transforms them into pointing device commands passed to the panel via serial link. The pointing commands have the same effect on the panel as the touch screen interactions performed by users.

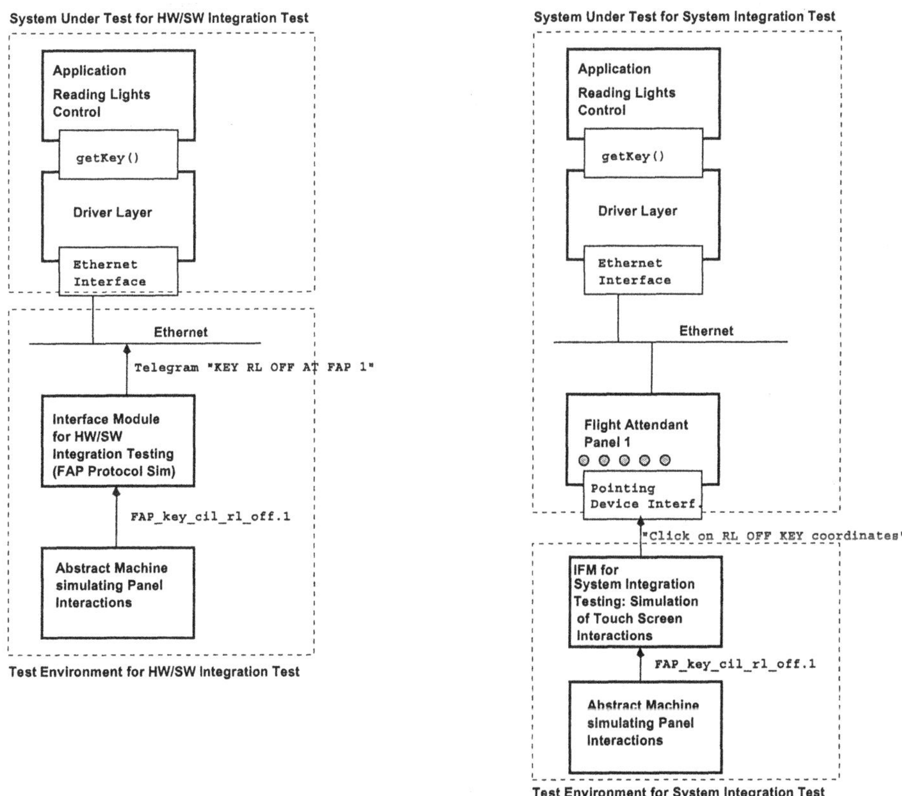

Figure 3. Interfaces for HW/SW integration and system integration test.

2.2 Automatic test data generation from specifications

Deficiencies of the conventional approach. Many severe errors in control systems are only detected when special sequences of inputs are exercised on the system. Typically, these sequences occur in real operational situations, but – due to a lack of application expertise – are overlooked or taxed as "unrealistic" by the developers and testers involved, so that these situations are neither covered properly in the design nor in the test suites. A major cause for this problem is given by the sequential programming language style of many test scripting languages, which makes the generation of combinatorial patterns for input sequences a very tedious and time-consuming task to perform.

State machine based test data generation. Instead of defining test data in an explicit way, it should be automatically created from a set of "generation rules", so that many different combinations of stimuli can be derived from a small set of rules. An appealing approach is to use state machines to specify these rules: The possible sequences of inputs and outputs which may be generated by the SUT interacting with its environment may be regarded as words of a formal language, and it is well known (see [8]) that automata can be used to check whether given words are members of a specific language. For test generation, we just turn this concept upside-down, starting with timed state machines modelling the environment behaviour to be used in a test case and interpreting a machine-readable representation of the state machine to generate legal words, that is, legal traces of inputs to the SUT which may also depend on SUT outputs and timing conditions before they are triggered. This basic approach has been investigated by several research groups (see the bibliography below) using various formalisms for timed state machines or transition systems. The results of Meyer [9] show that also in presence of real-time conditions the language generated by the timed traces (i. e. the sequence of communications tagged with time stamps) remains regular. Therefore these state machines can be interpreted without backtracking and in bounded time, so that the principle is suitable for hard real-time testing with on-the-fly test data generation.

Example: Creation of combinatorial event sequences. The following example has been developed for a situation where *"Reading Lights On"* and *"Reading Lights Off"* commands should be tested while choosing different panels for creation of the command inputs. These commands can be issued fro the flight attendant panels introduced above and additional attendant panels (AAP) residing on different flight decks at specific bus addresses and ports. The CSP process `RL_TEST` below performs the data generation in real-time, making use of two subordinate processes `SELECT_FAP_EVENT(chan)` and `SELECT_AAP_EVENT(chan)`: At first the process waits for a time interval specified by timer `rl_timer`. After this an event `FAP_key_cil_rl_on.<id>` is generated (in auxiliary process `SELECT_FAP_EVENT(chan)`), where the internal choice operator `|~|` denotes nondeterministic selection of an id parameter from the set `fap_id_t`. After another waiting interval, auxiliary process `SELECT_AAP_EVENT(chan)` selects an event `AAP_key_cil_rl_off.<d>.<b>.<a>`, where the triple (d, b, a) is chosen nondeterministically as specified by the nested `|~|` construct. After this, process `RL_TEST` starts another recursion.

In the RT-Tester system, the choice operators are evaluated to select data from the specified ranges in an automatic way. When a state is revisited, the test system selects new data tuples from the choice sets. The algorithm is designed as a combination of random choices and systematic coverage of branches which have not yet been chosen. As a consequence, `RL_TEST` will generate the more of ON/OFF events the longer it runs. Timers may be associated with random intervals, allowing to gain higher coverage in the time domain, if certain WAIT-situations are revisited.

```
channel FAP_key_cil_rl_on : fap_id_t
DECKS = { 0..1 }
ADDRESS = { 1..15 }
AAP_PORT = { 0..1 }
channel AAP_key_cil_rl_off : DECKS.ADDRESS.AAP_PORT

RL_TEST =
    WAIT(rl_timer);
    SELECT_FAP_EVENT(FAP_key_cil_rl_on);
    WAIT(rl_timer);
    SELECT_AAP_EVENT(AAP_key_cil_rl_off);
    RL_TEST

SELECT_FAP_EVENT(chan) =
    (|~| id : fap_id_t @ chan!id -> SKIP)

SELECT_AAP_EVENT(chan) =
    (|~| d:DECKS @ (|~| b:ADDRESS @ (|~| a:AAP_PORT @ chan!d.b.a -> SKIP)))
```

2.3 Automatic evaluation against specifications

Automatic generation of test data may lead to millions of communications between testing environment and SUT during a single test execution. While it is desirable to stimulate and record such large numbers of testing events, their manual evaluation will be infeasible in most cases. As a consequence, the success of the testing approach depends on possibilities for automatic evaluation. Formally speaking, correctness conditions can always be expressed by assertions about the timed traces (i. e. the sequence of communications tagged with time stamps) observed during test executions. These assertions may be expressed as logical formulae (e. g., a variant of temporal logic or trace logic) or equivalently as a collection of state machines admitting only those traces which are compliant with the assertions.

Observe that the most powerful assertion about the SUT is given by the requirements and design specifications. If they are available in a formal and machine-readable representation, the test evaluation problem is completely solved.

Observe further that for regression testing in the real-time domain, the test execution log (i. e., the recorded timed trace) of a previous test is unsuitable as a reference for regression testing: Especially in the case of complex controllers with many interfaces, the behaviour as it appears at the SUT interface will always be nondeterministic to a certain degree, for example due to timing jitters and internal scheduling decisions which cannot be observed during the test. As a consequence, a one-to-one comparison with previous execution results will nearly always fail. Instead, checking should be performed against assertions which are liberal enough to admit legal deviations in the regression run which are consistent with the applicable specifications.

2.4 Test configurations as distributed systems

A second problem with conventional test scripting languages consists in the fact that – similar to sequential programming languages – they encourage testers do elaborate test cases where one interface is stimulated or observed at a time. As a consequence, errors that only occur if certain events occur simultaneously will not be detected by the testing team. Moreover, it is often impossible to monitor large numbers of SUT output interfaces in parallel during the test execution. Under these circumstances, errors which are caused by instabilities at interfaces which should *not* be affected by certain operations are often overlooked. These observations motivate a testing approach where the testing environment is designed as a distributed system and where all forms of parallelism that are possible in the real operational environment can occur in the testing environment, too. This approach is modelled by a network of timed state machines operating in parallel. Each machine may act on certain SUT input interfaces, monitor and check SUT outputs and communicate with other state machines in order to exchange information about the current status of the test execution.

2.5 Generic test specifications

Today, many control systems can be configured by tables defining "software switches" which influence the behaviour of the system. For product certification, it is mandatory to demonstrate that the system handles a large variety of configurations correctly. From an object-oriented point of view, the control software may be regarded as a generic class. A concrete object of this controller class is generated by instantiating the software for a concrete configuration table. This observation leads to the requirements that test specifications should be generic as well: The configuration dependent rules for test data generation and evaluation are specified using generic parameters equivalent to the ones evaluated by the control software and are instantiated by the same tables. This allows to use a single set of test specifications for all test cases checking one generic aspect of SUT behaviour in presence of configuration data variations.

Example: Use of generic parameters in test specifications. The CIDS configuration table allows to configure the aircraft cabin zones which are affected by a *"Reading Lights Off"* key dependent on the specific panel where the key was pressed. For a specific test case with fixed configuration table T, the test system compiles T into parameter definitions using mathematical data types (constants, sets, sequences and combinations thereof). For *"Reading Lights Off"* keys, we use sets for each cabin zone z, containing the AAP identifications (deck, address, port) of those panels where the reading lights off key has an effect on z: Generic parameter

```
GENERIC_RL_RESET_AAP_ZONE_1 = { 0.1.1, 0.2.1 }
```

states that reading lights in zone 1 are switched off by *"Reading Lights Off"* keys pressed on AAPs with $(deck, address, port) = (0,1,1)$ and $(deck, address, port) = (0,2,1)$. The checker specifications are modularised by the cabin zone structure: `RLCHECKER_ZONE_1` checks timeliness and correctness of reading light state changes in zone 1:

```
RLCHECKER_ZONE_1 =
  . . .
  AAP_key_cil_rl_off?d.b.a
       -> ( if ( member(d.b.a,GENERIC_RL_RESET_AAP_ZONE_1) )
            then ( setTimer.1 ->
                        ...  wait for all reading lights in zone
                             1 to be switched off before timer 1
                             has elapsed ...)
            else ... disregard this AAP key ... )
  . . .
```

Whenever an AAP key event is simulated by the test data generator (such as process `RL_TEST` introduced above), the event is registered by all zone checkers as an input statement `AAP_key_cil_rl_off?d.b.a`. Using the `member()` condition in the `if`-statement above, the checker determines whether the panel affects the local zone. If this is the case, the checker sets a timer and waits for all reading lights to be switched off within the admissible time interval. If the panel does not affect the local zone, it is just ignored by the checker.

For a new configuration table, the checker specification is recompiled with the new definitions of `GENERIC_RL_RESET_AAP_ZONE_1` and other generic parameters. The specification source code remains unchanged. Note that the real checkers are also generic in the cabin zone number, so that a single source may be used for all zone-specific checkers and all configuration table settings.

3. HARDWARE-IN-THE-LOOP TEST CONFIGURATION

After having explained our testing approach on a conceptual level, we will now describe the test configuration for HW/SW integration testing in more detail (see Figure 4).

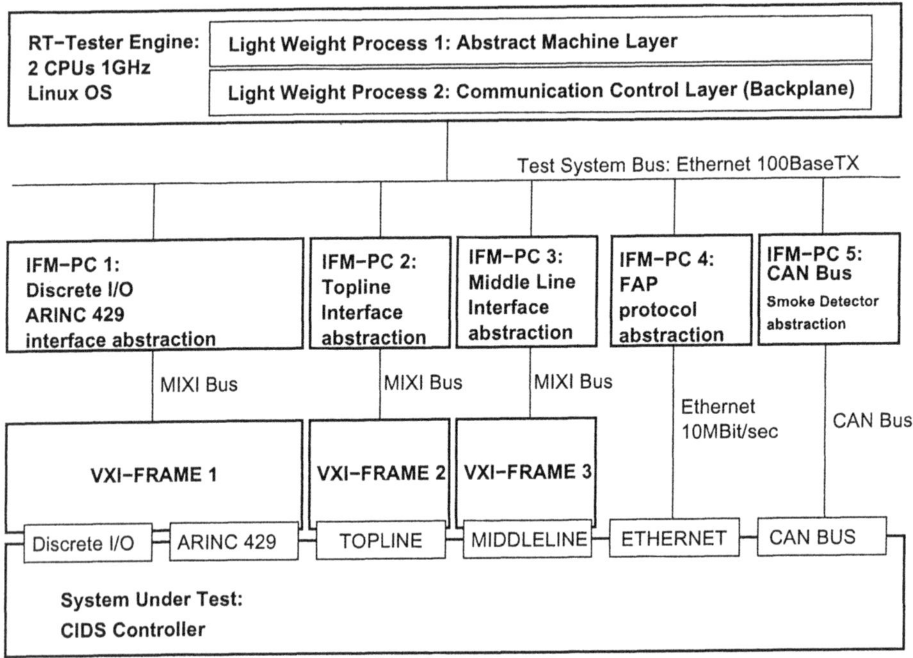

Figure 4. HW/SW integration test configuration.

The System Under Test is now given by the CIDS controller alone; panels and other CIDS devices outside the controller are not part of this configuration. The CIDS controller commands a variety of interfaces: Discrete I/O is used to switch external devices on/off (e. g., the flight warning buzzer in the cockpit) and to receive discrete state information (e. g., state of landing gears). The ARINC 429 bus is used to communicate with other controllers (e. g. , the environmental control system responsible for air conditioning). Topline and Middleline are proprietary busses developed by KID-Systeme which are used to control external devices (such as reading lights or AAPs) via intelligent bus interfaces. The Flight Attendant Panels (FAP) described in the examples above are connected to the CIDS controller via Ethernet. The CAN bus interface (A318 only) is used for communication with smoke detectors.

In the HW/SW integration test environment, VXI systems are used to read/write date on the first 4 interfaces described above. The interface module software is integrated in PCs acting as front ends to the VXI systems, so that only interface boards and low-level drivers are allocated inside the VXI frames. For Ethernet and CAN bus, standard PCI cards are used.

Test data generation and on-the-fly evaluation is performed in the test engine. To exploit the CPU power available in an efficient way, the RT-Tester system allows to allocate abstract machines and communication control layer on a configurable number of light weight processes (LWPs). Typically, each LWP will be executed on a separate CPU. Within each LWP, scheduling is performed by a specific cooperative multi-tasking technique developed for RT-Tester in order to optimise real-time performance: Context switches between abstract machines or CCL processes are implemented on user thread level and do not require the participation of the underlying operating system. In particular, an increasing number of AMs participating in a test execution will not compromise the performance since the effort needed for context switching is very close to that of a C function call.

Simple tests only need a small number of AMs, but more complex tests involving several applications (e. g. emergency evacuation system tested in cooperation with the telephone and passenger address systems) may utilise several hundred AMs, each stimulating or checking a specific logical aspect of the whole test execution.

For the whole set of software and HW/SW integration tests, about 3000 different generic CSP specifications are used. They access over 1500 different logical interfaces, which may refer to global variables or function call interfaces in software tests or to specific logical data items passed along one of the HW interfaces shown in Figure 4, when HW/SW or system integration testing is performed. The number of different discrete events which are passed along these logical interfaces and either generated or checked in at least one test case is about 1.1 million.

4. SUMMARY

4.1 Conclusion

In this article, we have presented the underlying concepts and architecture of a testing environment for the Cabin Management controllers in the new Airbus A318, A340-500/600 and A380 aircrafts. The distinguishing features in contrast to conventional testing approaches were (1) re-usability of tests on software integration test, HW/SW integration and system test level, (2) automatic test data generation and test evaluation based on networks of timed state machines and (4) utilisation of generic test specifications.

The main advantages of our approach are (a) Automatic test data generation often generates situations where errors are uncovered but which typically would not have been investigated in manual tests. (b) Identification of error causes is facilitated because tests can be replayed with small modifications on lower integration levels: If a system test uncovers an erroneous situation, it can be replayed on software integration level using auxiliary debugging tools for pinpointing software bugs. (c) The effort needed for regression testing is considerably reduced because tests can be automatically replayed and correctness checks are based on specification that do not reject legal deviations of the regression test execution from the reference test results. (d) The overall testing effort is considerably reduced because of the automatic generation/evaluation and documentation facilities and the re-use of concept, interfaces and specification parts on different integration levels.

4.2 Related Activities and Future Work

Due to the usual space limitations, several aspects of ongoing and future work which are related to the material presented above can only be mentioned briefly:

To improve the hard real-time testing capabilities, a new test engine concept based on PC clusters with a customised hard real-time variant of the Linux operating system is currently in its trial phase. All relevant hardware interfaces needed for testing avionics controllers are directly integrated as PCI boards in the test engine cluster. The cluster communication is performed via FireWire (IEEE 1394) or Myrinet. This activity is performed within the VICTORIA project, which is part of the current European R&D Framework Programmes and focuses on the development of novel technologies for avionics control and its validation, verification and test.

For software integration testing, a large portion of the overall testing effort has to be invested into interface module development, because often a large number of software interfaces has to be accessed during different software integration stages. It is currently investigated how the IFM generation can be (at least partially) automated by generating the abstraction mapping between software interfaces and CSP channels in an automatic way.

For practical testing in an industrial setting it is important to know how the tool-based testing approach fits into the project development approach defined by the underlying V-Model and other applicable standards. A publication elaborating these questions for the Avionics Software V-Model RTCA/D 178B [2] and the IEEE standard [6] on test documentation is currently under preparation.

The reader may have noticed that in the test setting described in this article, interfaces were considered to be discrete. This is true for the CIDS controller. However, in many embedded systems test applications, time-continuous data has to be generated and checked as well. To this end, we enhance the abstract machines introduced above by global real-valued state variables which may change "continuously" over time according to differential equations or similar specifications of time-continuous evolutions. The underlying semantic concept is given by Hennessy's *Hybrid Automata* [4].

Acknowledgments

The project described in this article would be unmanageable without the help and initiative of many people. The author would like to thank Manfred Endreß, Thomas Fritz, Manfred Kühnel, Sascha Marckwardt and Ute Meyer (KID-Systeme), Cornelia Zahlten, Christof Effkemann, Oliver Meyer, Raymond Scholz, Hauke Steenbock, Kai Thomsen (Verified Systems International), Markus Dahlweid, Dirk Meyer and Aliki Tsiolakis (Bremen University) for reliable and stimulating cooperation in this – sometimes rather challenging – project.

Last, but not least, the author would like to express his gratitude to the organisers of the TestCom2002 for granting him the possibility to deliver this presentation.

References

[1] Cardell-Oliver, Rachel. (2000). Conformance Testing of Real-Time Systems with Timed Automata. In *Formal Aspects of Computing.* (12):350-371

[2] RTCA DO178B: *Software Considerations in Airborne Systems and Equipment Certification.* (1993).

[3] Hennessy, M. C. (1988). *Algebraic Theory of Processes.* MIT Press.

[4] Henzinger, Th. A. (1996). in *Proceedings of the 11th Annual IEEE Symposium on Logic in Computer Science (LICS 1996)*, pp. 278-292.

[5] Hoare, C.A.R. (1985). *Communicating sequential processes.* Prentice-Hall International, Englewood Cliffs NJ.

[6] IEEE Std 829-1998. *IEEE Standard for Software Test Documentation.* The Institute of Electrical and Electronics Engineers, New York.

[7] KID-Systeme. *CIDS Digital Cabin Management System.* Information available under `http://www.kid-systeme.de`.

[8] Lewis, Harry R. and Papadimitriou, Christos H. (1981). *Elements of the Theory of Computation.* Prentice-Hall International, Englewood Cliffs, New Jersey.

[9] Meyer, Oliver. (2001). *Structural Decomposition of Timed CSP and its Application to Real-Time Testing.* Dissertation, Universität Bremen, FB 3.

[10] Nielsen, Brian. (2000). *Specification and Test of Real-Time Systems.* Ph. D. Thesis, Department of Computer Science, The Faculty of Engineering and Science, Aalborg University, Publication No. 12.

[11] Peleska, Jan and Siegel, Michael. (1996). From Testing Theory to Test Driver Implementation. In M.-C. Gaudel and J. Woodcock (Eds.): FME '96: Industrial Benefit and Advances in Formal Methods. LNCS 1051, Springer-Verlag, Berlin Heidelberg New York 538-556.

[12] Peleska, Jan. (1996). Test Automation for Safety-Critical Systems: Industrial Application and Future Developments. (invited keynote), In M.-C. Gaudel and J. Woodcock (Eds.): FME '96: Industrial Benefit and Advances in Formal Methods. LNCS 1051, Springer-Verlag, Berlin Heidelberg New York pp. 39-59.

[13] Peleska, Jan. (1997). *Formal Methods and the Development of Dependable Systems.* Habilitationsschrift, Bericht Nr. 9612, Dezember 1996, Institut für Informatik und praktische Mathematik, Christian-Albrechts-Universität Kiel.

[14] Peleska, Jan and Siegel, Michael. (1997). Test Automation of Safety-Critical Reactive Systems. *South African Computer Jounal* 19:53-77.

[15] Peleska, Jan. (1998). Testing Reactive Real-Time Systems. Tutorial, held at the FTRTFT '98. Danmark Technical University, Lyngby.

[16] Peleska, Jan and Buth, Bettina. (1999). Formal Methods for the International Space Station ISS. In E.-R. Olderog, B. Steffen (Eds.): Correct System Design, Springer LNCS 1710, pp. 363-389.

[17] Roscoe, A. W. (1998). *The Theory and Practice of Concurrency.* Prentice-Hall International, Englewood Cliffs NJ.

[18] Verified Systems International GmbH. (1998). *RT-Tester Test Automation System.* Information available under `http://www.verified.biz`.

[19] Sadeghipour, Sadegh. (1998). *Testing Cyclic Software Components of Reactive Systems on the Basis of Formal Specifications.* Schriftenreihe Forschungsergebnisse zur Informatik, Bd. 40. Verlag Dr. Kovaĉ, Hamburg.

[20] Schneider, Steve. (1995). An Operational Semantics for Timed CSP. *Information and Computation*, 116:193–213.

[21] Tretmanns, Jan. (1992). *A Formal Approach to Conformace Testing.* PhD Thesis, University of Twente, Haag.

SESSION IX

FSM-BASED TESTING

TEST GENERATION FOR CEFSM COMBINING SPECIFICATION AND FAULT COVERAGE

Sergiy Boroday[1], Alex Petrenko[1], Roland Groz[2], and Yves-Marie Quemener[2]
1 – CRIM, Montréal; 2 – France Telecom R&D

Abstract We discuss how specification coverage and fault coverage based test derivation strategies can be combined. In particular, the problem of deriving a test suffix, which raises tester confidence in the configuration of the system, reached after a test derived by a specification coverage criterion, is formalized and solved in the CEFSM setting. The traditional mutant-based test derivation approach is extended with nondeterministic mutants to cover more faults. An experimental tool and case study are reported.

Key words: communicating extended state machines, black box testing, SDL, model based testing, specification coverage, fault models, fault coverage, test derivation.

1. INTRODUCTION

1.1 Specification vs. Fault Coverage

In this section, we contrast two common strategies used for deriving tests from formal specifications in terms of state machines, in particular specification coverage driven approach and fault model/mutation driven approach. We consider here the model of communicating extended FSM (EFSM). There exist a number of tools that support software development activities around specifications based on this model.

Specification coverage: In [GCR96], it is argued that coverage of the extended transitions of an EFSM corresponds well to the preferred coverage implied in the conformance testing standard IS9646. As an example, the commercial tools available on SDL now offer test generation facilities, which were designed based on research for generating conformance tests

[EGHJ97], [KJG99]. Such tools may resort to reachability analysis to compute tests that will cover transitions of the EFSM and provide test preambles to reach specific configurations of the EFSM enabling the transitions to be tested. However, they currently do not check the tail state of transitions or the configuration reached after a test. As a result, faults in an implementation (known as Implementation Under Test), viz. faults whereby a transition in the IUT would reach a wrong tail configuration, may easily go undetected. Therefore, the current test generation methods used in tools for EFSM testing have very limited fault detection capabilities.

Fault coverage: Fault models have been used in many testing methods for the classical FSM model [Petr00]. Typical fault models for EFSM can include a wrong tail state and erroneous values of certain variables after a test execution. In mutation-based testing, a faulty implementation is assumed to be derived from a specification, while the difference between them could be explained in terms of the specification's elements or a mutation operator [BDDD91], [YPB94], [ABM98], [FMMD99]. In a more general view, a fault model could be derived from a higher level of testing requirements, than just structural mutations of the specification.

The question arises whether one could merge the two approaches into a test derivation strategy for communicating EFSM to incorporate both concerns, covering interesting portions of the specification and increasing the fault coverage of the resulting tests according to the user-defined fault models. In the next section, we discuss a framework for mutant-based test derivation which embraces both approaches.

1.2 Confirming configuration w.r.t. mutant set

Our idea is to start from an existing test suite as computed by the first approach. Instead of simply adding new tests, we consider that such a test suite exercises well the basic structure of the specification, and that likely residual faults are defined by the user. Then, as in traditional FSM test methods, we derive with a fault-based approach confirming sequences to check the tail configuration (state and data) of each test with respect to the given fault/mutation model. In [PBG99], we investigated such a combined approach for EFSM specifications and now we extend it to cover modular specifications in the form of CEFSM.

Given a (multi-module) specification, a few mutants, and a test sequence, it is required to find a confirming sequence of a given maximal length that distinguishes the specification from mutants when applied to each of the mutants after the test. All the potential implementation faults are modeled by the given mutants themselves that are somehow derived from the specification and their data configurations. Thus, there are two means for modeling faults, first by introducing some structural changes or mutations into the specification and second, by choosing the initial configuration (configuration reached after the prefix test sequence) of a mutant. Under a competent programmer hypothesis, mutants are usually supposed to differ from the specification only in a marginal way. Therefore, here we assume that the mutants inherit input and output ports of the specification and are defined over the set of inputs of the specification. The problem of building mutants from a given specification in the form of CEFSM is the task of the test expert working from test requirements.

A simple way of building a mutant is to take the CEFSM specification and initialize it into a (suspicious) configuration different from the final configuration reached after the test. An implicit fault model is that an implementation under test reproduces the reference reaction to the test, as it passes the test, but ends up in this erroneous configuration. A confirming sequence has to detect such a residual implementation fault if the fault is an error, in other words, if the mutant is distinguishable from the specification. In this scenario, the test is used only to determine the expected configuration to properly initialize the specification.

In the case of modular specifications, guessing suspicious configurations for each of the modules becomes a daunting task. Moreover, when a mutant structurally differs from the specification, it is not clear how to change the initialization inherited from the specification. We, therefore, assume that the test expert just builds a number of mutants that can pass the given test. This means that the specification and all the mutants are set in the initial configurations. We are required to determine an input sequence that confirms the initial configuration of the specification w.r.t. the initial configurations of mutants taking the given test as a predefined prefix or preamble. Note that this setting does not exclude the above scenario when the test expert just defines a suspicious configuration. In this case, the prefix becomes an empty sequence.

We believe that the process of deriving representative mutants is application-dependant and we do not attempt to give here any generic recipe. What we can suggest here is that to capture more faults with a single mutant the test expert could first mutate the specification according to his/her testing strategy and then choose states and/or variables in a few modules to abstract them. Such abstraction can be used to cover multiple faults instead of only single faults; moreover abstraction may reduce the configuration number and the "size" of configurations. Note that since the process of abstraction induces non-determinism, we allow for such mutants to be non-deterministic even when the specification is perfectly deterministic. The presence of non-deterministic mutants makes our problem statement more general than a classical mutation-based testing problem.

2. CEFSM MODEL

2.1 Extended finite state machine, EFSM

The EFSM model defined in [PBG99] is extended with multiple output signals, as this makes it easier to map languages such as SDL into CEFSM.

Definition 2.1. An *extended* finite state machine (EFSM) M is a pair (S, T) of a finite set of states S and a finite set of transitions T between states from S, such that each transition $t \in T$ is a tuple (s, x, P, op, w, up, s'), where $s, s' \in S$ are the initial and final states of the transition, respectively; $x \in X$ is input, X is a finite set of inputs, and each $x \in X$ is associated with a set of input vectors D_{inpx}, each component of an input vector corresponds to an input parameter associated with x, the sets of input parameters of different signals are mutually disjoint; $w \in Y^*$ is a sequence of output signals $y_1, y_2, \ldots, y_n$, $y_i \in Y$, where Y is a finite set of (elemental) outputs, disjoint from X, each $y \in Y$ is associated with a set of output vectors D_{outy}, each component of an output vector corresponds to an output parameter associated with y, the sets of output parameters of different signals are mutually disjoint; P, op, and up are functions, defined over input parameters and context variables V, namely:

- P: $D_{inpx} \times D_V \rightarrow$ {True, False} is a predicate, where D_V is a set of context vectors $\vec{v}$;
- op: $D_{inpx} \times D_V \rightarrow D_{outy_1} \times D_{outy_2} \times \ldots \times D_{outy_n}$ is an output parameter function that defines values of parameters of each signal in the output word;
- up: $D_{inpx} \times D_V \rightarrow D_V$ is a context update function.

We normally use $(s \text{—} x, P/op, w, up \rightarrow s')$ to denote a transition $t \in T$, we will also use the notation $(s \text{—} x, P/y_1(op_1), y_2(op_2), \ldots, y_n(op_n), up \rightarrow s')$. An empty output word will be dropped from a transition to simplify its notation and such a transition is called a *silent* transition.

A *parameterized* signal, input or output, is a pair of the signal itself and a vector of its parameters. It may also be defined as a pair of a signal and a mapping of its parameters into the parameter values. We will use notations for signals in the form of, for example, $y(2, 3)$ meaning the signal y whose two parameters are instantiated to 2 and 3.

Definition 2.2. A context vector $\vec{v} \in D_V$ is called a *context* of M. A *configuration* of M is a pair of state s and context $\vec{v}$.

A context may also be defined as a mapping of variables into variable values.

In the case of empty sets of context variables and parameters, we do not make a difference between configuration and state, in other words, the EFSM model includes the FSM model as a special case.

The EFSM operates as defined in [PBG99]. The machine usually starts from a designated configuration, called the *initial* configuration. A pair of an EFSM and the initial configuration is called an *initialized* EFSM. The *behavior* of an initialized EFSM is the set of all its input-output sequences.

Definition 2.3. An *input-output sequence* of an EFSM (or input-output word) is a sequence of parameterized inputs interleaved by parameterized outputs produced by the EFSM executing a finite sequence of transitions from a certain configuration in response to these inputs.

We target a class of specification EFSMs which are consistent, completely specified, deterministic, and observable [PBG99]. We use the abbreviation REFSM to refer to a machine from this Restricted class of EFSMs. At the same time, in our constructions, we will also use other types of EFSMs, which do not necessarily meet all these requirements.

2.2 Communicating EFSM, CEFSM

Now we define what we mean by a system of communicating EFSMs.

Definition 2.4. A finite set of consistent, completely specified EFSMs along with two disjoint sets of external parameterized input and output signals is called a system of *communicating* EFSMs (CEFSM), if the following conditions are satisfied:

a) the sets of output signals of any two EFSMs are mutually disjoint;
b) the external inputs are all inputs of communicating EFSMs that are not outputs of communicating EFSMs;
c) each external output is an output of an EFSM;
d) any signal is always associated with the same set of parameters, whenever it appears.

CEFSM functions as follows. Communications are performed via input (FIFO) queues, a single queue is associated which each communicating EFSM (as in SDL). External and internal inputs enter the corresponding queues, while each EFSM consumes signals from its queue. A signal may enter several queues at the same time. A global configuration of the system is defined as a tuple of configurations of component EFSMs and configuration (contents) of their queues. A global configuration of the system with empty queues is called *stable*. When the environment offers an external parameterized input signal to the system, which is in a stable configuration, this input enters queues of all EFSMs to which input alphabets it belongs, and the system goes into an unstable global configuration (a configuration with non-empty queues). In an unstable configuration of CEFSM, an EFSM (with non-empty queue) takes a signal from its queue and fires an enabled transition. The machine produces a (possibly empty) sequence of outputs, which are consequently put into input queues of corresponding machines, and/or sent to the environment if there are external outputs among these signals. Thus the system moves into a new global configuration, which is either stable or unstable. If a stable configuration is eventually reached the CEFSM can accept another external input, otherwise it falls into livelock.

We make certain assumptions about the environment and behavior of the CEFSM. First of all, we assume that the environment is slow, this means that it submits a next external input to the system only in a stable configuration, when all the queues are empty (this assumption is also known as the synchronization assumption). Test derivation and test execution with a slow testing environment is much simpler compared to an unrestricted one.

Our next assumption concerns only specifications of systems to be tested. We assume that there exists a maximal number of communications that can be triggered by an external input in a specification CEFSM. This implies that:

- the number of external outputs, which may be obtained in response to any external input, never exceeds a certain bound;
- a system always stabilizes in response to external input (it has no livelocks).

Under these assumptions, for a given CEFSM there exists an equivalent EFSM, except for pathologic nondeterministic CEFSMs that allow infinite set of alternative output parameter values for a pair of configuration and input signal. Such CEFSMs have no equivalent EFSMs, because our EFSM model supports only limited nondeterminism (between several transitions), and nondeterminism in output and update function (multifunctions) is not allowed. A system of communicating REFSMs is not necessarily equivalent to an REFSM, because its behavior in terms of external inputs and outputs can be nondeterministic. We rely on the existence of an EFSM equivalent to the given CEFSM in order to formally define input sequences that separate two CEFSM, i.e., that distinguish their external behavior.

2.3 Configuration separating and confirming sequences

We extend the definition of a separating sequence given in [PBG99] to cover multiple outputs.

Definition 2.5. Given two EFSMs *M* and *N*, two parameterized signals of *M* and *N* are said to be *compatible* if the names of the signals coincide and every common signal parameter has the same value in both parameterized signals. Two parameterized input-output sequences, $z_1...z_k$ of M and $z'_1...z'_{k'}$ of N, are *compatible* if $k' = k$ and for all $i = 1, ..., k$, z_i and z'_i are compatible.

Based on this notion, we now define separability of configurations.

Definition 2.6. Given a parameterized input sequence α of EFSMs M and N, configuration c of M and configuration c' of N are *separable* (*by* α) if every parameterized input-output sequence, produced by (M, c) in response to α, is not compatible with any parameterized input-output sequence that can be produced by (N, c') in response to α. α is said to be a sequence *separating* c from c'.

Configurations of REFSMs with the same sets of inputs, outputs, and their parameters that are not separable are also referred to as *equivalent* configurations. Two REFSMs are *equivalent* if their initial configurations are equivalent. Note that in this study, we assume that a given REFSM may have different configurations that are equivalent.

Definition 2.7. A parameterized input sequence α *confirms* a configuration c w.r.t. a set of configurations C (possibly of different machines) if it separates c from every configuration c' of the set C separable from c. Such a sequence is called a *complete configuration confirming sequence*.

In the above definition, the configuration c is usually assumed to be the one of the specification EFSM M and therefore called the *expected* configuration, while the configurations in the set C are referred to as *suspicious* configurations representing configurations of some faulty implementation machines to which an IUT may erroneously arrive having successfully passed some test case. Following a best-effort approach, as advocated in [PBG99], instead of aiming at finding complete configuration confirming sequence, we target *configuration-confirming sequence*, as a sequence of length l or lesser that confirms c w.r.t. a subset of maximal cardinality of C among all possible parameterized input sequences of that length. Here l is a predefined integer that indicates the acceptable length of the sequence. Whenever complete configuration confirming sequence of length l exists, any configuration-confirming sequence is complete and vice versa. The following proposition gives us sufficient conditions for the existence of configuration-confirming sequence.

Proposition 2.1. Given the expected configuration c and the set of suspicious configurations C, a configuration-confirming sequence exists if the set C, domains of input parameters, or domains of output parameters are finite.

We will restrict ourselves to finite suspicious configuration sets. So, in our problem setting, configuration-confirming sequence always exists. Derivation of a suspicious set (with the corresponding machines) is discussed in [PBG99]. These machines will be referred to as *mutants*. Unlike the traditional approach, our mutants are allowed to be nondeterministic to model more faults.

Configuration-confirming sequence for CEFSM is defined based on the corresponding equivalent EFSM.

3. TEST DERIVATION

Given an REFSM M, an expected configuration c_0 of M, a set C of k of suspicious configurations of k possibly different mutant (C)EFSMs, c_1 of N_1, c_2 of N_2, ..., c_k of N_k, and the maximal length l of sequences, we are required to determine a configuration-confirming sequence. The mutant machines are assumed to be observable and completely defined. The mutants share the same input signal set with the specification. However, mutant's signals could be abstracted from certain parameters of the specification. In this section, we discuss three approaches for deriving confirming sequences for EFSM and CEFSM.

3.1 Distinguishing machine

For the case of single output transitions a solution based on the reachability analysis of the distinguishing machines is proposed in [PBG99]. To determine a configuration confirming sequence, the reachability analysis of this machine should be performed with dedicated tools, e.g., simulators and model checkers. However, the transfer of this method onto real world EFSM languages, which do not follow our EFSM syntax and semantics, may be problematic and faces complexity issues. Therefore, in next section, we consider an alternative method, which reduces derivation of the confirming sequence to reachability analysis of a CEFSM defined from given specification and mutants.

3.2 Distinguishing system for EFSM

We now reduce the testing problem to the problem of analyzing the behavior of a CEFSM. The idea is to build a system of $k + 2$ communicating machines, called a *distinguishing system*. One machine is the original machine modified with the *eot* signal ("end of transition" signal). The *eot* signal is inserted at the end of the output word of each transition to facilitate the comparison of different machines' behavior caused by the same input. There are k machines of the system each of which represents an EFSM initialized in a corresponding suspicious configuration and signals a discrepancy between its behavior and that of the original machine by issuing a designated signal to the environment. The *Monitor* assists communications between machines. We formally define a distinguishing system as a CEFSM, that includes the following EFSMs: M_0, M_1, M_2, ..., M_k, *Monitor*. The set of external inputs of the system is defined as follows. For each input x of M there is an external input x^{ext} of the system with the same sets of input vectors and parameters, as the input x of the M. The system has elemental outputs $fail^1$, ..., $fail^k$.

The machine M_0 is a slightly modified machine M. It has the same state and input sets as the M. The set of outputs includes all the outputs of the M, as well as a designated output *eot*. All the parameters and their vectors are defined as in M. Transitions of M_0 are defined as follows. For every transition $(s\text{—}x,P_M/op_M,y_1y_2...y_h,up_M\rightarrow s')$ of M, there is a transition in M_0 $(s\text{—}x,P_M/op_M,y_1y_2...y_h\, eot,up_M\rightarrow s')$.

In other words, the only difference between M and M_0 is the *eot* signal appended to the output word of each transition. The initial configuration of the machine is c_0.

Next, we define the machines M_1, ..., M_k, corresponding to the mutants N_1, ..., N_k initialized in suspicious configurations c_1, ..., c_k, respectively. The machines M_1, ..., M_k are called the inverted mutants, as outputs of mutants become inputs in these machines. The transitions of M_i are also defined in such a way that any discrepancy in parameterized outputs produced by the machine (M_0, c_0) and the (N_i, c_i) in response to inputs is detected and signaled to the environment (the expected configuration c_0 is separated from the c_i). Speaking more formally, the inverted mutants are defined as follows.

Since, by definition, the sets of output signals of two different machines of any CEFSM must be disjoint, and signals are not allowed to have different sets of parameters, we rename signals. For every i, $1 \leq i \leq k$, the notation of signals of the machine M_i is decorated with the superscript i so that it becomes clear to which machine this signal belongs. The signal eot^i along with the sets of parameterized inputs and outputs of N_i (renamed as we described above) constitute the set of inputs of M_i. The output signal $fail^i$ is the only elemental output. For each variable of the machine N_i there is a variable of M_i with the same name and domain and for each input parameter vector inp_x of an input signal x of the machine the auxiliary context variables with the corresponding domains are defined. The projection of the context vector on these variables is denoted $\vec{u}_x$. There is a new state s_{fail} with the transitions $(s_{fail}\text{—}eot\rightarrow s_{fail})$, $(s_{fail}\text{—}x^i\rightarrow s_{fail})$, $(s_{fail}\text{—}y^i\rightarrow s_{fail})$, for all $x^i \in X^i$ and $y^i \in Y^i$.

For each transition $t = (s\text{—}x^i{}_t,P_M/op_M,y_1y_2...y_h\, eot,up_M\rightarrow s')$ of the N_i the machine M_i has the transition $(s\text{—}x^i{}_t,P_M/(\vec{u}_x := inp_x)\rightarrow q_{t,1})$, where inp_x is the input parameter vector of $x^i{}_t$. The state s also has the transitions $(s\text{—}y^i/fail^i\rightarrow s_{fail})$ for each $y^i \in Y^i$, and $(s\text{—}eot^i/fail^i\rightarrow s_{fail})$.

States $q_{t,j}$, $1 \leq j \leq h$, are new (compared to the states of N_i) and unique. They have the transitions $(q_{t,j}$—$y_j^i, inp_{y_j} \sim op_j(\vec{v}, \vec{u}_x) \rightarrow q_{t,j+1})$, $(q_{t,j}$—$y_j^i, \neg(inp_{y_j} \sim op_j(\vec{v}, \vec{u}_x))/fail^i \rightarrow s_{\text{fail}})$, where $inp_{y_j} \sim op_j(\vec{v}, \vec{u}_x)$ is a predicate that holds True iff the elements of vectors inp_{y_j} and $op_j(\vec{v}, \vec{u}_x)$ that correspond to same parameters are equal. The outgoing transitions of the states $q_{t,j}$ are $(q_{t,j}$—$y^i/fail^i \rightarrow s_{\text{fail}})$ for each $y^i \neq y_j^i$, $y^i \in Y^i$; and $(q_{t,j}$—$eot^i/fail^i \rightarrow s_{\text{fail}})$. In addition, for all $x \in X$, there are transitions $(q_{t,j}$—$x^i/fail^i \rightarrow s_{\text{fail}})$.

Finally, we define the outgoing transitions of the state $q_{t,h+1}$: $(q_{t,h+1}$—$eot^i/up_M \rightarrow s')$, $(q_{t,h+1}$—$y/fail^i \rightarrow s_{\text{fail}})$ for all $y \in Y$, and $(q_{t,h+1}$—$x^i/fail^i \rightarrow s_{\text{fail}})$ for all $x \in X$.

The initial configuration of M_i is defined by c_i and arbitrary values of the auxiliary context variables.

The machine *Monitor* has the only state s, input signals X, Y, eot, the output signals and their parameters are inputs and parameters of machines $M_1, \ldots, M_k$. The *Monitor* supports communications between the components with the transitions $(s$—$x^{\text{ext}}/op_x, xx^1 \ldots x^k \rightarrow s)$, $(s$—$y/op_y, y^1 \ldots y^k \rightarrow s)$, $(s$—$eot/eot^1 \ldots eot^k \rightarrow s)$, where op_x is a function that takes a parameter vector of x^{ext} and returns the parameter vectors for signals $x, x^1, \ldots, x^k$, preserving values of parameters. Similarly, the function op_y deals with the output parameter vector of y.

Proposition 3.1. An input sequence separates the expected configuration c_0 from the initial configuration c_i of the machine N_i iff the distinguishing system produces the external signal $fail^i$ when the environment applies the input sequence.

Consider the distinguishing system that consumes a certain (parameterized) input sequence. As it is clear from the former proposition, the number of outputs $fail^i$, produced by the distinguishing system in response to the last external input of the sequence is equal to the number of the configurations of C that this sequence separates from c_0. This leads us to the following corollary.

Corollary 3.2. An input sequence of length l or less is a configuration-confirming sequence of the expected configuration c_0 with respect to the set of suspicious configurations C iff the number of the *fail* signals produced by the distinguishing system in response to the sequence is maximal.

Thus, determining a configuration-confirming sequence amounts to finding a sequence that maximizes the number of *fail* in the distinguishing system.

The distinguishing system may be implemented in an EFSM-based language, such as SDL. A commercial model checker, such as ObjectGeode, can be applied to the distinguishing system to find confirming sequences.

The approach based on distinguishing system has its own limitations. First, mutant machines have to be observable, but transforming a mutant specification (in the form of SDL process) into an equivalent observable EFSM form, (as well as augmenting the specification with the *eot* signal), may be a challenging task. Second, the approach does not extend to treat modular specifications, CEFSM. These limitations are absent in the approach proposed in the next sections.

3.3 Distinguishing system for CEFSM

In order to apply the concept of the distinguishing system to the case of modular specifications, we could represent each mutant CEFSM in a distinguishing system by an EFSM such that has the same external behavior and produces the only output *fail* as an inverted mutant. The length of confirming sequence should never exceed the bound l, therefore, it is sufficient to partially unfold each mutant CEFSM by considering input sequences of the length l. This idea yields the following method:

1. Restrict the set of external parameterized inputs to a finite set.
2. For each mutant CEFSM, build a deterministic (mutant) LTS which represents the mutant's observable external behavior on all the input sequences of length l obtained from the above set of parameterized inputs.
3. For each mutant LTS, construct an inverted mutant machine. Build the distinguishing system as explained in Section 3.2.

We first build the reachability graph for a mutant CEFSM for the restricted input set, and remove in the resulting LTS internal actions, minimize, and determinize it. The obtained mutant LTS contains all the external traces of the corresponding mutant CEFSM that are produced by input sequences of length l from the restricted input set.

The procedure of inverting a mutant LTS is similar to that for the EFSM case, though it slightly differs because of

a) a transition of LTS is labeled with a single signal while an (E)FSM transition contains a sequence of an input and output signals;
b) LTS may have a state with outgoing transitions labeled with input and output;
c) absence of the *eot* signal.

Given a deterministic mutant LTS, the *inverted mutant machine* N^i is an EFSM with the only elemental output, $fail^i$. The input signals of the machine are all external input and output signals of the mutant CEFSM. For each transition (s—$x(p)$→t) of the mutant LTS, where $x(p)$ is a parameterized signal, the inverted mutant machine has a transition (s—x^i,P→t), where x^i is the signal with the same name as $x(p)$, decorated with i, and P is a predicate, which delivers True only when the parameterized signal is compatible with $x^i(p)$. In each state of the inverted mutant machine, transitions, which make the machine consistent and completely specified for all the signals of the mutant, produce a *fail* output and lead into the state s_{fail}, are defined.

In the distinguishing system, the specification CEFSM is used as it is, without introducing the *eot* signal. Accordingly, the monitor is simplified by removing this signal. The monitor ignores all the input signals x^{ext} that are not in the restricted input set. With these exceptions, the distinguishing system is as defined in the previous section. As in the previous section, the configuration-confirming sequence (for CEFSMs with the restricted input set) is the input sequence, which delivers the maximal number of *fails*; except the special case, when all the *fail* signal are produced on transitions, which are labeled with external inputs of the specification. In this case that input signal does not contribute to the separating sequence. This is the cost we pay for escaping from the *eot* signal.

Next, we describe how the distinguishing system can be implemented in the ObjectGeod environment.

3.4 Implementation with observers

To implement the above method in ObjectGeode we use so-called event observers, which are deterministic extended automata that are directly driven by events of a simulated system. Observers are defined in an SDL like language, GOAL. Observers are used to specify test purposes in the Object Geode TestComposer.

To automate the process of observer generation, we use the Aldebaran tool [CADP] along with a converter of an Object Geode graph into the Aldebaran LTS format GeodeParse. In addition, we have developed a number of shell and awk scripts that call the above programs in a proper order, and build observers. An auxiliary program [Wang01] for variable abstraction was also used in observer construction.

The environment we built allows us to deal with explicitly input complete SDL specifications, which are free from time constraints, timers could, e.g., be replaced by input signals. Additionally, specifications (but not mutants) are required to behave deterministically.

3.5 Extensions and enhancements

3.5.1 Handling multi-mutants

The ObjectGeode simulator can simulate a given SDL specification with several (mutant) observers. The developed script handles just a single mutant observer, but it does not take much time to extend it to process several observers and to eventually determine an input sequence that separates a maximal number of mutants. Since different mutants represent various faults, a goal function, which takes into account user-defined weights of mutants or mutant groups, could be defined. Derivation of a confirming sequence, which maximizes such a goal function, is possible with the Object Geode simulator.

3.5.2 Handling non-separable mutants

The question arises what can be done in the case when for a given specification and a mutant no conforming sequence exists. In terms of the FSM model, this means that the specification machine is a reduction (trace included into) of the mutant machine, hence no separating sequence. We call such a mutant *non-separable*. Note that a non-separable deterministic mutant is observationally equivalent to the specification, thus no useful test can be suggested in this case. However, a nondeterministic non-separable mutant could be used to choose a most "powerful" candidate sequence to be applied as a "quasi-confirming" sequence in this case.

The idea comes from interpreting a nondeterministic mutant as a compact joint representation of a number of potential implementation faults, see, e.g., [PeYe92]. Different faults create thus various executions of the mutant. Therefore, given a candidate input sequence, we may use the number of different executions or output sequences produced by the mutant in response to it to characterize the number of faults "covered" by the sequence. Note that in the case, when a mutant has a chaos state, capable of producing any output sequence in response to any input sequence, a transfer sequence to this state could be most powerful.

The introduced measure can also be used to handle several mutants, by appropriately modifying the goal function to incorporate both, separable and non-separable, mutants.

4. EXPERIMENTS

To validate the approach, experiments on the VTT2 protocol, which is proposed by FranceTelecom R&D, have been performed.

4.1 The VTT2 example

We use a receiving block of the VTT2 protocol, which is a simplified version of a video transmission protocol. The protocol consists of three processes, each of which has two to four states, three to six variables of types boolean, natural, and a set of naturals. Each process has three inputs (including a timer which we replace with an external signal) and two or three outputs. Some signals are parameterized.

4.2 Mutations and tests

We have defined two mutants from our SDL specification of the receiving block of the VTT2 protocol. For those two mutants, we use the same fault model: we suppress one assignment from the original specification. In the first case, it is the assignment of a boolean variable, in the second one, it is a natural variable. In addition, for each mutant, we have abstracted a boolean variable to cover more options for erroneous behavior. This induces nondeterminism in the mutants.

For each of those mutants, we found a test case which does not distinguish between a correct implementation and the mutant. For the first one, we used a test case of length 7, and for the second one of length 18. It is required, for each pair of the mutant and test case, to find a confirming sequence, which being applied to the mutant right after the test case delivers only output sequences different from output sequences of the specification.

4.3 Results

The simulation of the distinguishing systems, built for $l = 3$ (the maximal acceptable length of confirming sequences) is performed. As a result, complete confirming sequences for both test cases are found.

Table 1 provides the characterization of the experiments in terms of states (configurations) and transitions in the constructed objects for each of the two test cases and mutants. As expected, an LTS that describes the observable behavior of a mutant has much fewer states that the unfolded mutant itself. In our example, the number of states reduces by about 30 times. The final number of the configurations traversed during the search of confirming sequences is negligible in our example.

Table 1. Characterization of the experiments in terms of states and transitions

	Test case 1		Test case 2	
	States	**Transitions**	**States**	**Transitions**
OG graph of the mutant	3376	6402	3357	8297
Aldebaran LTS (sliced LTS)	6249	9275	5067	10007
Minimized τ-free LTS	238	1380	173	529
Determinized LTS	226	1308	158	514
OG graph of the distinguishing system (specification + observer)	66	76	59	80

5. CONCLUSION

We addressed the following testing scenario. Assume that some test generation tool has produced from a formal specification in the form of CEFSM/SDL a test case based on some specification coverage concerns. The efforts have to be made to improve the fault detection capability of the test case at a reasonable price by extending the test. The novelty and thus, the complexity of this scenario lie in the fact that fault/mutation coverage-driven testing approaches are traditionally considered incompatible or even orthogonal to specification coverage-driven approaches.

We present a solution to this problem based on which we conclude that fault/mutation and specification coverage approaches for communicating EFSMs are in fact compatible and can seamlessly be integrated into a common test derivation environment.

The specific contributions of our work are as follows.

We cast the problem of extending a given test in a formal setting, using the model of untimed CEFSM. The model is extended with multi-outputs such that a machine produces a sequence of elemental output signals in response to a single input signal. The idea behind this definition is to impose as few restrictions on the system as possible, e.g., multicast is allowed. This reduces the gap between the SDL and EFSM models. The operational semantics is also given based on a slow environment assumption. This implies that confirming sequences are to be applied to a system when it is in a stable state (with empty queues). The notion of configuration-confirming sequence for CEFSM is introduced.

The notion of the distinguishing system is introduced based on the ideas presented in [PBG99]. The distinguishing system allows us to determine a confirming sequence for a specification in the form of a single EFSM. We also extend the distinguishing system to cover CEFSM specification by replacing each mutant CEFSM with a single EFSM that models the behavior of the mutant CEFSM within a restricted scope. We rely on a model checker to eventually determine a most powerful confirming sequence. Thus, we follow a trend in the area to use a model checker engine to derive tests, see e.g., [WaLi93], [CaSc96], [HLS96], [ABM98], [KJG99], [JM99]. At the same time, the novelty of our approach is that nondeterministic mutants are used to reduce the state space needed to model faults/mutations, while covering more potential faults.

Using the ObjectGeode environment, we demonstrated that the proposed testing methodology is compatible and complementary to the existing test derivation facilities of the industrial SDL tools.

ACKNOWLEDGMENTS

This work was partly supported by France Telecom (research contract 001B341). The work of Yves-Marie Quemener was partly supported by the European Commission (FET project ADVANCE, contract No IST-1999-29082). We would like to thank D. Vincent for his contribution to an experiment on GOAL observers; Alain Kerbrat for the GeodeParse tool, and discussions; Telelogic for the ObjectGeode license given to CRIM, and the Vasy team of INRIA for the CADP tool license.

REFERENCES

[ABM98] Ammann P., Black P., and Majurski W. Using Model Checking to Generate Tests from Specifications. Proceedings of 2nd IEEE International Conference on Formal Engineering Methods (ICFEM'98); December 1998; Brisbane, Australia. IEEE Computer Society.

[BDDD91] v. Bochmann G., Das, A. Dssouli R., Dubuc M., Ghedamsi A., Luo G. Fault Model in Testing. Proceedings of the IFIP IV Workshop on Protocol Test Systems; October 1991; Leidschendam, The Netherlands.

[CADP] CADP (Caesar/Aldebaran Development Package). http://www.inrialpes.fr/vasy/cadp

[CaSc96] Callahan J. and Schneider F. Specification–Based Testing using Model Checking. Proceedings of the 2nd SPIN Workshop; August 1996; Rutgers, NJ.

[JM99] Jeron T. and Morel P. Test Generation Derived from Model-Checking. In Proceedings of the 11th Conference on Computer-Aided Verification (CAV'99); July 1999; Trento, Italy. LNCS 1633.

[FMMD99] Fabbri S.C.P.F., Maldonado J.C, Masiero P.C., and Delamaro M.E. Proteum/FSM: A Tool to Support Finite State Machine Validation Based on Mutation Testing. Proceedings of the 19th International Conference of the Chilean Computer Science Society; November 1999; Talca, Chile.

[EGHJ97] Ek A., Grabowski J., Hogrefe D., Jerome R., Koch B., Schmitt M. Towards the industrial use of validation techniques and automatic test generation methods for SDL specifications. Proceedings of the 8th SDL Forum; September 1997; Evry, France. Elsevier.

[GCR96] Groz R., Charles O., and Renévot J., Relating Conformance Test Coverage to Formal Specifications. Proceedings of the IFIP TC6/WG6.1 Joint International Conference on Formal Description Techniques (IX) for Distributed Systems and Communication Protocols, and Protocol Specification, Testing, and Verification (XVI); October 1996; Kaiserslautern, Germany. Chapman&Hall.

[HLS96] Huang S., Lee D., Staskauskas M., Validation-based test sequence generation for networks of extended finite state machines. Proceedings of the IFIP TC6/WG6.1 Joint International Conference on Formal Description Techniques (IX) for Distributed Systems and Communication Protocols, and Protocol Specification, Testing, and Verification (XVI); October 1996; Kaiserslautern, Germany. Chapman&Hall.

[KJG99] Kerbrat A., Jéron T., Groz R. Automated test generation from SDL specifications. Proceedings of the 9th SDL Forum; June 1999; Montreal, Canada. Elsevier.

[Petr00] Petrenko A. Fault Model-Driven Test Derivation from Finite State Models: Annotated Bibliography, LNCS 2067, Proceedings of the Summer School MOVEP'2000, *Modeling and Verification of Parallel Processes*; June 2000; Nantes, France.

[PBG99] Petrenko A., Boroday S., and Groz R. Confirming configurations in EFSM. Proceedings of the IFIP Joint International Conference on Formal Description Techniques for Distributed Systems (FORTE XII) and Communication Protocols, and Protocol Specification, Testing, and Verification (PSTV XIX); October 1999, China. Kluwer.

[PeYe92] Petrenko A. , Yevtushenko N. Test Suite Generation for a FSM with a Given Type of Implementation Errors. Proceedings of the IFIP 12th International Symposium on Protocol Specification, Testing, and Verification; 1992; USA. North-Holland.

[WaLi93] Wang C.–J., and Liu M. T., Generating test cases for EFSM with given fault model. Proceedings of the IEEE INFOCOM'93; 1993; San Francisco, USA.

[Wang01] Wang X. Abstraction of Variables in SDL, Master project in progress, McGill University, 2001.

[YPB94] Yao M. , Petrenko A., and v. Bochmann G. A Structural Analysis Approach to the Evaluation of Fault Coverage for Protocol Conformance Testing, Proceedings of the 7th IFIP WG 6.1 International Conference on Formal Description Techniques (FORTE'94) October 1994; Berne, Switzerland. Elsevier, 1995.

FSM BASED RE-TESTING METHODS

Khaled El-Fakih+, Nina Yevtushenko++ and Gregor v. Bochmann+++
+Department of Computer Science, American University of Sharjah, UAE, kelfakih@aus.ac.ae
++Tomsk State University, 36 Lenin Str., Tomsk, 634050, Russia, yevtushenko.rff@elefot.tsu.ru
+++ School of Information Technology and Engineering, University of Ottawa, Canada, bochmann@site.uottawa.ca

Abstract The selection of appropriate test cases is an important issue in software engineering. A number of methods are known for the selection of a test suite based on the specification and an implementation under test given in the form of a finite state machine (FSM). In realistic applications, this specification evolves incrementally throughout incorporating frequent modifications. In this paper, we adapt three well-known test derivation methods, namely the W, Wp, and HIS methods, for generating tests that would test the modified parts of the evolving specification. Application examples are provided.

Keywords: Conformance testing, finite state machines, test derivation, re-testing

1. INTRODUCTION

Many methods have been developed for deriving tests for a system represented by a Finite State Machine (FSM) model. The purpose of these tests is to determine whether an implementation of the system conforms to (i.e., is correct with respect to) its specification. Usually a conforming implementation is required to have the same I/O behavior.

In realistic applications, maintaining a system modeled by a given specification machine involves modifying its specification as a result of changes in the users' requirements and designers implement incrementally these modifications. Testing the whole system implementation after each modification is considered expensive and time consuming. Therefore, it is important to generate tests (called re-tests) that would only test the modified parts of the implementation that correspond to the modified parts of its specification. This would reduce the maintenance cost of such a system, which is about two-thirds of the cost of the software production [10].

In this paper, we present test generation methods (called henceforth as re-testing methods) that select tests (called re-tests) for testing the modified parts of the system specification, in order to check that these modifications were correctly implemented in the system implementation. Here we assume that the parts of the system implementation that correspond to the unmodified parts of the system specification are left intact. Moreover, we also reasonably assume that before modifying the system specification, its implementation was tested and found conforming to this specification. These methods are based on well-known test derivation methods called the W[1], Wp [3], and HIS [8] methods.

The problem of deriving re-testing sequences can be converted into the problem of test derivation from an FSM with a fault function [7] or from its generalization [5]. In this case, potential implementations are represented as all complete sub-machines of a given nondeterministic FSM that is called a mutation machine. However, the mutation machine from which re-testing sequences are derived, is special. Each unmodified specification transition is a deterministic transition of the mutation machine while each modified transition becomes chaotic; each pair (state, output) becomes possible as its tail state and output in a potential implementation. In other words, on one hand, the mutation machine has a number of deterministic transitions that can be used deriving a test suite, while on the other hand, a number of all possible paths that include modified transitions becomes exponential. Based on these features, we propose a proper technique for test derivation. First, we do not explicitly enumerate all possible implementation paths under an appropriate input sequence and secondly, we essentially use unmodified specification transitions that still remain deterministic in the mutation FSM. However, we always mention when our method delivers the same test suite as the methods for test derivation from an arbitrary mutation machine proposed in [7], [5].

This paper is organized as follows. Section 2, describes the finite state machine model, and Section 3 briefly describes the W, Wp, and HIS methods for generating tests from a given FSM specification. Based on these methods, our re-testing methods are presented in Section 4 with appropriate application examples. Section 5 concludes the paper.

2. FINITE STATE MACHINES

A deterministic *finite state machine* is a 7-tuple $M = (S, X, Y, \delta, \lambda, D_M, s_1)$, where: S is a finite set of states, s_1 is the *initial state*, X is a finite set of input symbols, Y is a finite set of output symbols, δ is a next state (or transition) function: δ: D_M --> S, λ is an output function: λ: D_M --> Y, and D_M is a specification domain: $D_M \subseteq S \times X$.

We use as in [3] the notation "(s_i -x/y-> s_j)" to indicate that the FSM M at state s_i responds with an output y and makes the transition to the state s_j when the input x is applied. State s_i is said to be the *head* or *starting* state of the transition, while s_j is said to be the *tail* or *ending* state of the transition. If we are not interested in the output we write "s_i-v->s_j" when an input sequence v is applied at state s_i. FSM M is said to be *completely specified* or simply a *complete* FSM, if $D_M = S \times X$; otherwise, M is said to be *partially specified* or simply a *partial* FSM. In the complete FSM, we omit the specification domain D_M, i.e. a complete FSM is a 6-tuple $M = (S, X, Y, \delta, \lambda, s_1)$. The concatenation of sequences v_1 and v_2 is the sequence $v_1.v_2$. For a given alphabet Z, Z^* is used to denote the set of all finite words over Z. Let V be a set of words over alphabet Z. The prefix closure of V, written ***Pref***(V), consists of all the prefixes of each word in V, i.e. ***Pref***$(V) = \{\alpha \mid \exists \gamma (\alpha.\gamma \in V)\}$. The set V is *prefix-closed* if ***Pref***$(V) = V$.

Let $M_S = (S, X, Y, \delta_S, \lambda_S, D_S, s_1)$ and $M_I = (T, X, Y, \Delta_I, \Lambda_I, D_I, t_1)$ be two FSMs. In the following sections M_S usually represents a protocol specification while M_I denotes an implementation, and thus, FSM M_I is further assumed to be complete. Given an input sequence $\alpha = x_1\ x_2 .. x_k \in X^*$, α is called a *defined input sequence*(**DIS**) at state $s_i \in S$, if there exist k states $s_{i1}, s_{i2}, ..., s_{ik} \in S$ such that there is a sequence of specified transitions s_i- x_1-> s_{i1} --> ... --> $s_{i(k-1)}$- x_k-> s_{ik} in the finite state machine M_S. Hereafter, **DIS**$(M_S|s_i)$ will be used to denote the set of all the defined input sequences at state s_i of machine M_S.

We say that states s_i of M_S and t_j of M_I are compatible if **DIS**$(M_S|s_i) \cap$ **DIS**$(M_I|t_j)=\emptyset$ or if $\forall\ \alpha \in$ **DIS**$(M_S|s_i) \cap$ **DIS**$(M_I|t_j)$ it holds that $\lambda_S(s_i, \alpha) = \Lambda_I(t_j, \alpha)$. Otherwise; we say that states s_i and s_j are distinguishable. Input sequence $\alpha \in$ **DIS**$(M_S|s_i) \cap$ **DIS**$(M_I|t_j)$ such that $\lambda_S(s_i, \alpha) \neq \Lambda_I(t_j, \alpha)$ is said to distinguish the states s_i and t_j. An FSM is said to be *reduced* if its states are pair-wise distinguishable. If the FSMs happen to be complete, then the definition of compatible states reduces to the definition of equivalent states (see for example, [4]).

3. REVIEW OF THE W, WP, AND HIS METHODS

In the following section we briefly describe test derivation methods where the specification is given as a reduced FSM M_S while an implementation under test (IUT) is modeled by a complete FSM M_I.

Let t_i be a state of M_I and s_j be a state of M_S. Consider set V of input sequences such that $V \subseteq \mathbf{DIS}(M_S|s_j)$. State t_i is said to be equivalent to s_j with respect to the set V (written as $t_i \cong_V s_j$), if $\Lambda_I(t_i, \alpha) = \lambda_S(s_j, \alpha)$ holds for any $\alpha \in V$. In other words, for each input sequence of V, a behavior of M_I at state t_i coincides with that of M_S at state s_j.

We say that M_I *conforms* to M_S if and only if $t_1 \cong_{\mathbf{DIS}(M_S|s_1)} s_1$, where t_1 and s_1 are the initial states of M_I and M_S, respectively. In other words, for each input sequence where a behavior of M_S is defined, M_I has the same behavior, i.e. the implementation is quasi-equivalent to the specification [4]. This conformance relation corresponds to the notion of weak conformance [9].

A set Q of input sequences is called a *state cover set* of FSM M_S if for each state s_i of S, there is an input sequence $\alpha_i \in Q$ such that s_1-α_i->s_i.

Usually the testing methods reviewed in this section use state identification facilities in order to check that each state and each transition defined in the specification also exists in the implementation. These facilities have certain input/output behaviors that can distinguish the states of an FSM. Given a reduced FSM M_S and a state $s_i \in S$, a set $W_i \subseteq \mathbf{DIS}(M_S|s_i)$ of defined input sequences at state s_i is called a *state identifier* of state s_i if for any other state s_j there exists $\alpha \in W_i \cap \mathbf{DIS}(M_S|s_j)$ such that $\lambda_S(s_i, \alpha) \neq \lambda_S(s_j, \alpha)$. We now define a collection of state identifiers that has been named a family of *harmonized identifiers* [6], [8] or a separating family [11]. A *separating family* is a collection of state identifiers W_i, $s_i \in S$, which satisfy the condition that for any two states s_i, and s_j, $i \neq j$, there exist $\beta \in W_i$ and $\gamma \in W_j$ which have common prefix α such that $\alpha \in \mathbf{DIS}(M_S|s_i) \cap \mathbf{DIS}(M_S|s_j)$, and $\lambda_S(s_i, \alpha) \neq \lambda_S(s_j, \alpha)$. A separating family exists for any reduced (partial or complete) machine.

A *characterization set* of the FSM M_S, often simply called a *W set*, is a set of input sequences which satisfies the following conditions:

(1) For any $s_k \in S$, $W \subseteq \mathbf{DIS}(M_S|s_k)$,
(2) For any two states s_i, and s_j, $i \neq j$, there exists $\beta \in W$ such that $\lambda_S(s_i, \beta) \neq \lambda_S(s_j, \beta)$.

A W set always exists for a reduced completely specified machine. However, the W set does not always exist for a reduced partially specified machine.

Given a specification reduced FSM $M_S = (S, X, Y, \delta_S, \lambda_S, D_S, s_1)$, $|S|=\boldsymbol{n}$, and a complete implementation FSM $M_I = (T, X, Y, \Delta_I, \Lambda_I, t_1)$ such that

$|T|=n$, let W be a characterization set of M_S (if exists) and $F = \{W_1,\ldots, W_n\}$ be a separating family of M_S.

All the methods have two phases. In the first so-called *state identification* phase, they establish a one-to-one mapping $h_{S\text{-}I}$: $S \rightarrow T$ by the use of a characterization set W or a separating family F. Given a prefix-closed state cover set $Q = \{\alpha_1, \alpha_2,\ldots, \alpha_n\}$ of the specification FSM, for each state $s_j \in S$, the state identification phase comprises the sequences: $r.\alpha_j.W_j$ (HIS method) or $r.\alpha_j.W$ (W and Wp methods).

We note that, if the specification FSM M_S is partial, a characterization set W may not exist; in this case, the W and Wp methods cannot be applied. However, the HIS method can be applied.

If FSM M_I passes the state identification test sequences, then there exists one-to-one mapping $h_{S\text{-}I}$: $S \rightarrow T$ such that: $h(s_j) = t \Leftrightarrow s_j \cong_{W_j} t$ in the HIS method, and $h(s_j) = t \Leftrightarrow s_j \cong_W t$ in the W and Wp methods.

The second so-called *transition testing* phase, assures that for each state $s \in S$, and input $x \in X$ that is defined at state s the mapping $h_{S\text{-}I}$ satisfies the following property:

$$\lambda_S(s, x) = \Lambda_I(h_{S\text{-}I}(s), x) \text{ and } h_{S\text{-}I}(\delta_S(s, x)) = \Delta_I(h_{S\text{-}I}(s), x) \qquad \textbf{(X-1)}$$

For this purpose, for each sequence $\alpha_j \in Q$ that takes the specification FSM to appropriate state s_j, and each $x \in X$ that takes the M_S from state s_j to state s_k, the testing transition phase includes the set of sequences:

$r.\alpha_j.x.W_k$ in the HIS and Wp methods, where W_k is a state identifier of the state s_k in the specification FSM (for the Wp method, we have $W_k \subseteq W$) or

$r.\alpha_j.x.W$ in the W method

If FSM M_I passes the test sequences of both testing phases, then it is quasi-equivalent to the specification FSM, i.e. is a conforming implementation. If the specification FSM is complete then the quasi-equivalence relation reduces to the equivalence relation, i.e. the specification FSM and its conforming implementation have the same Input/Output behavior.

4. FSM BASED RE-TESTING

4.1 Problem Definition

Let the reduced FSM $M_S = (S, X, Y, \delta_S, \lambda_S, D_S, s_1)$ be the specification of a given system. We assume that the complete implementation FSM $M_I = (T, X, Y, \Delta_I, \Lambda_I, t_1)$ of M_S with the same number of states has been tested and found conforming to M_S. Therefore, there exists a one-to-one mapping $h_{S\text{-}I}$: $S \rightarrow T$ such that for each state $s \in S$ and input $x \in X$ that is defined at state s, (X-1) holds.

Let the reduced $M_S' = (S, X, Y, \delta_S, \lambda_S, D_S', s_1)$ be the modified specification, and $M_I'=(T, X, Y, \Delta_I, \Lambda_I, t_1)$ be the modified implementation that must conform to M_S'. We assume that only transitions corresponding to the modified parts of M_S' have been changed in M_I' and we want to generate test sequences for the modified parts of the system specification, in order to check that these modifications were implemented correctly in the modified implementation M_I'. In other words, for each unmodified transition (s_j-x/y->s_k) of the M_S', we assume that transition ($h_{S\text{-}I}(s_j)$-x/y->$h_{S\text{-}I}(s_k)$) has not been changed in the modified implementation M_I'. We note that in case where new states are added (or deleted) to (or from) M_S, we let S' denote the set of states of M_S' and T' denote the set of states of M_I', respectively.

In general, we have the following types of modifications that can be made in M_S and implemented by a designer in M_I:

(1) outputs of some transitions are modified, (2) tail states of some transitions are modified, (3) outputs and tail states of some transitions are modified, (4) new transitions are added (5) some transitions are deleted, (6) new states are added, and (7) some states are deleted.

4.2 The Re-testing Methods

The re-testing methods adapted for the W, Wp, and HIS test derivation methods have also two phases. In the first phase, re-tests are selected in order to check (or re-identify) some states of the modified specification in the new implementation, and in the second re-testing phase, re-tests are selected to check each modified transition for correct output and tail state. Here, we examine different cases that can be used to generate short re-testing test sequences.

For convenience, hereafter, we use the input symbols a and b for unmodified transitions, and x and z for modified ones.

4.3 Case-1: The Unmodified Part of the Modified Specification is Reduced

Here we assume that the unmodified part $UP\text{-}M_S'$ of the modified specification M_S' is reduced. Then, there exist state identifiers $W_1, \ldots, W_n$, which satisfy the following conditions: 1) each W_i is a subset of the defined input sequences at state $s_i \in S$ in the $UP\text{-}M_S'$, 2) given two states s_i, and s_j, $i \neq j$, there exist sequences in W_i and W_j with the common prefix β such that $\lambda_S(s_i, \beta) \neq \lambda_S(s_j, \beta)$.

We note that since the unmodified part of the specification can be partial, a characterization set W may not exist. However, we can always select state identifiers with the above conditions.

4.3.1 General solution

For each modified edge (s_j-x/y->s_k), its corresponding re-testing test cases are formed as follows:

If we use the HIS or Wp methods: $r.\alpha_j.x.W_k$, **(1-a)**

where W_k is a state identifier of state s_k.

If a characterization set W exists and we use the W method: $r.\alpha_j.x.W$ **(1-b)**

Theorem 1. Given a modified specification M_S' and its implementation M_I', let the unmodified part of M_S' be reduced and have state identifiers W_1, ..., W_n. If implementation M_I' passes the re-testing test suite which consists of the union of the test cases over all modified transitions as given in Formulae (1-a) or (1-b), then the implementation M_I' is quasi-equivalent to M_S'.

We omit the proof of Theorem 1 since it is a particular case of Theorem 2.

We note that if the specification FSM is complete then the above case is a particular case of the advanced procedure in [7] since each state identifier is a so-called stable state identifier, i.e. is a state identifier of the corresponding state in each potential implementation.

4.3.2 An Optimized Solution

We observe that a sequence that distinguishes two states of the initial specification and traverses only unmodified transitions when applied at these states, also distinguishes the corresponding states of the modified implementation M_I'. Moreover, when the unmodified part of the modified specification is reduced, the mapping $h_{S\text{-}I}(s)$: $S \rightarrow T$ between the initial specification and its conforming implementation is the only candidate that can satisfy (X-1) for the modified specification and its implementation. Therefore, we do not need to re-identify states of the modified implementation. Moreover, the test suite constructed using the formulae of the general solution may be shortened if we use, when checking certain transitions, shorter state identifiers that pass through already tested transitions rather than those generated only from the unmodified part of the modified specification. In other words, instead of using state identifiers derived in advance, we can generate shorter state identifiers, as modified transitions are tested. For this purpose, we assume that a linear order "<" over modified transitions of the specification is given. This order satisfies the following property: If $\alpha_r.z \in Q$ is a prefix of $\alpha_j \in Q$, then for any two modified transitions (s_r-z->s_l) and (s_j-x->s_k), transition (s_r-z->s_l)<(s_j-x->s_k). In this case, when checking a modified transition, we can use lower order transitions (or already checked transitions) to generate shorter re-testing sequences. The reason is that if the implementation at hand passes retesting sequences for transition (s_r-z/y->s_l) then it has the corresponding transition ($h_{S\text{-}I}(s_r)$ -z/y-> $h_{S\text{-}I}(s_l)$), and this transition can be used for retesting a higher order transition. In this section, we illustrate by an example the advantage of using such a linear order. However, we do not discuss how to derive an order that provides the shortest re-testing sequences.

For each modified edge (s_j-x->s_k), its corresponding re-testing test cases are formed as in Formulae (1-a) or (1-b). However, as a state identifier of state s_k, we use state identifier W_k (or characterization set W in W method) of the part of M_S that comprises unmodified transitions or modified transitions (s_r-z->s_l) where (s_r-z->s_l) < (s_j-x->s_k). In other words, for testing transition (s_j-x->s_k) the state identifier W_k has sequences that if applied at state s_k only traverse unmodified transitions or modified transitions (s_r-z->s_l) < (s_j-x->s_k). This allows, when checking a modified transition, the use of already re-checked transitions (or lower order transitions) in order to generate shorter state identifiers.

Theorem 2. Given a modified specification M_S' and its implementation M_I', let the unmodified part of M_S' be reduced, and for each modified transition (s_j-x->s_k) W_k is a state identifier of state s_k in the part of M_S that comprises unmodified transitions or modified transitions (s_r-z->s_l) < (s_j-z->s_k). If implementation M_I' passes the re-testing test suite which consists of the union of the test cases over all modified transitions as given in Formulae (1-a) or (1-b), then the implementation is quasi-equivalent to M_S'.

Proof. A proof of Theorem 2 is given in [2].

As an example for the general and optimized solution methods based on the HIS method, we consider the modified specification FSM M_1 shown in Fig. 1. FSM M_1 has the input set $X=\{a, b, c\}$, output set $Y=\{y_1, y_2, y_3\}$. The labels of the modified transitions are shown in bold. The unmodified part of FSM M_1 has a separating family $\{w_1, w_2, w_3, w_4\}$ of state identifiers, where $w_1= \{bb\}$, $w_2= \{bb\}$, $w_3= \{bb, c\}$ and $w_4= \{bb, c\}$. In fact, for each state s_i of M_1 we have the following input/output sequences in response to w_i.

Table 1. Responses of M_1 to state identifiers (if defined)

	s_1	s_2	s_3	s_4
$b\,b$	$y_1\,y_2$	$y_2\,y_2$	$y_2\,y_1$	$y_2\,y_1$
c			y_2	y_1

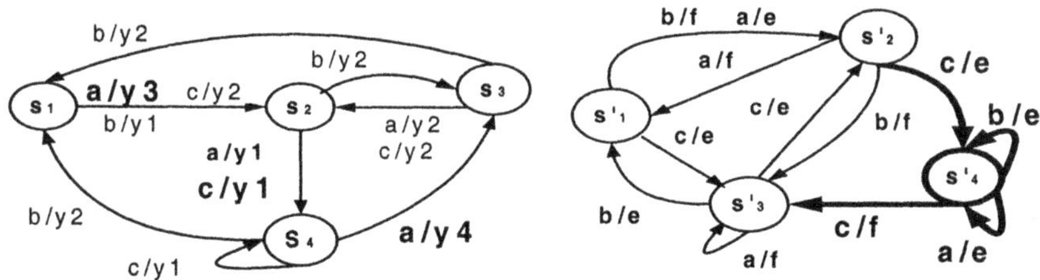

Figure 1. Specification M_1.

Figure 2. Specification M_S'.

None of the above state identifiers passes through a modified transition if applied at an appropriate state, and thus, the unmodified part of M_S' is reduced. According to the general solution, in order to re-test the modified transitions, the following re-testing sequences of length 24 are generated using Formula (1-a): $\{r.\alpha_1.a.w_2 + r.\alpha_2.c.w_4 + r.\alpha_4.a.w_3\} = \{r.\varepsilon.a.bb,\ r.b.c.bb,\ r.b.c.c,\ r.ba.a.bb,\ r.ba.a.c\}$, where $\alpha_1 = \varepsilon$, $\alpha_2 = b$ and $\alpha_4 = ba$ are the corresponding sequences of the state cover set .

We now use the following linear order over modified transitions (s_1-a->s_2) < (s_4 a->s_3) < (s_2-c->s_4). In order to re-test the modified transition (s_1-a-> s_2), the re-testing test sequence $\{r.a.w_2 = r.a.bb\}$ is used. If the implementation at hand passes this sequence, then we have the following responses to the input a :

At state $h_{S\text{-}I}(s_1)$: y_3, at state $h_{S\text{-}I}(s_2)$: y_1, and at state $h_{S\text{-}I}(s_3)$: y_2,

Consequently, in order to re-test transition (s_4-a->s_3), the re-testing test sequence $r.\alpha_4.a.a = r.b.a.a.a$ will be enough instead of $r.\alpha_4.a.w_3$, since $r.\alpha_4$ reaches state s_4 through unmodified transitions and if afterwards, the modified implementation produces the expected output y_4 to the input symbol a, then a becomes a distinguishing sequence for the part of the specification comprising unmodified transitions and transitions (s_1-a->s_2) and (s_4-a->s_3), where for the last transition only its output has been checked; therefore, a is a distinguishing sequence for the corresponding part of the modified implementation.

Afterwards, in order to check the ending state s_4 of the modified transition (s_2-c->s_4), the distinguishing sequence a can be used instead of the previous state identifier $w_4 = \{bb, c\}$. Hence, the re-testing test sequence of this transition is $r.\alpha_2.c.a = r.b.c.a$. Therefore, according to the optimized solution method, in order to re-test the modified transitions, the following re-testing sequences are generated using the above linear order and Formulae (1-a): $\{r.a.bb + r.b.a.a.a + r.b.c.a\}$.

The total length of these sequences is 13, where the total length of those generated using Formula (1-a) of the general solution method is 24. The HIS method generates a test suite of length 51 if the whole specification of M_S' is considered for test derivation.

4.4 Case-2: Each State of the Modified Specification is Reachable Through Unmodified Transitions and the Unmodified Part is Not Reduced.

In some cases, the unmodified part of the modified specification M_S' is not reduced. However, each state of M_S' is reachable through some unmodified transitions. Since each state of M_S' can be reached through unmodified transitions, the only possible correct mapping between the states of M_S' and M_I' is the old mapping established between the states of M_S and M_I. Therefore, in order to check that this mapping still holds for the states of the modified specification and implementation the only states that have state identifiers passing through modified transitions have to be re-identified in the new implementation. Moreover, in order to re-identify such a state, it is enough to apply only the sequences of the corresponding state identifier that pass through modified transitions.

Let Q be a prefix-closed state cover set such that its sequences do not traverse modified transitions if applied at the initial state of M_S'. Let also $F = \{W_1, ..., W_n\}$ be a separating family of the modified specification, and W be a characterization set (if exists).

i) State re-identification phase

For each state s_r such that some sequences of W_r traverse modified transitions if applied at s_r the state re-identification sequences are formed as follows:

$$r.\alpha_r.W_r' \qquad \textbf{(2-1a)}$$

where $W_r' \subseteq W_r$ (or $W_r' \subseteq W$ for the W and Wp methods) comprises each sequence of the state identifier W_r (of the characterization set W) that, if applied at state s_r of the modified specification, traverses a modified transition. We note that each state of M_S' for which all sequences of the state identifier traverse only unmodified transitions, does not need to be re-identified.

ii) Re-testing modified transitions phase

For each modified edge (s_j-x->s_k), its corresponding re-testing test sequences are formed as shown in Formulae (1-a) and (1-b).

Theorem 3. Given the modified specification M_S' and its implementation M_I', let $F = \{W_1, ..., W_n\}$ be a separating family of M_S' and W be a characterization set of M_S' (if exists). Let also Q be a prefix-closed state cover set of M_S' such that each sequence of the set Q does not traverse a modified transition if applied at the initial state. If implementation M_I' passes the re-testing test suite which is the union of the re-testing test sequences given in Formula (2-1a) and Formulae (1-a) or (1-b), then the implementation is quasi-equivalent to M_S'.

We omit the proof of Theorem 3 since it is a particular case of Theorem 4.

We note that union of the test cases given in Formula (2-1a) and Formula (1-a) coincides with the test suite returned by procedures in [7], [5], since both methods return a test suite without input sequences that traverse only unmodified transitions. However, here we underline the advantage of selecting a state cover set and state identifiers with sequences that do not traverse any modified transition. In this case, the old image of a corresponding state of a modified specification must be preserved and therefore, there is no need to check unmodified transitions at the corresponding state.

4.5 Case-3: Some States are only Reachable Through Modified Transitions

In some cases, the unmodified part of the modified specification M_S' is not reduced and some states of M_S' are only reachable through modified transitions. This case always holds when additional states are introduced when modifying the specification. Here, for the subset of states, say $S_{r\text{-}m}$ of the modified specification that are only reachable through modified transitions, the old conforming mapping might not be preserved between the new specification and its implementation, i.e. some $s_k \in S_{r\text{-}m}$ of the modified specification might be mapped to a new state of its implementation (say $t_l \in T_{r\text{-}m}$), different from t_k. Each such state must be re-identified in the new implementation and moreover, differently from former two cases, we have to check unmodified transitions from this state.

As an example, we modify the specification M_S shown in the upper part of Fig. 3 and obtain the FSM M_S' shown in the upper of Fig. 4. The modified transitions are shown as bold lines. We note that the mapping between states of M_S and its conforming implementation M_I, shown in the lower part of Fig. 3, is $h_{S\text{-}I}(s_k) = t_k$ for k= 1,...,4. Moreover, we let M_I', shown in the lower part of Fig. 4, be the implementation of M_S'. M_S' has $W = \{aa\}$ as a characterization set which is a state identifier of each state. In fact, we have the following output responses to *aa*. For state s_1, *xx*. For state s_2, *xy*. For state s_3, *yy*, and for state s_4, *yx*.

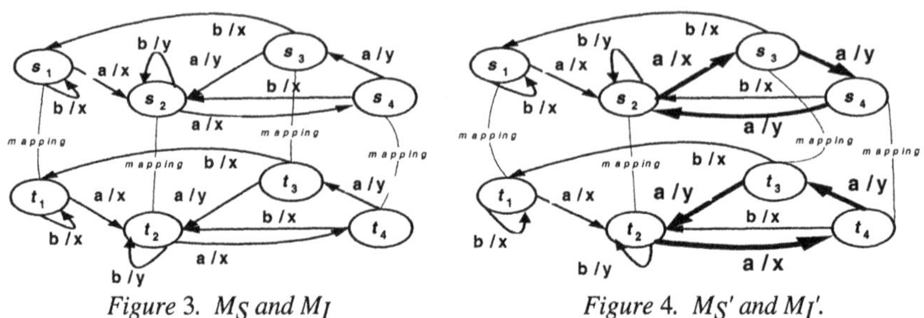

Figure 3. M_S and M_I

Figure 4. M_S' and M_I'.

We note that the modified implementation state t_4 of M_I' has the output response *yy* to *aa*, i.e. state s_3 of M_S' is *W*-equivalent to t_4 of M_I' while state s_4 of M_I' is *W*-equivalent to t_3 of M_I'. States t_1 and t_2 of M_I' are *W*-equivalent to s_1 and s_2 of M_I'. The mapping is preserved for the modified transitions from states t_3 and t_4 under input *a*. However, it is not preserved for the unmodified transitions at states s_3 of M_S' and s_4 of M_S' under input b, i.e. M_I' is a wrong implementation of M_S'. Therefore, appropriate unmodified transitions also need to be checked in order to kill such a wrong mapping.

As in the previous section, we select a prefix-closed state cover set with the following property. Given state $s_j \in S$ of M_S' reachable through unmodified transitions, we select the sequence $\alpha_j \in Q$ that does not traverse any modified transition.

The re-testing method has two phases. In the first phase, some states of the modified specification are re-identified in the new implementation. It may occur that for some states of the modified specification that are only reachable through modified transitions their old image must still be preserved in the new implementation. In particular, those are the states that have a so-called stable identifier [7] that distinguishes a state from any other state in each possible implementation. For each such state, we derive a state identifier (if it exists) that kills, through the re-identification phase, implementations where the state has a new image. We start from the set of states that are reachable through unmodified transitions. As in Case-2, the old mapping must still be valid for these states and only modified transitions from these states need to be checked. Moreover, given such a state, if the sequences of its state identifier do not traverse modified transitions then the state does not need to be re-identified. Otherwise, we select state re-identification sequences using Formula (2-1a) of Case-2, where in order to check the new mapping of a state, say s_j, we concatenate the sequence $r.\alpha_j$ with each sequence of the state identifier of the s_j that passes through a modified transition. Then, we iteratively identify all other states for which the old mapping must be preserved; however, their state identifiers are derived in a proper way as described below. Afterwards, since each remaining state, say $s_j \in S_{r-m}$, of the modified specification could have a new image, i.e. s_j could be mapped to say $t_k \in T_{r-m}$ instead of the old image $h_{S\text{-}I}(s_j) = t_j$, re-tests are selected to re-identify the image of s_j in the new implementation, i.e. check (or establish) that s_j is W-equivalent to t_k, and to check that this mapping is conforming. In order to re-identify s_j, re-tests are selected by concatenating $r.\alpha_j$ with each sequence in the state identifier of state s_j including sequences which traverse only unmodified transitions Moreover, in order to check that this mapping is a valid one (i.e. kill wrong mappings), re-tests are selected to check each outgoing transition from s_j for correct output and ending state in the new implementation.

In order to implement the above steps, we determine a subset S_u of the set of states of the modified specification such that for the states in S_u the old mapping between the states of the modified specification and its conforming modified implementation must still be preserved. The set S_u enjoys a nice property. For each state in S_u, we do not need to check its outgoing unmodified transitions. In the following paragraph, we determine which states may be in the set S_u and derive the set S_u together with a separating family $F=\{W_1, \ldots, W_n\}$ (or characterization set W) so that if the implementation passes the re-identification test sequences, then there exists one-to-one mapping $h: S \rightarrow T$ such that the following property holds.

$$\text{For each state } s_i \in S_u \text{ we have: } s_i \cong_{W_i} t \Leftrightarrow t = h_{S\text{-}I}(s_i). \qquad \textbf{(X-2)}$$

First, we add to the empty set S_u each state s_j that is reachable from the initial state through unmodified transitions. As in Case-2, the images of these states have to be still preserved in the new implementation. Then, for state s_j and each state $s_i \in S$, $s_i \neq s_j$, we include in the state identifiers W_j and W_i a sequence that distinguishes the states s_j and s_i in the modified specification. We note that, as discussed for Case-2, we recommend, while building the state identifier W_j, to select the sequences that do not pass through modified transitions if applied at state s_j, since we do not need to apply these sequences while re-identifying s_j.

Afterwards, we iteratively include in S_u each state $s_j \in S \backslash S_u$, such that for each state $s_i \in S \backslash S_u$, $s_i \neq s_j$, there exists sequence β_{ij} that does not traverse modified transitions if applied at states s_i and s_j and $\lambda_S(s_i, \beta_{ij}) \neq \lambda_S(s_j, \beta_{ij})$, or there exists input x such that transitions (s_j-x->s_k) and (s_i-x->s_r) are unmodified, $s_k \neq s_r$ and $s_k, s_r \in S_u$. In the former case, we include sequence β_{ij} in W_i and W_j. Since β_{ij} does not traverse modified transitions if applied at states s_i and s_j we have that $\Lambda_I(h_{S\text{-}I}(s_i), \beta_{ij}) = \lambda_S(s_i, \beta_{ij})$, and $\lambda_S(s_j, \beta_{ij}) \neq \Lambda_I(h_{S\text{-}I}(s_i), \beta_{ij})$. Thus, if β_{ij} is included into W_i and W_j and the implementation passes the corresponding state re-identification sequences, then s_j is not W-equivalent to $h_{S\text{-}I}(s_i)$ (i.e $h_{S\text{-}I}(s_j) \neq h_{S\text{-}I}(s_i)$). In the latter case, we include into W_i and W_j the sequence $x\beta$ where β is a common prefix of the appropriate sequences in W_i and W_j such that $\lambda_S(s_k, \beta) \neq \lambda_S(s_r, \beta)$. Thus if $\Lambda_I(h_{S\text{-}I}(s_i), x.\beta)=\lambda_S(s_i, x.\beta)$, then $\lambda_S(s_j, x.\beta) \neq \Lambda_I(h_{S\text{-}I}(s_i), x.\beta)$. If $x.\beta$ is included in W_i and W_j and the implementation passes the corresponding state re-identification sequences, then s_j is not W-equivalent to $h_{S\text{-}I}(s_i)$. Due to the definition of state identifiers for states in S_u, such a sequence exists. If any sequence of each state identifier is defined at each state then we derive the set W as the union of all state identifiers. We note that in order to kill for s_j any mapping h_I where $h_I(s_j) \neq h_{S\text{-}I}(s_j)$, the corresponding state re-identification sequences are derived by concatenating $r.\alpha_j$ with every sequence of the set W_j (or W for the Wp and W methods).

Finally, we derive state identifiers for the remaining states in $S \backslash S_u$. For each state s_j in $S \backslash S_u$ and for each state $s_i \in S$, $s_i \neq s_j$, we include a sequence β_{ij} in W_i and W_j (if it does not already exist) such that $\lambda_s(s_i, \beta_{ij}) \neq \lambda_s(s_j, \beta_{ij})$. In order to re-identify s_j in the new implementation and kill its possible wrong images, the corresponding re-testing sequences include all re-identification sequences and re-testing sequences for testing all outgoing transitions from state s_j.

The characterization set W (for the W, and Wp methods) can be obtained as the union of state identifiers W_i, i=1, ..., n (if possible). We note that in order to reduce the number of transitions which need to be checked we use another technique than that based on stable state identifiers [7]. The main idea behind our approach is based on the observation that for each state reachable through unmodified transitions and some other states, the old image must be preserved in each conforming modified implementation. Our technique can also be used to reduce a test suite derived from a mutation machine [5] if the latter has many deterministic transitions.

i) Phase of state re-identification

For each state s_j of the modified specification that needs to be re-identified in the new implementation, we derive its state re-identification test sequences as follows:

If α_j does not traverse a modified transition, the re-identification sequences are formed as in Formula (2-1a).

If α_j traverses a modified transition then there are test sequences

$r.\alpha_j.W_j$ (HIS method); **(3-1a)**

$r.\alpha_j.W$ (W and Wp methods). **(3-1b)**

Every sequence of the set W_j (or W) must be applied after α_j, whether the sequence applied at state s_j traverses a modified transition or not.

ii) Phase of re-testing modified transitions

For each modified edge (s_j-x->s_k), where $s_j \in S_u$, its corresponding test cases are formed as in Formulae (1-a) or (1-b). For each state $s_j \notin S_u$,

Formula (1-a) or (1-b) are applied for each outgoing transition from state s_j including those which are unmodified.

Theorem 4. Given the modified specification M_S' and implementation M_I', let Q be a prefix-closed state cover set of M_S' and $F = \{W_1, \ldots, W_n\}$ and W be a separating family and a characterization set (if exists) of the modified specification M_S' derived as described above. If implementation M_I' passes the re-testing test suite derived for Case-3, then the implementation is quasi-equivalent to M_S'.

Proof. As we demonstrated by the example, in Case 3, a one-to-one mapping h: $S \rightarrow T$ such that state s_i of M_S' is W_i-equivalent to state $h(s_i)$ of M_I' can be different from $h_{S\text{-}I}$. We first need to check whether the one-to-one mapping h exists at all.

We consider a relation $h \in S \times T$ such that: $(s_j, t_j) \in h \Leftrightarrow s_j \cong_{W_j} t_j$. If the implementation passes the re-identification test cases given by Formulae (2-1a), (3-1a) and (3-1b) then h is a one-to-one mapping h: $S \rightarrow T$. We next show that $h(s_j) = h_{S\text{-}I}(s_j)$ holds for each $s_j \in S_u$.

Given state $s_j \in S$ of M_S' such that the sequence $\alpha_j \in Q$ does not traverse modified transitions, if M_I' passes the test sequences given in Formulae (3-1a) then the state $h_{S\text{-}I}(s_j) = h(s_j)$. The initial state s_1 is in the set S_u, i.e. the base of induction holds.

Let us assume that $h(s) = h_{S\text{-}I}(s)$ holds for each state s of a current set S_u and that state s_j is the next state we are going to include into S_u using the procedure described above. Since h is a one-to-one mapping, for each state $s \in S_u$ it holds that $h(s_j) \neq h_{S\text{-}I}(s)$. On the other hand, for each state $s_i \in S \setminus S_u$, $i \neq j$, by construction of the state identifier, $\exists$ a sequence $\beta_{ij} \in W_j \cap W_i$ such that β_{ij} does not traverse modified transitions if applied at states s_i or s_j and $\lambda_S(s_i, \beta_{ij}) \neq \lambda_S(s_j, \beta_{ij})$, or $\exists$ a sequence $x\beta \in W_j \cap W_i$ such that the final states of unmodified transitions (s-x->s_k) and (s_i-x->s_r) are different and $\lambda_S(s_k, \beta) \neq \lambda_S(s_r, \beta)$. In the former case, M_I' has different output responses to the sequence $\beta_{ij} \in W_j \cap W_i$ at the states $h(s_j)$ and $h_{S\text{-}I}(s_i)$, i.e. $h(s_j) \neq h_{S\text{-}I}(s_i)$. In the latter case, M_I' at states $h_{S\text{-}I}(s_k)$ and $h_{S\text{-}I}(s_r)$ has different output responses to the sequence $\beta \in W_k \cap W_r$, i.e. M_I' has different output responses to the sequence $x\beta \in W_k \cap W_r$ at the states $h(s_j)$ and $h_{S\text{-}I}(s_i)$, i.e. $h(s_j) \neq h_{S\text{-}I}(s_i)$. Therefore, by induction, $h(s_j) = h_{S\text{-}I}(s_j)$ for each state $s_j \in S_u$.

For each unmodified transition (s_j-a ->s_l) from state $s_j \in S_u$ it holds that $\lambda_S(s_j, a) = \Lambda_I(h_{S\text{-}I}(s_j))$ and $h_{S\text{-}I}(s_l) = \Delta(h_{S\text{-}I}(s_j), a)$.

If M_I' passes the test cases $r.\alpha_j.x.W_k$ for a modified transition (s_j-x ->s_k) then $\lambda_S(s_j, x) = \Lambda_I(h_{S\text{-}I}(s_j), x)$ and the ending state of the transition ($h_{S\text{-}I}(s_j)$-x ->t_k) is W_k-equivalent to s_k.

Due to the construction of retesting sequences, we also check that (X-1) holds for each transition from each state $s_j \notin S_u$. Thus, if M_I' passes the test, then the mapping h satisfies (X-1), i.e. M_I' is quasi-equivalent to M_S' □

As an application example for Case-3 with the HIS method, we add to the given specification a new state s'_4 and its corresponding incoming and outgoing edges producing the modified specification M_S' shown in Fig. 2.

The state cover set of M_S' is $Q'=\{\varepsilon, b, c, bc\}$. We consider each incoming and outgoing transition of the added state (here s'_4) as a modified transition. Therefore, the modified transitions of M_S' are (s'_2-*c*/*f*->s'_4), (s'_4-*b*/*f*->s'_4), (s'_4-*a*/*e*->s'_4), and (s'_4-*c*/*f*->s'_3).

According to Case-3, we add to the set S_u states s'_1, s'_2, and s'_3 since these states are reachable through unmodified transitions and there exists a state identifier for each of these states that does not pass through modified transitions. In this example, the sequence *bb* is such an identifier. In fact, we have the following input/output sequences in response to *bb*. For state s'_1, *ff*. For state s'_2, *fe*. For state s'_3, *ef*, and for state s'_4, *ee*.

These states, i.e., s'_1, s'_2, and s'_3 , do not need to be re-identified in the new implementation. In order to re-identify the added state s'_4, the re-test sequence $r.\alpha_4.W_4 = r.bc.bb$ is selected using Formula (3-1a). If the modified implementation passes this sequence then there is a one-to-one mapping between states of the modified specification and implementation that are *bb*-equivalent.

Afterwards, in order to test the modified transition (s'_2-*c*/*f*->s'_4) whose head state s'_2 is in S_u, the sequence $r.\alpha_2.c.W_4 = r.b.c.bb$ is selected using Formula (1-a). Moreover, the following re-testing test sequences are selected using Formula (3-1c) in order to check the outgoing transitions from state $s'_4 \in S \backslash S_u$: $r.\alpha_4.a.W_4+r.\alpha_4.b.W_4+r.\alpha_4.c.W_3 = r.bc.a.bb+r.bc.b.bb+r.bc.c.bb$

Consequently, the re-testing test suite has sequences of total length 18. The traditional HIS method derives a test suite of length 32 if the whole specification of M_S' is considered for test derivation.

5. FURTHER RESEARCH WORK

We have extended the re-testing methods presented in this paper for the case when the system implementation may have more states than its specification. Moreover, we are adapting these methods for a system modeled as an Extended Finite State Machine (EFSM). The problem here is to find an appropriate way for re-testing both the control flow and the data flow parts of a modified EFSM. Finally, we are investigating how the re-testing methods can be applied to a labeled transition system (LTS).

REFERENCES

[1] T. S. Chow, 'Test design modeled by finite-state machines'. *IEEE Trans. SE*-4, No.3, pp. 178-187, 1978.

[2] K. El-Fakih, N, Yevtushenko, and G. v. Bochmann, 'Re-testing Based on Finite State Model', Technical Report, University of Ottawa, 2001.

[3] S. Fujiwara, G. v. Bochmann, F. Khendek, M. Amalou, and A. Ghedamsi, 'Test selection based on finite state models', *IEEE Trans. SE*-17, No. 6, 591-603, 1991.

[4] A. Gill, *Introduction to the Theory of Finite-State Machines.* McGraw-Hill, 1962.

[5] I.Koufareva, A.Petrenko, N.Yevtushenko. Test generation driven by user-defined fault models. In *Proc. of the IFIP TC6 12th International Workshop on Testing of Communicating Systems*, Hungary, pp. 215-233, 1999.

[6] A. Petrenko, *Checking experiments with protocol machines*, Proceedings of the IFIP Fourth International Workshop on Protocol Test Systems, the Netherlands, 1991, pp. 83-94.

[7] A. Petrenko and N. Yevtushenko,'Test suite generation for a FSM with a given type of implementation errors', *Proc. of the 12th IWPSTV*, pp. 229-243, 1992.

[8] A. Petrenko, N. Yevtushenko, A. Lebedev, and A. Das, 'Nondeterministic state machines in protocol conformance testing', In *Proc. of the IFIP Sixth International Workshop on Protocol Test Systems*, France, pp. 363-378, 1993.

[9] K. Sabnani and A. Dahbura,'A protocol test generation procedure'. *Computer Networks and ISDN Systems*, Vol. 15, No. 4, 285-297, 1988.

[10] S. Schach, *Software Engineering*, Boston:Aksen Assoc., 1992.

[11] M. Yannakakis and D. Lee, 'Testing finite state machines: fault detection', *Journal of Computer and System Sciences*, 50, 1995, pp. 209-227, 1995.

A NEW APPROACH TO CHECKING SEQUENCE GENERATION FOR FINITE STATE MACHINES *

Burak Serdar, Kuo-Chung Tai
North Carolina State University
Computer Science Department
Raleigh, North Carolina, USA 27695-7534
bserdar@ieee.org, kct@eos.ncsu.edu

Abstract A formal model for generating checking sequences for finite state machines is proposed. The model is based on the machine identification problem, which deals with determining the internals of an unknown machine by performing experiments on it. This approach provides a formal framework which can be used to reason about properties of checking sequences in general. Based on this model, a new method called the U_γ-method employing UIO sequences is developed. The method assumes that the specification machine possesses a compound distinguishing sequence. The U_γ-method does not rely on the existence of the reset feature, and constructs checking sequences that can identify all faults of an implementation provided that the implementation has the same number of states as the specification. Empirical results are given to compare the U_γ-method with existing methods. These results show that the U_γ-method generates shorter checking sequences than existing U-methods for most cases.

Keywords: Conformance testing, checking sequences, finite state machines, machine identification, unique input/output sequences

1. INTRODUCTION

Conformance testing is the process of testing an implementation with respect to its specification. A specification of a system in diverse areas can be modeled by a finite state machine (FSM). An FSM models the system as a set of transitions between states. Usually, the implementation under test is treated as a black-box. A tester gives an input

*This work was supported in part by NSF Grant CCR-9901004.

sequence to a machine, and observes the produced output sequence. The applied input sequence is called a **test sequence** [9] [2] [3] or a **checking sequence** [6] [5] [15].

In this work, we deal with preset checking sequences for FSM specifications. A preset checking sequence is constructed using the specification machine before the test. Usually, the process involves constructing an input sequence which verifies transitions of the implementation. This is achieved by bringing the implementation to a known state, applying a test input, verifying the output, and verifying that the implementation is in the expected state. This approach is called **transition checking**.

Popular test generation methods include the D- [5] [11], W- [2] and U-methods [3] [11]. These methods utilize distinguishing sequences (DS), W-sets and unique input/output (UIO) sequences to verify the states of an implementation. The basic D- [11] and W-methods [2] assume the existence of reliable reset feature and provide guaranteed fault coverage, where methods given in [5] and [15] achieve the same goal without using the reset feature. The basic U-method [3] [11] also utilizes the reset feature, but cannot detect all faults of an implementation [14]. The UIO-v method [1] provides guaranteed fault coverage using the reset feature, by applying each UIO sequence to all the states of the implementation. The UIOG method [17] also provides guaranteed fault coverage without using the reset feature, by applying each UIO sequence to all states using an approach similar to locating sequences [6].

In this paper, we first develop a formal model for checking sequence generation based on the machine identification problem. The machine identification problem deals with determining the internals of an unknown machine by performing experiments on it [12]. This model is an extension of the ideas introduced in [6]. Then we develop a checking sequence generation method called the U_γ-method using UIO sequences without using the reset feature. This method offers guaranteed fault coverage provided that the implementation has the same number of states as the specification. The applicability of the U_γ-method is limited to the class of machines having a compound DS [7].

The rest of the paper is organized as follows: Section 2 gives some basic definitions and the notation we use. Section 3 introduces our formal model for checking sequence generation. Section 4 presents the U_γ-method. Section 5 provides empirical results and compares the U_γ-method with some of the existing methods. Section 6 gives the concluding remarks.

2. NOTATION AND BASIC DEFINITIONS

A **deterministic FSM** is a 6-tuple $M = (Q_M, \Sigma_{IM}, \Sigma_{OM}, \delta_M, \lambda_M, q_{0M})$ where Q_M is the finite set of states, Σ_{IM} is the input alphabet, Σ_{OM} is the output alphabet, $\delta_M : Q_M \times \Sigma_{IM} \to Q_M$ is the state transition function, $\lambda_M : Q_M \times \Sigma_{IM} \to \Sigma_{OM}$ is the output function and $q_{0M} \in Q_M$ is the initial state. M is said to be **completely specified** if δ_M and λ_M are total functions. $\delta_M(q,x) = p$ and $\lambda_M(q,x) = y$ mean that the FSM M at state q makes a transition to state p with input x and produces the output y. We use the same notation to denote the transitive closures of these functions: $\delta_M : Q_M \times \Sigma_{IM}^* \to Q_M$ and $\lambda_M : Q_M \times \Sigma_{IM}^* \to \Sigma_{OM}^*$. We further extend δ_M to denote the forward image of a set of states under an input string s, i.e. for $P \subseteq Q_M$, $\delta_M(P,s) = \{\delta_M(q,s) \mid q \in P\}$. An FSM M is said to have the **reset feature** if there is a special input symbol *reset* such that for every state $q \in Q_M$, $\delta_M(q, reset) = q_{0M}$. The **language of an FSM** M is defined to be $\mathcal{L}(M) \subseteq (\Sigma_{IM} \times \Sigma_{OM})^*$ such that $x/y \in \mathcal{L}(M) \iff \lambda_M(q_{0M}, x) = y$.

Two states q and p of an FSM M are said to be **equivalent** (or $q \equiv p$) if for all $s \in \Sigma_{IM}^*$, $\lambda_M(q,s) = \lambda_M(p,s)$. Let M and N be two machines with disjoint state sets and identical alphabets. $q \in Q_M$ is said to be **equivalent** to $q' \in Q_N$ if and only if $\lambda_M(q,s) = \lambda_N(q',s)$ for all $s \in \Sigma_{IM}^*$. N is said to be equivalent to M ($N \equiv M$) if and only if $q_{0N} \equiv q_{0M}$. A machine M is said to be **minimal** if $\forall q, p \in Q_M$, $q \neq p \Rightarrow q \not\equiv p$.

Let M be a minimal FSM. An input sequence d is called a **distinguishing sequence** (DS) if no two states of M respond to d with identical outputs. There may not exist a distinguishing sequence for every FSM [8]. An input sequence u is called a **unique input-output sequence** (UIO sequence) for a state q if $\lambda_M(q,u) \neq \lambda_M(p,u)$ for all $p \neq q$. Existence of UIO sequences are not guaranteed for every FSM [3]. The set $U = \{u_q\}_{q \in Q_M}$ is called a **UIO suite** for machine M where each u_q is a UIO sequence corresponding to the state q. A **characterizing set** or **W-set** is a set of input sequences for which the output sequences produced by M in response to the set of input sequences are different for each state of M.

Define the function $\Delta_M : 2^{Q_M} \times \Sigma_{IM}^* \to 2^{2^{Q_M}}$ as

$$P \in \Delta_M(R,x) \iff \exists y \in \Sigma_{OM}^* \; (q \in P \iff q \in R \; and \; \lambda_M(q,x) = y)$$

Intuitively, every $P \in \Delta_M(R,x)$ is the set of states in R that give the same output to x. A **compound DS** of a machine M is a set of input sequences D having a common prefix s such that for each $P \in \Delta_M(Q_M, s)$, there is a sequence in D that distinguishes the states in P [7]. If d is a

DS for M, then $\{d\}$ is a compound DS for M, but there exist machines having a compound DS but not a DS.

An FSM M can also be viewed as an edge labeled directed graph $G = (V_G, E_G)$ where V_G is the set of vertices corresponding to the set Q_M of states and E_G is the set of edges corresponding to the set of transitions of M. Each edge $e = (q, p, x/y)$ is a state transition from state q to state p with input symbol x and output symbol y. We let $head(e) = p$, $tail(e) = q$ and $label(e) = x/y$. A **walk** is a finite sequence $W =< v_0, e_1, v_1, \ldots, e_k, v_k >$ of vertices and edges such that, for $1 \leq i \leq k$, $tail(e_i) = v_{i-1}$ and $head(e_i) = v_i$. We use $tail(W) = v_0$ and $head(W) = v_k$. The **label** of a walk W ($label(W)$) is the concatenation of labels of consecutive edges of W. G is called **strongly connected** if there exists a walk between every pair of vertices.

3. A FORMAL MODEL FOR CHECKING SEQUENCE GENERATION

In this section, we develop a formal model for checking sequence generation based on the ideas discussed in [12] and [6]. First, we define checking sequences in terms of a machine identification function. Then, we introduce the abstract DS and abstract UIO concepts, which will be necessary to construct algorithms using the transition checking approach.

Let Σ_I and Σ_O denote an input and output alphabet respectively. An **abstract experiment** $\chi = y/z$ is an input/output string where $y \in \Sigma_I^*$ and $z \in \Sigma_O^*$. Given an FSM M with $\chi \in \mathcal{L}(M)$, every prefix of y transfers M from q_{0M} to a certain state. Define $A_M : \Sigma_I^* \rightarrow Q_M$ as $A_M(v) = \delta_M(q_{0M}, v)$ where $v \leq y$. A prefix of y is called an **abstract state** relative to χ. We show the output string corresponding to an abstract state ω as $O_\chi(\omega)$, i.e. $O_\chi(\omega)$ is the prefix of z with $|O_\chi(\omega)| = |w|$.

Let Φ_n be the set of equivalence classes of all deterministic FSMs having at most n states in their minimal machine, with Σ_I and Σ_O as the common input and output alphabets respectively. Let $[R] \in \Phi_n$ represent the equivalence class of Φ_n such that $M \in [R] \iff M \equiv R$. The **machine identification function** $\mathcal{I}_n : (\Sigma_I \times \Sigma_O)^* \rightarrow 2^{\Phi_n}$ is defined as $[M] \in \mathcal{I}_n(\chi) \iff \chi \in \mathcal{L}(M)$.

Definition 1 *For an abstract experiment $\chi = y/z$, y is called an* **abstract checking sequence** *relative to χ if $|\mathcal{I}_n(\chi)| = 1$.*

Definition 2 *If y is an abstract checking sequence relative to the abstract experiment $\chi = y/z$, then y is called a* **checking sequence** *for M where $[M] \in \mathcal{I}_n(\chi)$.*

Let $\chi = y/z$ be an abstract experiment, v and ω be two abstract states relative to χ.

Definition 3 *v and ω are called* **congruent** *relative to χ ($v \cong_\chi \omega$) if $\forall[M] \in \mathcal{I}_n(\chi)$, $A_M(v) \equiv A_M(\omega)$. A set of abstract states C is called a* **congruent set** *relative to χ if $\forall v, \omega \in C$, $v \cong_\chi \omega$.*

The set of all maximal congruent sets associated with χ is denoted by $\mathcal{C}_\chi$.

Definition 4 *v and ω are called* **incongruous** *relative to χ ($v \ncong_\chi \omega$) if $\forall[M] \in \mathcal{I}_n(\chi)$, $A_M(v) \not\equiv A_M(\omega)$. C_1, $C_2 \in \mathcal{C}_\chi$ are called incongruous relative to χ if and only if $\exists v \in C_1$, $\omega \in C_2$ such that $v \ncong_\chi \omega$.*

Proposition 1 *If $v \cong \omega$, then $v.s \cong \omega.s$ for every input string s.*

The following example illustrates the congruence concept: Let $\chi = a.b.a.a.b.a/c.d.d.c.d.d$ be generated by a machine with two states ($n = 2$). The following can be deduced:

- a/c, $a.b.a/c.d.d \Rightarrow \lambda_M(q_{0M}, a) = c$ and $\lambda_M(\delta_M(q_{0M}, a.b), a) = d$ for all $[M] \in \mathcal{I}_2(\chi)$. So, $q_{0M} \not\equiv \delta_M(q_{0M}, a.b)$ for all $[M] \in \mathcal{I}_2(\chi)$, hence $\epsilon \ncong_\chi a.b$.
- Two different outputs are observed for the input symbol a. Since only two-state machines are considered, we conclude that the input a is a DS for all $[M] \in \mathcal{I}_2(\chi)$. Now consider the abstract states $v_1 = a.b$ and $v_2 = a.b.a.a.b$. $v_1.a/o_1.d \leq \chi$ and $v_2.a/o_2.d \leq \chi$. Then, states $A_M(v_1)$ and $A_M(v_2)$ respond with the same output to the DS for all $[M] \in \mathcal{I}_2(\chi)$. This implies that $A_M(v_1) \equiv A_M(v_2)$ for all $[M] \in \mathcal{I}_2(\chi)$. By definition, $v_1 \cong_\chi v_2$.

We extend the mapping A to congruent sets by letting $A_M(C)$ to denote $A_M(v)$, $v \in C$. Now let $v.\sigma/o_v.o_\sigma \leq y/z$ for some input symbol $\sigma \in \Sigma_I$, and let $v \in C_1$ and $v.\sigma \in C_2$ where C_1, $C_2 \in \mathcal{C}_\chi$. From this abstract experiment, we can conclude that $\delta_M(A_M(C_1), \sigma) = A_M(C_2)$ and $\lambda_M(A_M(C_1), \sigma) = o_\sigma$ for all $[M] \in I_n(\chi)$. Based on this observation, we can define the **abstract transition function** and **abstract output function** relative to $\chi = y/z$ as follows:

$$\delta_\chi(C_1, \sigma) = C_2 \iff \exists v \in C_1,\ v.\sigma \in C_2$$

$$\lambda_\chi(C_1, \sigma) = o_\sigma \iff \exists v \in C_1,\ v.\sigma/o_v.o_\sigma \leq y/z$$

Definition 5 *The* **congruence machine** *relative to an abstract experiment χ is defined to be $M_\chi = (\mathcal{C}_\chi, \Sigma_I, \Sigma_O, \delta_\chi, \lambda_\chi, C_0)$ where $\mathcal{C}_\chi$ is the* *set of all congruent sets relative to* χ, Σ_I *is the input alphabet,* Σ_O *is the output alphabet,* δ_χ *is the abstract transition function,* λ_χ *is the abstract output function and* $C_0 \in \mathcal{C}_\chi$ *is the congruent set containing the empty prefix.*

It should be noted that the congruence machine is not only defined relative to the abstract experiment χ, but also to a specific instance of the identification function $\mathcal{I}_n$ as well. But, the number of states of the congruence machine can exceed n. Furthermore, there is no guarantee that the congruence machine will be completely specified. The following theorem sets the necessary and sufficient conditions for the completeness of the congruence machine.

Theorem 1 *Given an abstract experiment* $\chi = y/z$ *and the identification function* $\mathcal{I}_n$, *the congruence machine* M_χ *is complete with* $|\mathcal{C}_\chi| \leq n$ *if and only if* y *is an abstract checking sequence relative to* χ.

Proof Assume that M_χ is complete with $|\mathcal{C}_\chi| \leq n$. Then for any $s \in \Sigma_I^*$, there exists a corresponding $t \in \Sigma_O^*$ such that $s/t \in \mathcal{L}(M_\chi)$. Observe that for some $\chi = y/z$, $\chi \in \mathcal{L}(M)$ for all $[M] \in \mathcal{I}_n(\chi)$. Then, $s/t \in \mathcal{L}(M)$ for all $[M] \in \mathcal{I}_n(\chi)$, which means that $\lambda_M(q_{0M}, s) = t$. So, for $[M], [M'] \in \mathcal{I}_n(\chi)$, $\lambda_M(q_{0M}, s) = \lambda_{M'}(q_{0M'}, s)$, which implies that $M \equiv M'$. Then, $|\mathcal{I}_n(\chi)| = 1$, and y is an abstract checking sequence relative to χ.

Now assume that y is an abstract checking sequence relative to χ. Then, $\mathcal{I}_n(\chi) = \{[M]\}$ where $M \equiv M_\chi$. By definition, $|Q_M| \leq n$, so $|\mathcal{C}_\chi| \leq n$. If M is not complete, then there exists M' such that $\mathcal{L}(M) \subset \mathcal{L}(M')$. Then, $\chi \in \mathcal{L}(M')$, which means that $[M'] \in \mathcal{I}_n(\chi)$. This contradicts with the fact that $|\mathcal{I}_n(\chi)| = 1$, therefore M is complete.

3.1 Abstract DS and Abstract UIO

DS and UIO sequences can be used to recognize the states of an implementation: If it is known that the implementation under test possesses the same DS (or UIO sequences) with the specification, then any two abstract states with identical outputs to the DS (UIO sequences) are congruent.

Definition 6 *A string* $s \in \Sigma_I^*$ *is called an* **abstract distinguishing sequence** *relative to* $\chi = y/z$ *if* s *is a distinguishing sequence for all* $[M] \in \mathcal{I}_n(\chi)$.

Proposition 2 *For a given abstract experiment* $\chi = y/z$ *and an input string* s, *if* $\mathcal{C}_\chi$ *contains* n *congruent sets* $\{C_i\}_{i=1,\dots,n}$ *that are pairwise* *incongruous such that for* $j, k = 1, \ldots n$, $j \neq k \iff \lambda_\chi(C_j, s) \neq \lambda_\chi(C_k, s)$, *then* s *is an abstract distinguishing sequence relative to* χ.

Intuitively, for an FSM M with a distinguishing sequence s, if an input sequence y is constructed which applies s to every state of M, then the sequence s is an abstract distinguishing sequence for the abstract experiment $y/\lambda_M(q_{0M}, y)$.

The similar argument can be applied to UIO sequences:

Definition 7 *A string* $u \in \Sigma_I^*$ *is called an* **abstract UIO sequence** *for an abstract state* v *relative to* $\chi = y/z$ *if* u *is a UIO sequence for the state* $\delta_M(q_{0M}, v)$ *for all* $[M] \in \mathcal{I}_n(\chi)$. *We also call* u *an abstract UIO sequence for a congruent set* C *if* u *is an abstract UIO sequence for an abstract state* $v \in C$.

Proposition 3 *Let* $\chi = y/z$ *be an abstract experiment. A string* $u \in \Sigma_I^*$ *is an abstract UIO sequence for the congruent set* C *if there exist* n *congruent sets* $\{C_i\}_{i=1,\ldots,n}$ *relative to* χ *that are pairwise incongruous such that* $C = C_i$ *for some* i, $1 \leq i \leq n$, *and for* $1 \leq k \leq n$, $k \neq i \iff \lambda_\chi(C_k, u) \neq \lambda_\chi(C_i, u)$.

4. AN ALGORITHM FOR CHECKING SEQUENCE GENERATION USING UIO SEQUENCES

4.1 Motivation

Several algorithms have been developed for generating checking sequences using UIO sequences. The basic UIO method [16] [3] assumes the existence of the reset feature, and offers limited fault coverage. The UIO-v method [1] extends the basic UIO method by validating that the UIO sequences are correctly implemented by the implementation, therefore providing guaranteed fault coverage. The validation is performed by applying each UIO sequence to every state. The UIOG method [17] provides guaranteed fault coverage without using the reset feature. This method validates that the UIO sequences are correctly implemented using state and UIO verification subsequences. The UIOG method usually results in longer checking sequences than the other methods due to the structure of the verification subsequences.

In this paper, we propose a new method called the U_γ-method, which provides guaranteed fault coverage without using the reset feature. The method is developed based on the observation that if a UIO sequence u_q corresponding to a state q is known to be valid for an implementation, u_q can be used to obtain a reference point in the experiment: All abstract states arrived after observing the output $\lambda_M(q, u_q)$ to the input u_q are pairwise congruent.

4.2 The U -Method

The U_γ-method generates a checking sequence of the form $\gamma.\alpha.\beta$. The γ-sequence verifies that the implementation correctly implements the UIO sequences that will be used to construct the rest of the checking sequence. The α-sequence recognizes the states arrived after applying a UIO sequence to its corresponding state. The β-sequence verifies the transitions of the implementation [5].

The assumptions of the U_γ-method are:

1 The specification machine M is deterministic, minimal, completely specified and strongly connected,

2 M has a UIO suite U which contains a UIO sequence for each state,

3 The specification machine possesses at least one compound DS with some $u \in U$ being the common prefix,

4 The implementation has the same number of states as the specification.

4.2.1 Construction of the γ-sequence.

The γ-sequence applies each $u \in U$ to all states in Q_M. Consider a particular UIO sequence $u_q \in U$ corresponding to a state $q \in Q_M$. The sets $P \in \Delta_M(Q_M, u_q)$ contain states that give the same output to u_q. The γ-sequence should be constructed such that for each P, at least $|P|$ distinct states are applied the input sequence u_q.

Definition 8 *An input sequence d is called a* **restricted DS** *for the state set $P \subseteq Q_M$ if d distinguishes all the states in P.*

Lemma 1 *If D is a compound DS of M with u being the common prefix, there exists a restricted DS for each $P \in \Delta_M(Q_M, u)$ and $\delta_M(P, u)$.*

Lemma 2 *Let d be a restricted DS for $\delta_M(P, u)$ where $P \in \Delta_M(Q_M, u)$. Also let $\chi = y/z$ be an abstract experiment obtained from M by applying $u.d$ to all $q \in P$. Then u is applied to $|P|$ pairwise incongruous abstract states relative to χ.*

Lemma 3 *Let D be a compound DS of M with the UIO sequence u being the common prefix. If y is an input sequence constructed such that for each $P \in \Delta_M(Q_M, u)$, all $q \in P$ are applied d_P where $d_P \in D$ is a*

restricted DS for P, then u is an abstract UIO sequence for the abstract experiment $y/\lambda_M(q_{0M}, y)$.

Following these properties, we have the first construction rule: For each $u \in U$ and for each $P \in \Delta_M(Q_M, u)$, if $\delta_M(P, u)$ has a restricted DS d_P, the γ-sequence should contain applications of $u.d_P$ to all states in P.

Definition 9 *A set of input sequences W_P is called a* **restricted W-set** *for the state set $P \subseteq Q_M$ if for every pair of states q, r in P, W_P contains an input sequence to distinguish q and r.*

Lemma 4 *Let u_r be a UIO sequence for the state r of M. For some input sequence u, consider the state set $P \in \Delta_M(Q_M, u)$. For each $q \in P$, let t_q denote a transfer sequence from $\delta_M(r, u_r)$ to q. Construct an input sequence y such that r is applied $u_r.t_q.u$ and $u_r.t_q.w$ for all $q \in P$ and $w \in W_P$ where W_P is a restricted W-set for P. If u_r is an abstract UIO sequence for $\chi = y/\lambda_M(q_{0M}, y)$, then u is applied to $|P|$ pairwise incongruous abstract states relative to χ.*

The second construction rule is as follows: Let u_r be a UIO sequence, which is also the common prefix of a compound DS of M. For each $u \in U$ and for each $P \in \Delta_M(Q_M, u)$, if $\delta_M(P, u)$ does not have a restricted DS, the γ-sequence should be constructed such that for each $q \in P$, r is applied $u_r.t_q.u$ and $u_r.t_q.w$ where t_q is a transfer sequence from $\delta_M(r, u_r)$ to q and $w \in W_P$.

Table 1. The machine M_1

Present State	Next State, Output		
	$x = 0$	$x = 1$	$x = 2$
A	B, 1	D, 0	A, 1
B	A, 1	D, 0	A, 0
C	C, 0	B, 1	B, 0
D	C, 2	C, 2	B, 0

As an example, consider the machine M_1, whose state table is given in Table 1. Let $U = \{0.2, 0, 2\}$. The input sequence 0 is a UIO sequence for C and D. A and B respond with 1 to the input 0, and go to B and A respectively. 2 is a restricted DS for the set $\{A, B\}$, therefore if the γ-sequence contains the input/output strings 0.2/1.0 (for A), 0.2/1.1 (for B), 0/0 (for C) and 0/2 (for D), then 0 will be an abstract UIO sequence for the abstract experiment $\gamma/\lambda_M(q_{0M}, \gamma)$.

The input sequence 2 is a UIO sequence for A. The states C and D give the output 0 to the input 2, and go to B. C can be used as a reference point: At any moment in the test, observing a 0/0 guarantees that the implementation was in a state equivalent to C before the application of 0. The set $\{2\}$ is a restricted W-set for $\{C, D\}$, therefore the γ-sequence should be constructed such that C is applied 0.0/0.0 (which applies the sequence 0 to distinguish C from D), 0.1.1.0/0.1.0.2 (which brings the implementation to D by applying 1.1, and applies 0 to distinguish D from C), 0.2/0.0 (which applies 2 to C), and 0.1.1.2/0.1.0.0 (which brings the implementation to D by applying 1.1, and applies 2 to D).

As a result of the above discussion, we have the following algorithm:

Algorithm 1 (γ-sequence): *Let u_r be the common prefix of a compound DS of M. Construct the graph $G_\gamma = (V, E \cup E')$ where V corresponds to Q_M, E corresponds to the transitions of M and E' is constructed as follows:*

For each $u \in U$
For each $P \in \Delta_M(Q_M, u)$
For each $q \in P$
if $\delta_M(P, u)$ has a restricted DS d then
$(q, \delta_M(q, u.d), u.d) \in E'$
else
$(r, \delta_M(r, u_r.t_q.u), u_r.t_q.u) \in E'$,
$(r, \delta_M(r, u_r.t_q.w), u_r.t_q.w) \in E'$
where $t_q \in \Sigma_{IM}^*$ such that $\delta_M(r, u_r.t_q) = q$ and $w \in W_P$

The γ-sequence is the input label of the walk on G_γ which traverses all elements of E' at least once.

Theorem 2 *Let U be a UIO suite for machine M. Assume that M possesses a compound DS with $u_r \in U$ being the common prefix. If γ is an input sequence generated by Algorithm 1, U is an abstract UIO suite for the abstract experiment $\gamma/\lambda_M(q_{0M}, \gamma)$.*

4.2.2 Construction of the α- and β-sequences.

The α- and β-sequences are constructed using the algorithms given in [5]. The α-sequence is used to recognize the state arrived *after* a UIO sequence is applied to its corresponding state. To construct the α-sequence each state q is applied $u_q.u_p$ where $\delta_M(q, u_q) = p$. The β-sequence verifies each transition of the implementation. To construct the β-sequence each state q is applied $\sigma.u_p$ when q is recognized, where σ is an input symbol and $\delta_M(q, \sigma) = p$. The state q is recognized if it is arrived by the application of a UIO sequence to its corresponding state, or if it is arrived from a recognized state using only verified transitions. Since the β-sequence is concatenated to the α-sequence, the β-sequence starts from a recognized state. In [5], it is shown that for completely specified and strongly connected machines, it is always possible to construct a β-sequence that verifies all the transitions.

Theorem 3 *Let s be an input sequence generated by the U_γ-method for a machine M. Then, s is an abstract checking sequence relative to the abstract experiment $\chi = s/\lambda_M(q_{0M}, s)$.*

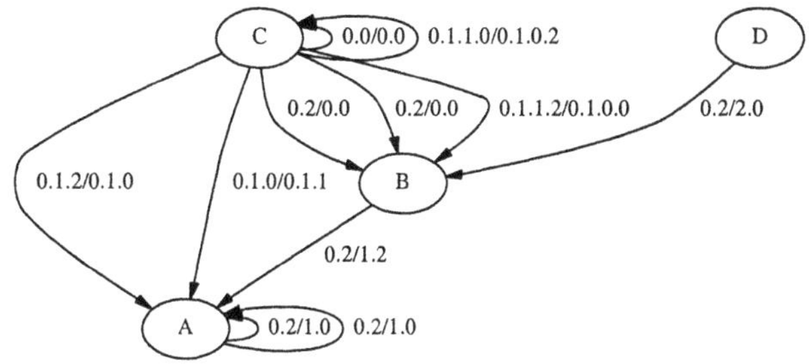

Figure 1. G_γ for the machine M_1 (only E' edges are shown)

The G_γ graph for machine M_1 is given in Figure 1. The segments of the checking sequence are:
$\gamma = 0.2.0.2.0.2.0.2.1.0.2.1.0.0.1.2.1.0.0.2.1.0.0.0.0.1.1.0.0.1.1.2.1.0.0.1.0$
$\alpha = 0.2.2.2.1.0.0.0$
$\beta = 0.0.2.1.0.0.0.1.0.2.2.2.0.0.2.0.1.0.2.0.2.0.2.2.1.0.0.1.1.2.0.2.1.1.0$
The length of the resulting checking sequence is 80.

5. COMPARISON WITH OTHER METHODS

We performed experiments using randomly generated machines to compare the lengths of the checking sequences generated by different methods. We generated a total of 117000 random minimal machines having 3 to 15 states, and having 2 to 10 symbols in their alphabets. For each machine, we compared the lengths of checking sequences generated by the U-method, U_γ-method and UIOG method. We also generated checking sequences using Gönenç's method for machines with a DS.

We excluded the machines that do not have a suitable compound DS to be used with the U_γ-method. We also excluded the machines for which computing a compound DS required a long time ($|Q| > 10$ and $|\Sigma| < 5$). As a result, we only used 94460 machines to generate checking sequences.

For each machine M, we constructed a UIO suite U such that the use of the first construction rule is maximized. This choice gives shorter

γ-sequences. Table 2 gives the average lengths of checking sequences generated by the U-method and U_γ-method.

Table 2. Average lengths of checking sequences generated by the U-method and the U_γ-method

$\|\Sigma_M\|$		$\|Q_M\|$											
		3	4	5	6	7	8	9	10	11	12	13	14
2	l_U	24	37	50	66	80	97	114	130	-	-	-	-
	l_{U_γ}	37	61	109	143	209	261	348	399	-	-	-	-
4	l_U	45	65	86	109	134	159	184	209	236	-	-	-
	l_{U_γ}	39	64	96	128	164	199	241	279	330	-	-	-
6	l_U	66	92	120	149	180	213	248	284	319	356	394	432
	l_{U_γ}	51	74	103	135	174	214	253	296	337	378	422	465
8	l_U	88	121	156	192	229	267	308	350	393	438	484	531
	l_{U_γ}	64	89	119	151	187	227	272	320	366	411	460	509
10	l_U	110	151	193	236	281	326	373	420	469	520	570	626
	l_{U_γ}	77	107	140	174	210	252	293	341	390	442	495	551

These results show that the U_γ-method developed in this work can generate checking sequences that are comparable in length with the checking sequences generated by the U-method, with guaranteed fault coverage. For machines with large state sets and small alphabets, the U-method generates shorter checking sequences. On the other hand, for machines with large alphabets, the U_γ-method generates shorter checking sequences.

We also generated checking sequences using the UIOG method [17]. For machines having a small number of states, the lengths of the checking sequences generated are similar to those obtained by the U-method and U_γ-method. As the number of states increase, the length of the state verification sequences increase significantly–to the order of several thousands for machines having more than 7 states.

The U-method described in [9] generates checking sequences similar to the β-sequence portion of the U_γ-method. For certain cases, this method can generate significantly shorter checking sequences than the U_γ-method, but does not provide guaranteed fault coverage.

We also applied Gönenç's method to the machines possessing a DS [5]. When the UIO suite is constructed with the DS, the U_γ-method is equivalent to Gönenç's method. For the purpose of this experiment, we used UIO suites that do not contain the DS. We observed that Gönenç's method generates shorter checking sequences than the U_γ-method even if the UIO sequences are shorter than the DS. In fact, Gönenç's method appears to be the most efficient method for larger machines having a DS, but it applicability is limited than that of the U-methods.

6. CONCLUSION

In this paper we presented a new model for checking sequence generation for FSMs. This model defines the checking sequence generation problem based on the machine identification problem. This approach can be used to formally reason about properties of checking sequence generation methods.

Based on our model, we developed the U_γ-method. The U_γ-method generates relatively short checking sequences without relying on the reset feature. The checking sequences generated by the U_γ-method can detect all possible faults of an implementation provided that the implementation has the same number of states as the specification. Unfortunately, U_γ-method is only applicable to a restricted class of FSMs–namely to those machines having a UIO sequence for each state, and possessing a compound DS with one of the UIO sequences being the common prefix.

We also performed experiments to compare the U_γ-method with several other methods. We observed that the checking sequences generated by the U_γ-method are comparable to those generated by the U-method with improved fault coverage. The U_γ-method generates shorter checking sequences than the UIOG method, but the UIOG method is applicable to all machines having a UIO sequence for each state.

As future work, we wish to improve the applicability of the U_γ-method. The U_γ-method relies on the existence of a compound DS to verify at least one of the UIO sequences, and then using it as a reference point. It is possible to verify one of the UIO sequences without using a compound DS, but the overhead is significant. We are working on efficient methods to verify one UIO sequence. We also have not dealt with the problem of selecting an appropriate UIO suite for the U_γ-method in depth. Efficient algorithms are needed to make the U_γ-method more practical.

References

[1] W. Chen C. Y. Tang S. T. Vuong. Improving the UIOv-method for protocol conformance testing. *Computer Communications*, 18(9):609–619, Sep 1995.

[2] T. S. Chow. Testing software design modeled by finite state machines. *IEEE Transactions on Software Engineering*, 4(3):178–187, May 1978.

[3] A. Dahbura K. Sabnani. A protocol test generation procedure. *Computer Networks and ISDN Systems*, 15:285–297, 1988.

[4] S. Fujiwara et al. Test selection based on finite state models. *IEEE Transactions on Software Engineering*, 17(6):591–603, Jun 1991.

[5] G. Gönenç. A method for the design of fault detection experiments. *IEEE Transactions on Computers*, 19(6):551, Jun 1970.

[6] F. C. Hennie. Fault detecting experiments for sequential circuits. *Proc. of the 5th Annual Symposium on Switching Circuits Theory and Logical Design*, pages 95–110, Nov 1964.

[7] E. P. Hsieh. Checking experiments for sequential machines. *IEEE Transactions on Computers*, C-20(10):1152–1166, Oct 1971.

[8] Z. Kohavi. *Switching and Finite Automata Theory.* McGraw–Hill, 1978.

[9] D. Lee A. V. Aho, A. T. Dahbura and M.Ü. Uyar. An optimization technique for protocol conformance test generation based on UIO sequences and rural chinese postman tours. *IEEE Transactions on Communications*, 39(11):1604–1615, Nov 1991.

[10] D. Lee M. Yannakis. Testing finite state machines: State identification and verification. *IEEE Transactions on Computers*, 306–320, 1994.

[11] T. K. Leung D. P. Sidhu. Formal methods for protocol conformance testing: A detailed study. *IEEE. Transactions on Software Engineering*, pages 413–426, 1989.

[12] E. F. Moore. *Gedanken-Experiments on Sequential Machines, in Automata Studies.* Princeton University Press, 1956.

[13] B. Serdar. A new approach to checking sequence generation for finite state machines. Master's thesis, Computer Science Department, North Carolina State University, Available on-line at http://www.lib.ncsu.edu/etd/, 2001.

[14] Y. N. Shen F. Lombardi. Evaluation and improvement of fault coverage of conformance testing by uio sequences. *IEEE Transactions on Communications*, pages 1288–1293, 1992.

[15] H. Ural A. Rezaki. Construction of checking sequences based on characterization sets. *Computer Communications*, 18(12):911–920, 1995.

[16] M. Ü. Uyar A. T. Dahbura, K. K. Sabnani. Formal methods for generating protocol conformance test sequences. *Proceedings of IEEE*, 78(8):1347–1325, Aug 1990.

[17] M. Yao A. Petrenko G. Bochmann. Conformance testing of protocol machines without reset. *Proceedings of the 13th International Symposium on Protocol Specification, Testing and Verification*, pages 241–253, May 25–28 1993.

SESSION X

TTCN-3

*TIMED*TTCN-3 – A REAL-TIME EXTENSION FOR TTCN-3*

Zhen Ru Dai, Jens Grabowski, Helmut Neukirchen
Institute for Telematics, University of Lübeck
Ratzeburger Allee 160, D-23538 Lübeck, Germany
Tel.: +49 451 500 3721 Fax: +49 451 500 3722
{dai,grabowsk,neukirchen}@itm.mu-luebeck.de

Abstract The *Testing and Test Control Notation* (TTCN-3) was originally developed as successor of the second edition of the *Tree and Tabular Combined Notation*. TTCN-3 is a standardized test specification and implementation language to test functional behaviour of distributed systems. *TIMED*TTCN-3 is a real-time extension for TTCN-3 that supports the test and measurement of real-time requirements. *TIMED*TTCN-3 introduces absolute time, allows the definition of synchronization requirements for test components and provides possibilities to specify online and offline evaluation procedures for real-time requirements.

Keywords: Distributed systems testing, Test specification, TTCN-3, Real-time testing, Test evaluation, Non-functional requirements

1. INTRODUCTION

One of the most challenging research areas in testing is the testing of distributed real-time systems. Such systems are becoming ever more importance in daily life, such as for business and administration (e.g., E-Commerce), for home use (e.g., home brokerage), teaching (e.g., teleteaching and -tutoring) and process control (e.g., air traffic control). Testing is the most important means to assure the correctness of distributed real-time systems with respect to functional and real-time behaviour.

The procedures for testing functional behaviour are defined in the international ISO/IEC standard 9646 *Conformance Testing Methodology and Framework* (CTMF) [12]. Even though CTMF focuses on conformance testing of OSI protocol entities, CTMF has been applied successfully to other types of functional testing. Part 3 of CTMF defines the test specification language *Tree*

*Parts of this work have been funded by the European Commission contract IST-1999-11557 INTERVAL.

and Tabular Combined Notation (TTCN). The latest version of TTCN has been published in 1999 as European technical report by the European Telecommunications Standards Institute (ETSI) [3]. With *PerfTTCN* (*Performance TTCN*) [15] and *RT-TTCN* (*Real-Time TTCN*) [16, 17] two approaches exist to extend TTCN for real-time and performance testing.

PerfTTCN extends TTCN with concepts for performance testing. These concepts are: (1) *performance test scenarios* for the description of test configurations, (2) *traffic models* for the description of discrete and continuous streams of data, (3) *measurement points* as special observation points, (4) *measurement declarations* for the definition of metrics to be observed at measurement points, (5) *performance constraints* to describe the performance conditions that shall be met, and (6) *performance verdicts* for the judgement of test results. The PerfTTCN concepts are introduced mainly on a syntactical level by means of new TTCN tables. Their semantics are described in an informal manner only.

RT-TTCN is an extension of TTCN in order to test *hard* real-time requirements. On the syntactical level, RT-TTCN supports the annotation of TTCN statements with two timestamps for earliest and latest execution times. On the semantical level, the TTCN snapshot semantics has been refined and, in addition, RT-TTCN has been mapped onto timed transition systems [8].

The *Testing and Test Control Notation* (TTCN-3) [4, 7] has been developed from 1998 to 2001 by an ETSI experts team as successor language for TTCN. TTCN-3 is based on a textual core notation that has the look and feel of a common programming language. In comparison to TTCN, TTCN-3 includes no OSI and conformance testing specific constructs, but provides several additional concepts like, e.g., *dynamic test configurations*, *procedure-based communication* and *module control part*. The development of TTCN-3 concentrated on features for functional testing. Thus, some major concepts needed for real-time and performance testing are missing.

This paper tries to close this gap by proposing *Timed*TTCN-3 as a real-time extension for TTCN-3. *Timed*TTCN-3 introduces (1) a *new test verdict* to judge real-time behaviour, (2) supports *absolute time* as a means to measure time and to calculate durations, (3) allows to *delay* the execution of statements for defining time dependent test behaviour, (4) supports the specification of *synchronization conditions* for test components and (5) provides a means for the *online and offline evaluation* of real-time properties. Our first experiments give evidence that *Timed*TTCN-3 covers most PerfTTCN and RT-TTCN features while being more intuitive in usage. Moreover, the *Timed*TTCN-3 extensions are more unified than the other extensions by making full use of the expressiveness of TTCN-3 . Thus only a few changes to the language are needed.

2. AN INRES-BASED EXAMPLE

The concepts of *TIMED*TTCN-3 will be explained by a test case for the *Inres* protocol [9]. As shown in Figure 1a, the test case is written for the distributed test method of CTMF [12]. The *Implementation Under Test* (IUT) is an *Initiator* implementation. The *Upper Tester* (UT) function plays the role of an Initiator user and the *Lower Tester* (LT) function plays the role of a Responder entity. The UT has a direct connection with the IUT whereas the LT only has indirect access to the lower interface of the IUT via a *Medium Service.* UT and LT coordinate themselves by *Test Coordination Procedures* (TCP).

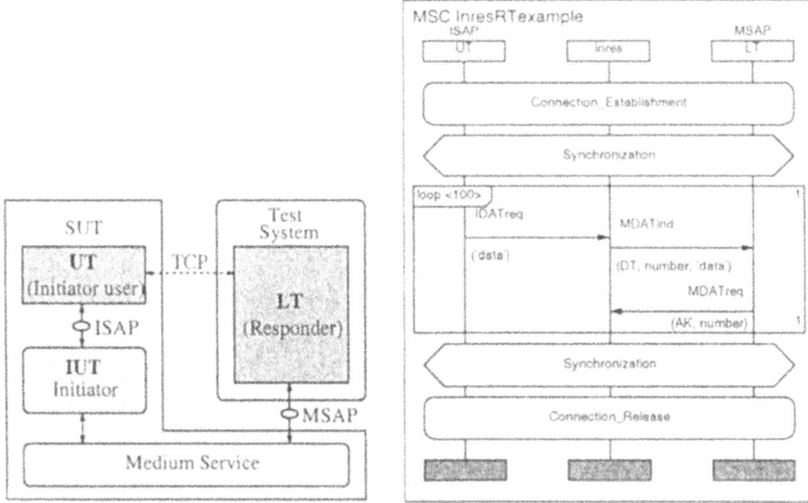

(a) Distributed test architecture (b) Control flow and message exchange

Figure 1. Test architecture and control flow for the Inres test case example

The example is designed to test the real-time properties *latency* and *mean arrival time* for the exchange of 100 data packets.[1] Its principle control flow and message exchange is presented by the Message Sequence Chart in Figure 1b. The test case starts with a preamble that establishes a connection between UT and LT. Afterwards, UT and LT synchronize in order to ensure that both tester functions are in a correct state to execute the test body. The test body includes the sending of 100 data packets from UT to LT. The LT must acknowledge the correct reception of each data packet. Otherwise, the SUT will retransmit the data packet or, after three retransmissions, release the connection.[2] At the

[1]Please note that in order to perform meaningful non-functional testing as described in this paper, it is necessary that an IUT has passed the related functional test cases.

[2]The retransmission of data packets and the exceptional connection release are not shown in Figure 1b.

```
(1)  testcase InresRTexample(integer sequenceStartNum)
(2)  runs on InitiatorUserType system InresSystemType {
(3)    var ResponderType responder := null;
(4)    var float sendTime := 0.0;
(5)    var default myDefault := null;
(6)    myDefault := activate(InitiatorDefault); // Default activation
(7)    map(self:ISAP, system:ISAP);
       // Creating/mapping/connecting/starting the Responder PTC
(8)    responder := ResponderType.create(self.timezone)
(9)    map(responder:MSAP, system:MSAP);
(10)   connect(self:CP, responder:CP);
(11)   responder.start(ResponderBehaviour(SequenceStartNum));
(12)   InitiatorPreamble(); // Preamble for connection establishment
(13)   CP.send(boolean:true); // Initial synchronization
(14)   CP.receive(boolean:true);
(15)   sendTime := self.now + 5.0; // Send the first time in 5.0s
       // Sending of 100 data packets in a loop
(16)   for (var integer i := 1; i <= 100; i := i + 1) {
(17)     resume(sendTime); // Wait until 'sendTime'
(18)     log (TimestampType:{self.now, self.timezone, IDATreq});
(19)     ISAP.send(IDATreqType:{self.now});
(20)     sendTime := sendTime + 0.01; // Send periodically every 10ms
(21)   }
(22)   CP.send(boolean:true); // Final synchronization
(23)   CP.receive(boolean:true);
(24)   verdict.set(pass); // Everything is OK
(25)   InitiatorPostamble(); // Postamble for connection release
(26) }
```

Figure 2. *TIMED*TTCN-3 test case description

end of the test body, UT and LT synchronize again and perform a postamble to release the connection.

The *TIMED*TTCN-3 code for the behaviour of the *main test component* (**mtc**) is shown in Figure 2. The **mtc** is the UT and plays the role of an Initiator user. Lines 1 and 2 provide the test case interface, i.e., name, formal parameters, component types for **mtc** (**runs on** clause) and *abstract test system interface* (**system** clause). Lines 3-7 describe variable declarations, a default activation and the mapping of **mtc** ports onto ports of the abstract test system interface.

The creation of the LT component, the mapping of LT ports onto ports of the abstract test system interface, the connection of LT and **mtc** ports, and the start of the LT component are specified in lines 8-11. The preamble *InitiatorPreamble* is called in line 12 and the initial synchronization by means of an UT-initiated handshake with boolean synchronization messages is shown in lines 13 and 14. The time for sending the first data packet is determined in line 15. The body of the test case consists of the **for** loop specified in lines 16-21. The loop body

```
(1)  function ResponderBehaviour(integer expectedNum) runs on ResponderType {
(2)    var float receiveTime := 0.0, sendTime := 0.0;
(3)    var MDATindType receivedMessage;
(4)    myDefault := activate(ResponderDefault); // Default activation
(5)    ResponderPreamble(); // Preamble for connection establishment
(6)    CP.receive(boolean:true); // Initial synchronization
(7)    CP.send(boolean:true);
       // Receiving 100 data packets in a loop
(8)    for (var integer i := 1; i <= 100; i := i + 1) {
(9)      alt {
(10)       [ ] MSAP.receive(MDATindType:{DT, expectedNum, ?})
                                              -> value receivedMessage {
(11)             receiveTime := self.now;
(12)             log(TimestampType:{receiveTime, self.timezone, MDATind});
(13)             sendTime := receivedMessage.data; // Extract the send time
(14)             // Latency online evaluation
(15)             if (evalLatency(sendTime, receiveTime, 0.001, 0.005) ==conf) {
(16)               verdict.set(conf);
(17)             }
(18)             MSAP.send(MDATreqType:{AK, expectedNum, 0.0});
(19)             expectedNum := toggle(expectedNum);
(20)           }
(21)       [ ] MSAP.receive(MDATindType:{DT, toggle(expectedNum), ?})) {
(22)             MSAP.send(MDATreqType:{AK, toggle(expectedNum), 0.0});
(23)             repeat;
(24)           }
(25)     }
(26)   }
(27)   CP.receive(boolean:true); // Final synchronization
(28)   CP.send(boolean:true);
(29)   verdict.set(pass); // Everything is OK
(30)   ResponderPostamble(); // Postamble for connection release
(31) }
```

Figure 3. *TIMED*TTCN-3 behaviour of the Responder test component

is repeated 100 times and specifies that a data packet is sent every 10ms (lines 19 and 20). The test case terminates with the final synchronization (lines 22 and 23), the setting of a **pass** verdict (line 24) and the call of the postamble *InitiatorPostamble* (line 25).

The behaviour of the LT is specified by the *TIMED*TTCN-3 function shown in Figure 3. The function can be structured into three parts. The first part consist of declarations (lines 2 and 3), a default activation (line 4), the call of the preamble *ResponderPreamble* (line 5) and the initial synchronization (lines 6 and 7).

The second part (test body) consists of a **for** loop (lines 8-26). The loop body is repeated 100 times and includes an **alt** statement with two alternatives. The first alternative (lines 10-20) describes the expected message exchange: A correct data packet is received (line 10), the actual time is retrieved and recorded (lines 11 and 12), the send time is extracted from the received message (line 13), the latency is checked (line 15), if the latency requirement is violated, the new test verdict **conf** (Section 3) is set (line 16), finally, the data packet is acknowledged (line 18) and the sequence number of the next correct data packet is computed (line 19). The second alternative describes the case when the previous acknowledgement got lost and, therefore, the previous data packet is re-transmitted by the IUT. The reception of the re-transmitted data packet is described in line 21 and its re-acknowledgement is specified in line 22.

The third part describes the final synchronization (lines 27 and 28), the setting of the **pass** verdict (line 29) and the call of *ResponderPostamble* (line 30).

The test case specifies the expected message exchange only. Erroneous and unexpected responses received from the SUT are considered to be handled by defaults (line 6 in Figure 2 and line 4 in Figure 3).

The *TIMED*TTCN-3 code in Figure 2 and Figure 3 includes the real-time extensions **self.now**, **resume**, **self.timezone**, the new verdict **conf**, a modified syntax for the **log** statement and a new parameter for the **create** operation. These extensions will be explained in the following sections.

3. NON-FUNCTIONAL VERDICTS

The TTCN-3 verdicts indicate whether a test case was successful (**pass**), inconclusive (**inconc**) or faulty (**fail**) with respect to functional requirements. By introducing the possibility to test non-functional requirements, additional information concerning the test outcome is needed: A test case may *pass* with respect to both functional and non-functional behaviour or it may *pass* only with respect to the functional behaviour while the non-functional requirements are violated.[3]

Since non-functional behaviour can be observed only in combination with functional behaviour on which the non-functional requirements are imposed, it is not meaningful to make any statements on non-functional test results if the functional behaviour is not conforming to the functional requirements.[4]

Even in case of a *functional inconclusive*, no statement can be made on non-functional test results, since such an inconclusive case may have other non-functional requirements than the pass case which is subject of testing. Hence, distinctive verdicts are just needed in case of a *functional pass*.

Besides the existing **pass** verdict which is used to indicate a *functional pass* with an associated *non-functional pass*, *TIMED*TTCN-3 introduces the new verdict **conf** (as abbreviation for *conforming*) to indicate a *functional pass* with an

[3] In the following, the terms *functional pass*, *non-functional pass*, etc. are used to describe the test outcome with respect to functional and non-functional behaviour.

[4] In the special case of a tester malfunction which may lead to a wrong real-time measurement, the **error** verdict will be set by the tester.

Current value of verdict	New verdict assignment value pass	conf	inconc	fail	none
pass	pass	conf	inconc	fail	pass
conf	conf	conf	inconc	fail	conf
inconc	inconc	inconc	inconc	fail	inconc
fail	fail	fail	fail	fail	fail
none	pass	conf	inconc	fail	none

Figure 4. *TIMED*TTCN-3 overwriting rules for the test verdicts

associated *non-functional fail.* Due to the introduction of the new verdict, the overwriting rules for verdicts are refined. They are presented in Figure 4. The new verdict **conf** is inserted between the verdicts **pass** and **inconc**.

An example for the usage of the new **conf** verdict can be found in Figure 3. If the latency requirement is violated (checked in the **if** statement in line 15), **conf** is assigned to the local verdict of the Responder test component (line 16). Due to the overwriting rules of *TIMED*TTCN-3, a **conf** verdict will not be overwritten by the **verdict.set(pass)** statement in line 29 (see also row 2, column 1 of Figure 4). The existing verdict **fail** is still available to express a *functional fail* (see Figure 11, lines 13 and 24).

4. TIME EXTENSION FOR TTCN-3

For the handling of time, TTCN-3 provides a *timer* mechanism. This timer mechanism is designed for supervising the functional behaviour of an IUT, e.g., to prevent the blocking of a test case or to provoke exceptional behaviour. But, it is too slow and too clumsy for the test and measurement of real-time properties, because the measurement of durations is influenced by the TTCN-3 snapshot semantics and by the order in which the port queues and the timeout list are examined. TTCN-3 makes no assumptions about the duration for taking and evaluating a snapshot. Thus, exact times can not be measured.

Furthermore, TTCN-3 has no concept of *absolute time*, i.e., a test component cannot read and use its local system time. In real-time testing, the absolute time is necessary to check relationships between observed test events and to coordinate test activities. In case of synchronized clocks in a distributed test environment, the system time may be exchanged among test components to check real-time requirements that cannot be measured locally or for the timely coordination of test activities.

As a consequence of these considerations, *TIMED*TTCN-3 has the concept of *absolute time* in order to support real-time testing. In case of a distributed test environment, the test cases may define the requirements for the synchronization of clocks of different test components.

4.1 Absolute Time

Absolute time is related to *clocks* that provide the actual value of time. We assume that each test component has access to such a clock, but make no assumptions about the number and the synchronization of these clocks[5]. Furthermore, we assume that the resolution of such clocks and the speed of the tester are adequate for the real-time requirements which are subject of testing.

For the handling of time values either a new type is needed, or the time values have to be mapped onto an existing basic type. Due to numerous possible time representations, e.g., the UNIX approach to count the seconds since 1.1.1970 [10] or a structured type with fields for year, month, day, hour etc., a common new type for time values is not easy to define.

For simplicity, *TIMED*TTCN-3 uses the existing **float** type and follows the UNIX approach, i.e., time is counted in seconds and the absolute time is represented by the number of seconds since a fixed point in time. In contrast to the UNIX scheme, *TIMED*TTCN-3 does not define a fixed starting point for the time measurement. For that, *TIMED*TTCN-3 supports the usage of absolute time by the operations **now** and **resume**:

- The **now** operation is used for the retrieval of the current *local time.* The local character of the **now** operation is reflected by its application to the **self** handle, i.e., **self.now** is the expected call statement for the **now** operation. Operation **now** returns a float value that equals the current absolute time when the operation is called. The mapping of the float value onto a concrete daytime, e.g., year, month, day, hour, etc., is considered to be outside the scope of *TIMED*TTCN-3 and has to be provided by the test equipment, e.g., in form of additional conversion functions.

- The **resume** operation provides the ability to delay the execution of a test component. The argument of the **resume** operation is considered to be an absolute time value, i.e., the point in time when the test component shall resume its execution. If required, a relative time can easily be specified by using the current time as reference time, e.g., waiting for 3 seconds can be described by **resume(self.now** + 3.0).

An example for the usage of the absolute time extension is shown in Figure 2. The current time is retrieved in line 15. It is used to calculate the sending time of the first data packet. The sending time is used by the **resume** operation in line 17. The test component will resume when the specified time is reached.

[5]From a conceptional point of view, synchronized test components share the same clock, even though in a real implementation, the clocks are synchronized by using a synchronization protocol [13, 14].

4.2 Synchronization of Clocks

Time values are observed and used locally by the test components. Time values that are observed in different test components may be exchanged and used for further computations. But this only makes sense if the clocks of the involved test components are synchronized. The synchronization itself is outside the scope of *Timed*TTCN-3 and should be guaranteed by the test equipment, but requirements for clock synchronization may very well be expressed in *Timed*TTCN-3. These requirements may be used by a *Timed*TTCN-3 compiler to distribute test components in an adequate manner or by a *Timed*TTCN-3 runtime environment to execute synchronization procedures for the test devices.

Timezones. Most specification and implementation languages either support *local time* or *global time.* Local time means that each behavioral entity, e.g., an SDL process or a TTCN-3 test component, has its own local time. Global time means that all behavioral entities share the same *global* time. Global time is perfect for the purpose of real-time testing, because all test components have by definition the same global time and are synchronized.

However, neither local nor global time are realistic assumptions for real-time testing situations. A real-time test environment typically consists of several devices. If synchronization among two or more test components is required to reach the goal of a test case, the components have to be executed either on the same device or on synchronized devices.

The developer of real-time test cases should not care about synchronization procedures and the distribution of test components himself, but he can support their implementation by identifying test components which have to be synchronized. For this purpose, *Timed*TTCN-3 supports the *timezones* concept.

A timezone is an (optional) attribute that can be assigned to a test component when the component is created. Test components with the same attribute are considered to be synchronized, i.e., they have the same absolute time. A test component can only have one timezone attribute. Components without timezone attributes are considered to be not synchronized with other components.

Implementation of the Timezones Concept. *Timed*TTCN-3 implements the timezones concept by using an enumeration type with the reserved name **timezones**. The user has to specify the timezone attribute values by defining the **timezones** type in the module definitions part of a *Timed*TTCN-3 module. This type has an implicit member of name **none** which indicates no clock synchronization. The usage of an enumeration type only makes sense if the number of timezones is finite and known. We believe that this is a realistic assumption. In *Timed*TTCN-3, a timezone attribute is associated with a test component when the component is created, i.e., the timezone attribute is an optional parameter of the **execute** and the **create** operations. The timezone attribute of an **mtc** is assigned by using an **execute** operation. Attributes of all other test components are assigned by means of the **create** operations.

The flexibility of the timezones concept can be improved by making the timezones visible to the test components. This is implemented in *TIMED*TTCN-3 by means of a special **timezone** function which returns the timezone of the component that called the function. In the case of a non-synchronized test component, the value **none** is returned. Like the **now** operation, the **timezone** operation is always applied to the **self** handle of a test component, i.e., **self.timezone** is the expected call statement for the **timezone** operation. The timezone information may be exchanged among test components to check if synchronization conditions are satisfied, or used to create several synchronized components.

```
(1)  type enumerate timezones {
(2)          Hamburg, Luebeck, Berlin
(3)  }
```

Figure 5. Definition of timezones

The usage of the timezone concept is shown in Figures 2, 5 and 10. Figure 5 presents the definition of timezones *Berlin*, *Hamburg* and *Luebeck*. In our test case example, the **mtc** is created by the **execute** statement in line 5 of Figure 10 and receives the timezone attribute *Luebeck*. The behaviour of the **mtc** is shown in Figure 2. The **mtc** creates the test component *Responder* (line 8) and assigns its own timezone to the new component, i.e., **mtc** and *Responder* are considered to be synchronized.

5. EVALUATION OF REAL-TIME PROPERTIES

While functional behaviour is basically tested by using sequences of **send** and **receive** operations, real-time requirements can be tested by relating particular points in time to each other [1, 2, 11]. The essence of the various real-time requirements can be broken down to the relationship of points in time. Mathematical formulae can be used to evaluate whether the points in time of interesting events fulfill a certain real-time requirement or not.

To obtain those points in time, functional TTCN-3 test cases are instrumented by statements which generate timestamps. *TIMED*TTCN-3 implements this approach by making use of the possibility to read absolute time values which serve as timestamps. The mathematical formulae which are applied on the timestamps can be coded as TTCN-3 functions. Those *evaluation functions* return a judgement which indicates whether a requirement is fulfilled or not. An *online* or an *offline evaluation* of timestamps is possible:

- *Online evaluation* is needed if it is not possible to separate functional and non-functional requirements, i.e., a non-functional property directly influences the functional behaviour of a testcase. In such a case, evaluation of non-functional observations must be performed during the testrun in order to react on the result of the evaluation. Online evaluation has the drawback of cluttering the testcase and slowing down the performance of the testcase which may be undesirable for time-critical testcases.

- *Offline evaluation* may be used if the non-functional requirements which are subject of testing have no influence on the functional reaction of a testcase. In this case, the code just needs to be instrumented by statements that log the relevant timestamps. Based on the timestamps in the logfile, the non-functional properties can be evaluated when the testrun has finished. Offline evaluation has the advantage of having a low impact on the performance of a testcase, since timestamps have to be logged only during the testrun.

5.1 Online Evaluation

For performing online evaluation, timestamps have to be evaluated during the testrun, e.g., by calling a special evaluation function with timestamps as actual parameters. In a distributed test architecture, non-functional requirements may involve timestamps which have been collected by different test components. In this case, the evaluating component needs to obtain timestamps from other components. To achieve this, timestamps can either be piggybacked in the payload of some IUT signals or be communicated directly among test components by using coordination messages. For implementing online evaluation, the new concepts of *TIMED*TTCN-3 which have been introduced so far, are sufficient.

In our example (Section 2), online evaluation is used to check the fulfillment of a non-functional *latency* requirement. In case of a violation, the local test verdict of the Responder test component is set to **conf** (line 16 in Figure 3).

The online evaluation of the latency requirement covers timestamps of several test components. Hence, the remote timestamps have to be transferred to the evaluating component. The evaluation function is called in the Responder test component (line 15). The **receive** operation for the *MDATind* signal (line 10) is local to the Responder component. The related timestamp is obtained by calling **now** and stored in variable *receiveTime* (line 11). In contrast, the corresponding **send** operation is performed by the **mtc** and the associated timestamp is piggybacked to the payload of the *IDATind* signal (line 19 in Figure 2).[6]

[6]In our Inres example, the payload of the *IDATind* signal is considered to be of type **float**. In the more general case, the **float** value has to be encoded into the particular payload type.

```
(1)  function evalLatency(float timeA, float timeB,
                          float lowerbound, float upperbound) return verdicttype {
(2)    var float latency:=timeB-timeA;
(3)    if ((latency<upperbound) and (latency>lowerbound)) {
(4)      return pass;      // non-functional pass
(5)    }
(6)    else {
(7)      return conf;      // non-functional fail
(8)    }
(9)  }
```

Figure 6. *TIMED*TTCN-3 online evaluation function

The Responder component extracts the piggybacked timestamp from the received signal and assigns it to variable *sendTime* (line 13 in Figure 3). Afterwards, *evalLatency* (line 15) is called. The actual parameters of this online evaluation function call are send and receive time as well as the boundaries 1ms and 5ms which describe the incarnation of the latency real-time requirement.

The evaluation function *evalLatency* (Figure 6) checks the condition related to latency ($lowerbound < t_{receive} - t_{send} < upperbound$) of related timestamps (line 3). Depending on the result, it returns either a **pass** or a **conf** verdict (lines 4 and 5) which may be used by the calling entity for further decisions.

5.2 Offline Evaluation

When using offline evaluation, the evaluation function is merely called after the test execution. *TIMED*TTCN-3 offers a means to record timestamps in a logfile during a testrun in order to evaluate them afterwards. The final test verdict is a composition of the functional test verdict and result of the subsequent offline evaluation. To enable offline evaluation of real-time requirements, *TIMED*TTCN-3 refines the existing logfile concept of TTCN-3.

TTCN-3 assumes that one global or several local logfiles exist and provides a **log** statement to enable logging of comments. The number of logfiles is not specified, the logging mechanism is not described and neither module control nor test components can access the global or local logfiles. For an efficient offline evaluation, module control and test components need access to the logfiles and the contents of the logfiles have to be specified more formally.

The Logfile Concept. A *TIMED*TTCN-3 logfile is basically a list of values of arbitrary TTCN-3 types. A logfile is of type **logfile** and it is possible to handle logfiles by means of variables or to pass them into functions.

Each *TIMED*TTCN-3 test component has its own local logfile. A local logfile is initialized when the owning component is created. When test execution finishes, i.e., the main test component terminates, the local logfiles are merged

Operation name	*Return type*	*Function*
first(*sortkey, value*)	**boolean**	Select and sort logfile by *sortkey* and move to first matching entry in the logfile
next(*value*)	**boolean**	Move to the next matching entry
previous(*value*)	**boolean**	Move to the previous matching entry
retrieve	type of *sortkey* used as parameter of **first**	Retrieve entry from current logfile position

Figure 7. Overview of *TIMED*TTCN-3 *logfile* operations

into a global one. *TIMED*TTCN-3 does not specify the internal mechanisms that are needed for storing and maintaining logfiles[7], but defines four functions for accessing the entries of a logfile (Figure 7).

Logging of Events. *TIMED*TTCN-3 refines the TTCN-3 **log** statement in order to write information into logfiles. In TTCN-3, the argument of the **log** statement is an arbitrary fixed string, in *TIMED*TTCN-3, the argument can be the value of any arbitrary valid type. For offline evaluation, a special structured type with a timestamp field may be specified. A corresponding offline evaluation function may only consider logfile entries of the special type in order to judge the fulfillment of the real-time requirement.

Logfile Operations. For retrieving entries of a logfile, *TIMED*TTCN-3 offers means for sorting a logfile by a certain field of the logfile's entries. Since a logfile may contain values of arbitrary types, sorting and retrieving is only possible for a certain type which has to be specified. According to the order which is imposed by sorting, the first, the next or the previous logfile entry may be retrieved. For this purpose, *TIMED*TTCN-3 uses an internal cursor which points to an entry in the logfile. This cursor can be moved and the value at the current cursor position may be retrieved.

The operation **first** serves two purposes: It selects the entries of the logfile by their types and sorts them. In addition, it moves the cursor to the first matching entry in the logfile. The first parameter of **first** specifies the field which is used as a sorting key. This is done using the TTCN-3 template notation: A "**?**" indicates the field which is used as sorting key, all other fields must be set to "**-**". The type of the template is used to select the type of entries which are regarded by the logfile operations presented in Figure 7. The second parameter can be used to further restrict the value of the entry, i.e., the internal cursor is

[7]The mechanisms for storing and maintaining logfiles are considered to be implementation specific and therefore outside the scope of *TIMED*TTCN-3.

Operation name	*Return type*	*Description*
getlog	**logfile**	Get logfile
getverdict	**verdicttype**	Get global verdict
setverdict(*verdict*)	–	Set global verdict

Figure 8. Overview of *TIMED*TTCN-3 operations for testrun handles

```
(1)  type record TimestampType {
(2)     float logtime;
(3)     timezones componentzone;
(4)     Messages messagename;
(5)   }
(6)  type enumerate Messages {
(7)     IDATreq, MDATind;
(8)   }
```

Figure 9. Data types used for offline evaluation in the Inres example

moved to the first entry that matches the second parameter. The same matching mechanisms which are available for TTCN-3 **receive** statements apply.

The operations **next** and **previous** place the internal cursor to the next matching entry before or after the current cursor position. The order to which **next** and **previous** refer to is imposed by the sorting resulting from operation **first**. The parameter of **next** and **previous** is used in the same way as the second parameter of **first**. More complex search operations may be build from these basic search operations. The three operations **first**, **next** and **previous** return **true** when the matching entry is found in the logfile, otherwise **false**. The value of the last matched entry, i.e., the value at the current cursor position, can be retrieved by the **retrieve** operation.

The Testrun Handle. For the handling of global logfiles, *TIMED*TTCN-3 introduces the concept of *testrun handles* and changes the semantics of the **execute** statement. A testrun handle is basically a pointer of type **testrun** which is returned by the **execute** statement and which gives access to the results of a testrun, i.e., the test verdict and global testlog. The operations which can be applied on a testrun handle are shown in Figure 8. The **getlog** operation is used to retrieve the logfile of a testrun. The operations **getverdict** and **setverdict** are used to retrieve and set the global verdict after a testrun. The change of the final testrun verdict might be necessary, if an offline evaluation shows that a non-functional property is not fulfilled. For the **setverdict** operation the same overwriting rules as defined in Section 3 apply.

Local Handling of Logfiles. Global logfiles can be retrieved by applying the **getlog** function to testrun handles (Figure 8). *TIMED*TTCN-3 also allows to apply the **getlog** function to **self** handles, i.e., a test component may access its own logfile in order to perform a local offline evaluation after the collection of timestamps.

Example. The smooth interworking of all *Timed*TTCN-3 concepts for offline evaluation will be explained by means of our test case example (Section 2). For logging test events, the data types shown in Figure 9 have been defined. Values of type *TimestampType* will be logged. Its field values describe the logtime (line 2), the timezone of the logging component (line 3) and the type of the message which causes the log event (line 4). The message type is described by an enumeration type (lines 6-8).

Local logfile entries are written by the **mtc** before sending an *IDATreq* message (line 18 in Figure 2) and by the Responder test component after the reception of a correct *MDATind* message (line 12 in Figure 3).

Figure 10 shows the *Timed*TTCN-3 module control part for the Inres example. The control part starts with variable declarations for the handling of a testrun, a logfile and a verdict value (line 2-4). The testcase *InresRTexample* is executed with *Luebeck* as timezone attribute for the **mtc** (line 5) and the **execute** statement returns a testrun handle which is assigned to variable *myTestrun*. The verdict is retrieved from the testrun and stored in variable *myVerdict* (line 6).

If *myVerdict* is **pass** (checked in line 7), the logfile is retrieved (line 8) and the offline evaluation function *evalMeanArrivalTime* is called (line 9). The actual parameters are the message identifier *MDATind* for which the mean arrival time should be checked, the timezone value *Luebeck* for the identification of relevant logfile entries, the time bounds of 10ms and 15ms that define the requirement to be checked, the integer value 100 that defines the number of relevant timestamps and the reference to the logfile to be evaluated. Finally, the result of the offline evaluation is assigned to the final verdict of the testrun (line 10).

```
(1)   control {
(2)     var testrun myTestrun; // Variable for testrun handling
(3)     var logfile myLog; // Variable for testlog handling
(4)     var verdicttype myVerdict; // Variable for global verdict
(5)     myTestrun := execute(InresRTexample(0), Luebeck);
(6)     myVerdict := myTestrun.getverdict; // Retrieval of verdict
(7)     if (myVerdict == pass) {
(8)       myLog := myTestrun.getlog; // Retrieval of testlog
(9)       myVerdict := evalMeanArrivalTime(MDATind, Luebeck,
                     0.01, 0.015, 100, myLog); // Offline evaluation
(10)      myTestrun.setverdict(myVerdict); // Change of testrun verdict
(11)    }
(12)  }
```

Figure 10. *Timed*TTCN-3 control part for the offline evaluation

```
(1)  function evalMeanArrivalTime(Messages messageId, timezones zone, float lowerbound,
             float upperbound, integer count, logfile timelog)    return verdicttype {
(2)    var float timeSum:=0, averageArrivalTime;
(3)    var TimestampType stampA, stampB;
(4)    if (timelog.first(TimestampType:{?,-,-},
               TimestampType:{?, zone, messageId}) == true) { // search
(5)      stampA := timelog.retrieve; // Get current timestamp entry
(6)      for (var integer i := 2; i <= count; i := i + 1) {
(7)        if (timelog.next(TimestampType:{?, zone, messageId}) == true) { // search
(8)          stampB := timelog.retrieve; // Get current timestamp entry
(9)          timeSum:= (stampB.logtime - stampA.logtime) + timeSum;
(10)         stampA := stampB;
(11)       }
(12)       else {
(13)         return fail; // Wrong number of messages indicates functional problem
(14)       }
(15)     }
(16)     averageArrivalTime := timeSum / (count-1);
(17)     if ((averageArrivalTime < upperbound) and (averageArrivalTime > lowerbound)) {
(18)       return pass; // return non-functional pass
(19)     }
(20)     else {
(21)       return conf; // return non-functional fail
(22)     }
(23)   }
(24)   return fail; // Wrong number of messages indicates functional problem
(25) }
```

Figure 11. TIMEDTTCN-3 offline evaluation function

The offline evaluation function *evalMeanArrivalTime* is shown in Figure 11. It implements the mathematical formula for mean arrival time based on timestamps, namely $\left[\sum_{i:=2}^{n}(t_i - t_{i-1})\right] / (n-1)$ and subsequently verifies that the mean arrival time falls within the range (*lowerbound, upperbound*).

In order to iterate through the timestamps of *MDATInd* messages, **first** (line 4 in Figure 11) and **next** (line 7) are used. Since the **first** operation in line 4 sorts the logfile by the *logtime* field, the timestamp entries are matched in ascending order. If **first** or **next** fails, the logfile contains less matching timestamps than expected. This is an indication for a non-conforming behaviour of the IUT. Hence, evaluation is aborted with a **fail** verdict (lines 13 and 24).

The **retrieve** operation (lines 5 and 8) yields the value of the last successfully matched entry, which is used to calculate the mean arrival time. Based on the final value of the calculation, either **pass** or **conf** is returned (lines 18 and 21).

6. SUMMARY AND OUTLOOK

We presented *TIMED*TTCN-3, a real-time extension for TTCN-3, and demonstrated its usage by applying it to a testcase for the Inres protocol. By introducing absolute time for test components, it is possible to wait until an absolute point in time and to collect timestamps. Timestamps may be evaluated online during the testrun or offline afterwards. For offline evaluation, *Timed*TTCN-3 offers a flexible log mechanism with local and global logfiles. The log mechanism also enables an evaluation of non-functional properties which are not real-time related. For example, failure rates for a fixed amount of data packets can be checked offline by logging correct as well as erroneous message receptions without any time information. *Timed*TTCN-3 can also be used for distributed test architectures, since it supports the specification of synchronization conditions for clusters of clock-synchronized test components. This allows to compare timestamps captured at different, but synchronized test components.

A module of pre-defined timestamp type definitions and evaluation functions can be provided in order to facilitate the usage of *Timed*TTCN-3. In this way, the real-time testcase developer simply needs to select the appropriate evaluation function from the pre-defined library and instrument the testcase accordingly.

In this paper we did not address the formal semantics of the new *Timed*TTCN-3 constructs. Most *Timed*TTCN-3 extensions can be explained by an extension of the existing TTCN-3 semantics. Only the concept of absolute time in combination with the notion of synchronized components and the **resume** operation requires new real-time semantics. These features allow the description of time dependencies among test components, i.e., absolute time values influence the behaviour in different test components.

We also did not cover load generation. For most real-time tests, it is necessary to establish some background load to obtain a realistic environment. This may easily be achieved by using either an external load generator or by explicitly implementing a load generator using *Timed*TTCN-3 statements. As described in [6], an external load generator may be controlled from TTCN-3 by abstract service primitives which are passed to the load generator by an adaptor port.

Furthermore, we did not address the issue of online evaluation functions with memory, i.e., variables of evaluation functions keep their values between subsequent calls. Such "static" variables are valuable for the online evaluation of real-time requirements like floating average. A simple workaround for "static" variables is possible by declaring such variables as component variables.

A further open issue is the graphical presentation of *Timed*TTCN-3 test cases. In the same manner as a graphical format (GFT) is currently developed for TTCN-3 [5], extensions of GFT are needed for a graphical presentation of *Timed*TTCN-3.

Our current work concentrates on applying the proposed extensions in a larger case study in order to assess the capabilities of *Timed*TTCN-3. This includes also the implementation of the language extensions in our TTCN-3 toolset. Our future work will focus on the mentioned open issues, especially on the real-time semantics and the graphical representation of *Timed*TTCN-3 test cases.

References

[1] ATM Forum Performance Testing Specification (AF-TEST-TM-0131.000). The ATM Forum Technical Committee, 1999.

[2] Traffic Management Specification Version 4.1 (AF-TM-0121.000). The ATM Forum Technical Committee, 1999.

[3] ETSI Technical Report (TR) 101 666 (1999-05): Information technology - Open Systems Interconnection Conformance testing methodology and framework; The Tree and Tabular Combined Notation (TTCN) (Ed. 2++). ETSI, 1999.

[4] ETSI European Norm (EN) 101 873-1 (2001-06): The Tree and Tabular Combined Notation version 3; Part 3: TTCN-3 Core Language. ETSI, 2001.

[5] ETSI Technical Report (TR) 101 873-3 (2001-06): The Tree and Tabular Combined Notation version 3; Part 3: TTCN-3 Graphical Presentation Format (GFT). ETSI, 2001.

[6] Roland Gecse, Péter Krémer, and János Szabó. HTTP Performance Evaluation with TTCN. In H. Ural, R.L. Probert, and G. von Bochmann, editors,*Testing of Communicating Systems*, volume 13. Kluwer Academic Publishers, 2000.

[7] J. Grabowski, A. Wiles, C. Willcock, and D. Hogrefe. On the Design of the New Testing Language TTCN-3. In H. Ural, R.L. Probert, and G. von Bochmann, editors,*Testing of Communicating Systems*, volume 13. Kluwer Academic Publishers, 2000.

[8] T. Henzinger, Z. Manna, and A. Pnueli. Timed Transition Systems. In*Real-Time: Theorie and Practice*, volume 600 of *Lecture Notes in Computer Science*, 1991.

[9] D. Hogrefe. Report on the Validation of the Inres System. Technical Report IAM-95-007, Universität Bern, November 1995.

[10] IEEE Standard 1003.1: Information technology – Portable Operating System Interface (POSIX) – Part 1: System Application: Program Interface (API) [C Language]. IEEE, 1996.

[11] Request for Comments 1193: Client requirements for real-time communication services. Internet Engineering Task Force (IETF), 1990.

[12] Information technology – Open Systems Interconnection – Conformance testing methodology and framework. ISO/IEC, 1994-1997. International ISO/IEC multipart standard No. 9646.

[13] L. Lamport. Time, Clocks, and the Ordering of Events in a Distributed System. *Communications of the ACM*, 21, 1978.

[14] P. Ramanathan, K.G. Shin, and R.W. Butler. Fault-Tolerant Clock Synchronization in Distributed Systems. *IEEE Computer*, 23, 1990.

[15] I. Schieferdecker, B. Stepien, and A. Rennoch. PerfTTCN, a TTCN Language Extension for Performace Testing. In M. Kim, S. Kang, and K. Hong, editors,*Testing of Communicating Systems*, volume 10. Chapman & Hall, 1997.

[16] T. Walter and J. Grabowski. Real-Time TTCN for Testing Real-Time and Multimedia Systems. In M. Kim, S. Kang, and K. Hong, editors,*Testing of Communicating Systems*, volume 10. Chapman & Hall, 1997.

[17] T. Walter and J. Grabowski. A Framework for the Specification of Test Cases for Real-Time Distributed Systems. *Information and Software Technology* (41), 1999.

IMPLEMENTATION OF TTCN-3 TEST SYSTEMS USING THE TRI

S. Schulz and T. Vassiliou-Gioles
Nokia Research Center, P.O. Box 407, FIN-00045 NOKIA GROUP, Finland
Stephan.Schulz@nokia.com

Testing Technologies IST GmbH, Bernburger Str. 24-25, D-10963 Berlin, Germany
vassiliou@testingtech.de

Abstract This paper discusses the implementation of test systems, which are specified based on Testing and Test Control Notation version 3 (TTCN-3). TTCN-3 has recently been standardized by [4] European Telecommunications Standards Institute (ETSI) as a new test specification language beyond protocol testing. TTCN-3 source code however constitutes only the first step in the development of a TTCN-3 test system. A complete test system implementation also requires the specification of a test and platform specific adaptation layer. This issue is addressed in the TTCN-3 Runtime Interface (TRI) draft standard also developed at ETSI which is intended to define this interface for all future TTCN-3 test system implementations. We present in this paper different kinds of test systems which can be built from the conceptual model provided by the TRI. Next to a discussion on the application of these concepts for classic conformance testing, we also propose a new approach to test system construction, which significantly simplifies the specification and implementation of TTCN test systems for IP-based applications. We illustrate this approach with the presentation of a TTCN-3 test system for a SIP proxy.

Key words: TTCN Standards, Conformance Testing, Test System Implementation, Communication Protocols, Testing of IP-based Applications

1. INTRODUCTION

TTCN (which originally referred to Tree and Tabular Combined Notation) was first published as a standard in 1992 by the International Organization for Standardization (ISO). Since then the notation has grown into wide spread use and popularity, especially for conformance testing for telecommunication protocols. Nevertheless, the tight integration of previous versions of TTCN [2] with the classical OSI (Open Systems Interconnection) conformance architecture [1] and their lack of flexibility [6] have made test specification cumbersome for applications which use text-based protocols, e.g., IP-based applications. Another shortcoming of this testing language so far has been its tabular specification format.

These shortcomings have now been addressed in the third version of this testing language called TTCN-3 [4]. Arguably the most visible change compared to its predecessor TTCN-2 [2] is the extension of test specification to a wider range of presentation formats. TTCN-3 is based on a textual core notation, which has a similar look and feel of a regular programming language. It offers a number of additional new features that make it more powerful and capable of testing in a wider range of application areas, e.g., procedure-based communication, and dynamic testing configurations during the execution of test cases [7].

TTCN-3 enables the abstract specification of test cases. In a second step a TTCN test specification needs to be integrated with some other test specific parts and a TTCN-3 execution environment to arrive at a complete test system implementation. Concepts for the implementation of such test systems have recently been addressed in the context of the TTCN-3 Runtime Interface (TRI) draft standard [8] which has been accepted as a technical report by ETSI in October 2001. A revision of the document is expected to upgrade it to an ETSI technical standard by the end of the year. The purpose of the TRI is to specify a small and well-defined runtime interface for all future TTCN-3 test system implementations. The TRI defines this interface as a set of operations which are either to be offered by a TTCN-3 execution environment or implemented by the user in a test specific adaptation layer.

A similar run-time interface has previously also been introduced for TTCN-2 test system implementations, i.e., the Generic Compiler/Interpreter Interface (GCI) [3,5]. The lack of acceptance of the GCI within the TTCN community has shown that the GCI had been formulated inadequately as it forced developers to use one particular test system implementation style. The definition of the TRI attempts to address the shortcomings of its TTCN-2 counterpart by excluding test execution management, test component communication and a value interface from the standard, and by specifying the runtime interface independent of a target implementation language.

In this paper we will first show the user perspective of a TTCN-3 test system and follow with a discussion of the implementation perspective, i.e., the conceptual model for TTCN-3 test system implementations on which the TRI is based. We follow with the presentation of two possible test system implementations, i.e., a conformance and a network tester, which arise from the TRI, and illustrate the construction of TTCN-3 Network Testers for a SIP proxy server. Finally, we emphasize the likely impact of this standard for future TTCN-based testing in our conclusions.

2. THE USER PERSPECTIVE OF A TTCN-3 TEST SYSTEM

Prior to discussing the TRI and a implementation perspective for test system implementation it is worthwhile to briefly review the user perspective of a TTCN-3 test system. Figure 1 shows an abstract view of a TTCN-3 test case as it is presented in the TTCN-3 standard [4]. It shows a test configuration during the execution of a test case consisting of a main (MTC) and a parallel test component (PTC). Notice that the figure depicts only a snapshot of a test system during the execution of a test case as the creation of test components as well as connections between components are dynamic in TTCN-3.

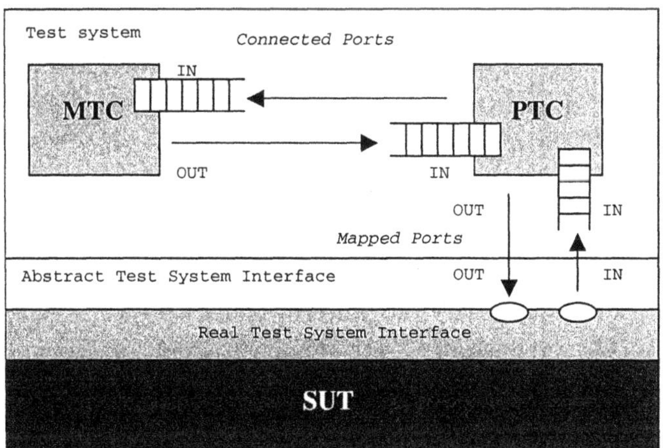

Figure 1. Conceptual view of a TTCN-3 test configuration.

A TTCN-3 test case is specified by the user in the form of TTCN-3 source code. A collection of such test cases is also known as the Abstract Test Suite (ATS). A test case specifies the instantiation of test components and their behavior. Test components can interact with each other after they connect via communication ports. Notice that new TTCN-3 feature is the possibility to specify one-to-many test component connections.

Secondly, a **system** component is generally used in each test case to specify an abstract test system interface. This abstract test system interface provides a means for test components to communicate with the System Under Test (SUT) via the real test system interface. The real test system interface can be understood as a test specific adaptation layer which establishes and handles the interaction between an executable form of the TTCN-3 ATS and the SUT [4].

In the TTCN-3 source code, the abstract test system interface is specified as a collection of communication ports, also called test system interface (TSI) ports, which are declared for the **system** component. During the execution of a test case ports of test components can be mapped dynamically to test system interface ports to establish either message or procedure based communication channel to the real test system interface.

Notice that Figure 1 (or the TTCN-3 standard) does not make any statement about the implementation of communication with the SUT, TTCN-3 external functions, timers, or SUT operations. These issues are nevertheless of relevance in an actual test system implementation or the implementation perspective of a TTCN-3 test system.

3. A CONCEPTUAL MODEL FOR TTCN-3 TEST SYSTEM IMPLEMENTATIONS

Concepts for a general TTCN-3 test system implementation, also commonly referred to as "tester", have been developed recently to define the TTCN-3 Runtime Interface (TRI). Figure 2 shows the conceptual model of a TTCN-3 tester proposed in the TRI standard which also serves as the basis for discussion in this paper.

In this figure, the TRI can be considered to be the most important interface in a test system implementation as it is located between a given or general part, i.e., the TTCN-3 test execution environment, and test specific parts, which implement communication with the system under test and aspects specific to the underlying processing platform of the test system. From this figure, Test Management, TTCN-3 Executable, and even parts of the Platform Adapter entities would be provided by vendors of TTCN-3 development tools whereas SUT Adapter and the remaining Platform Adapter functionality are specified by a test system developer.

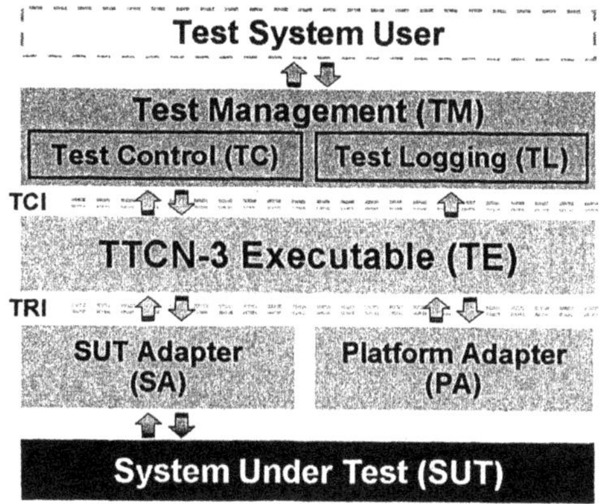

Figure 2. General Structure of a TTCN-3 Test System.

3.1 TTCN-3 Test System Overview

A TTCN-3 test system can be conceptually thought of as a set of interacting entities where each entity corresponds to a particular aspect of functionality required in a test system implementation. The part of the test system which implements interpretation or execution of a TTCN-3 test specification is represented by the TTCN-3 Executable (TE) entity. In a TTCN-3 tester this entity corresponds either to an interpreter or an executable test suite (ETS) produced by a compiler from a TTCN-3 ATS.

The remaining part of the TTCN-3 test system, which deals with any aspects that can not be concluded from information being present in the original ATS alone, can be decomposed into Test Management (TM), SUT Adapter (SA), and Platform Adapter (PA) entities.

As depicted in Figure 2, a TTCN-3 test system has two major interfaces, the TTCN-3 Control Interface (TCI) and the TTCN-3 Runtime Interface (TRI), which specify the interface between Test Management (TM) and TTCN-3 Executable (TE) entities, and TE and Adapter entities, respectively. Notice that current standardization efforts only focus on the definition of a TRI to allow TTCN-3 tool vendors a greater flexibility in their implementation of test execution environments. The real test system interface shown in previously Figure 1 is implemented by TRI operations which implement the interface between TE and SA.

3.2 Test System Entities and the TRI

This section briefly outlines the functionality associated with the entities depicted previously in Figure 2 and shows their relation to the TRI. The focus here is on a general understanding of these entities. For a more detailed discussion we refer to [8].

3.2.1 The Test Management Entity

Within the Test Management (TM) entity, we can distinguish between test execution control and logging related functionality. The TM entity is responsible for general tester management and includes the implementation of a user interface and general test execution management, e.g., the preparation of the test system for a test execution, the collection of final verdicts, and propagation of module parameters to the TTCN-3 Executable (TE) [4]. In addition, the TM maintains a log of test execution. This test system entity does not interact via the TRI.

3.2.2 The TTCN-3 Executable Entity

The TTCN-3 Executable (TE) is responsible for the interpretation or execution of the TTCN-3 ETS. We can think of the TE as implementing three separate tasks or aspects in the execution of a TTCN-3 test specifications: control of test case execution, proper execution of TTCN-3 behavior, and TTCN snapshot semantics [2].

The control aspect mainly implements the control part specified in a TTCN-3 ATS. It addresses, e.g., the proper sequencing of test cases or functions, collecting and resolving intermediate verdicts, and interacting with the TM to obtain module parameters. Other tasks include the initialization SUT and Platform Adapters prior to the execution of a test case as well as possibly the invocation of TRI operations for SUT operations, TTCN-3 external functions, and timer implementations.

The behavioral aspect of the TE implements the execution or interpretation of test cases and functions as defined in the corresponding TTCN-3 modules [4]. It also includes propagation and matching of test events, and management of TTCN-3 test configurations. Other tasks include the invocation of TRI operations for mappings of test component ports to test system interface ports, message or procedure based communication with the SUT, TTCN-3 external functions, SUT operations, and timer operations.

Notice that the TE entity is responsible for encoding test data prior to the invocation of TRI communication operations and decoding test data when receiving test data from the SUT Adapter according to the encoding rules specified in the TTCN-3 ATS. The implementation of the behavioral aspect also addresses message and procedure based communication operations between TTCN-3 test components. In addition, only TTCN-3 semantics of procedure based communication with the SUT need to be implemented in the TE. All remaining parts of procedure based communication operations with the SUT are implemented outside of the TE, i.e., in the SUT Adapter [8]. Similarly, all timers are implemented in the Platform Adapter.

Finally, a TTCN-3 Executable (TE) needs to maintain its own port queues for receiving operations and a list for timeouts to properly implement TTCN snapshot and timer semantics [2,4]. These queues store test events that the TE has been notified of by the SUT Adapter but which have not yet been processed. Similarly, the timer list stores timeouts that the TE has been notified of by the Platform Adapter.

3.2.3 The SUT and Platform Adapter Entities

The purpose of the SUT Adapter is to implement all message and procedure based communication of the TTCN-3 test components with the SUT. This entity serves as a means to properly propagate send requests to the SUT as well as SUT operations invoked by the TTCN-3 executable (TE) and to notify the TE of any received test data. It also realizes TTCN-3 SUT operations. Notice that implementation of procedure based communication in the SUT Adapter is responsible to distinguish between the different messages types (i.e., call, reply, and exception).

The Platform Adapter (PA) implements TTCN-3 external functions and provides a TTCN-3 test system also with one notion of time. Notice that although timers can be instantiated in the TE they are implemented in the PA [8].

4. TTCN-3 TESTER CONSTRUCTION

The specification of TTCN-3 ATS is only the first step in the construction of a TTCN-3 tester. A complete tester requires also the implementation of SUT and Platform Adapters. We focus here in our discussion on the implementation of the SUT Adapter as it always needs to be specified by a TTCN-3 user. As stated before, it can be assumed that Platform Adapters are for the most part (i.e., platform specific timer implementations) provided by vendors of TTCN-3 development tools.

We identify and describe in the following sections two types of TTCN-3 testers, which can be derived from the conceptual model presented in the previous section. The classical application of TTCN so far has been protocol conformance testing. This type of tester specification and implementation is still possible in TTCN-3 and will be outlined in the next section. In the following section we then introduce concepts for a second type of tester, called a network tester. Network testers promise a much simpler specification of TTCN-3 testers for, e.g., IP-based applications, by abstracting away the details of protocol based conformance testing.

4.1 Classic Conformance Testers

The construction of TTCN-3 conformance testers follows straight from the methodology provided by ISO standard 9646 [1,2]. Communication of the TTCN-3 test suite with the real test system interface, i.e., the protocol stack, is achieved via points of control and observation (PCOs). Here, the executable test suite communicates with the top layer of the protocol stack by sending and receiving Abstract Service Primitives (ASPs), which may contain Protocol Data Units (PDUs), via PCOs. This approach is illustrated in Figure 3.

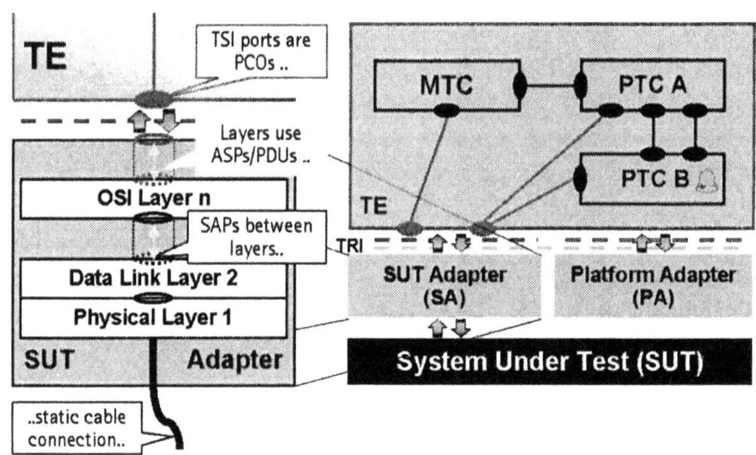

Figure 3. A Classic TTCN-3 Conformance Tester Example.

In TTCN-2, PCOs represented component ports and access points to the protocol stack at the same time. In TTCN-3, they are specified slightly differently. Here, Test System Interface (TSI) ports take the role of PCOs. TSI ports still represent access points to an underlying protocol stack but they are no longer directly associated with a specific test component. Notice that many-to-one test component mappings to a PCO, i.e., TSI port, allow now multiple test components to share one protocol stack implementation. A TTCN-2 like tester structure, however, can still be achieved by only specifying dedicated (one-to-one) mappings of test component ports to TSI ports in the TTCN-3 ATS.

SUT Adapters (SAs) for classic conformance testers are implemented similar to TTCN-2 protocol, e.g., based on the well known OSI protocol layer model [9]. Whereas protocol stacks have usually been tightly integrated in a tool dependent manner with test components in TTCN-2 testers, they are implemented separately in TTCN-3 testers, i.e., all protocol stacks are implemented in the SA. A set of TRI operations provides the required interface for executable test suite in the TE to access stacks in the SA and vice versa. The main motivation for such a definition of the TRI was to reflect the new TTCN-3 feature of an abstract test system interface (i.e., the **system** component).

TRI operations which need to be implemented by the test system developer for conformance testers as the bare minimum include the **triExecuteTestCase()** operation to initialize protocol stacks or establish required connections to the SUT, **triSend()** to implement ASPs or process and send PDUs to the SUT which have been received from the TTCN-3 ATS via a TSI port. Messages, which have been received by the tester from the SUT, are processed in the SA, eventually packaged within an ASP, and then passed from the SA to the executable test suite via a TSI port by invoking the **triEnqueueMessage()** operation. The information provided by **triMap()** and **triUnMap()** operations can be used by the SA to determine the appropriate destination test component for test data in the executable test suite when many test components have been mapped to one TSI port.

4.2 Network Testers

One of the key incentives in the design of TTCN-3 was to relieve this testing language from the peculiarities specific to conformance testing and to bring TTCN-3 to a larger audience, e.g., developers interested in a general approach to testing with no previous background in conformance testing. We identified a second type of tester, a network tester, which can be derived using the new features of the TTCN-3 language and operations defined in the TRI draft standard. Network testers are intended for the testing of protocols or applications which operate at an abstraction level above the network layer, i.e., Layer 3 in the OSI model.

4.2.1 Abstracting Protocol Stack Interaction

In protocol-based conformance testing PCOs have been defined as access points for test components to protocol stack implementations. ASPs have enabled users to access information via PCOs or influence the propagation of information in the protocol stack as explained in the previous section.

This test specification approach introduces unnecessary overhead and implementation complexity to testers where the executable test suite only use a minimal set of ASPs to interact with a protocol stack: establishing and closing a connection, and sending or receiving information via this connection. Testers for applications which use computer network protocols, most importantly internet protocols, fall into this category. Similarly, testers for applications in early stages of development (e.g., for which no protocol has been selected yet) such an interaction abstraction would suffice in many situations.

Since the TTCN-3 language already offers constructs to establish and close connections to a TSI port, and to send or receive data via a TSI port, the specification and implementation of testers for applications which use such protocols can be significantly simplified. Notice that the SA then establishes connections to the SUT dynamically based on TTCN-3 components *mapping* to a TSI port instead of a static association of each TSI port (or PCO) with a single SUT connection.

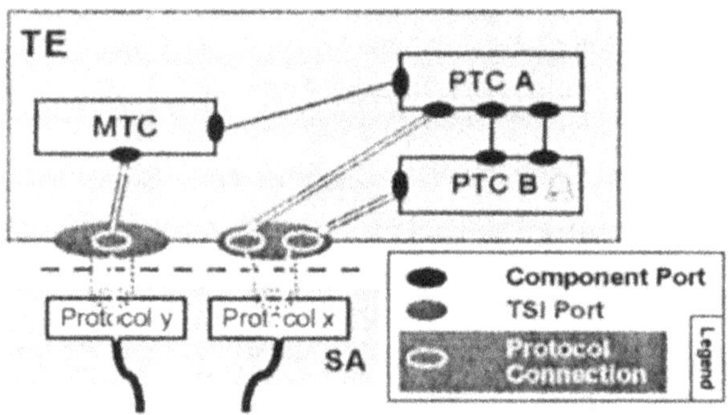

Figure 4. TTCN-3 Network Tester Example.

4.2.2 Implementation of TTCN-3 Network Testers

The result of the interaction abstraction is that TSI ports can be interpreted as complete protocol implementations. Mapping a test component port to a TSI port here implies the opening of a new connection with this protocol. Similarly, unmapping from this TSI port corresponds to closing that connection. Since the invocation of the TTCN-3 operations **`map()`** and **`unmap()`** has been directly correlated in the TRI standard with invocations of **triMap()** and **triUnmap()** operations the execution of such TTCN-3 operations serves in essence as a signal for the SA to take an action. The mapping of multiple components to the same TSI port simply results in several connections to the SUT using one specific protocol. Notice that in the specification of our TTCN-3 ATS we can ignore the details of how exactly this connection is established. An example network tester is shown in Figure 4.

SUT Adapters for network testers consist in this case mainly of complete protocol implementations. As in TTCN-3 conformance testers the user may implement in the SA the **triExecuteTestCase()** operation to initialize these protocol implementations or to establish a physical connection to the SUT statically for the duration of a test case if necessary. In network testers, however, **triMap()** and **triUnmap()** operations are used to administer protocols and connections, e.g., they invoke protocol specific operations to open or close a connection. Notice that this connection to the SUT is here more likely to be a virtual as opposed to a physical connection. **triMap()** and **triUnmap()** operate on component and TSI port types and allow therefore a flexible dynamic test configuration, if so desired.

Similarly, the **triSend()** operation is used now to invoke in the SA the actual protocol specific send primitive with the proper parameters. Messages, which have been received by the tester from the SUT on a connection are sent from the SA to the test suite via a TSI port by invoking again the **triEnqueueMessage()** operation. In this invocation the desired destination test component in the TTCN-3 ETS is determined from the information generated in previous mappings.

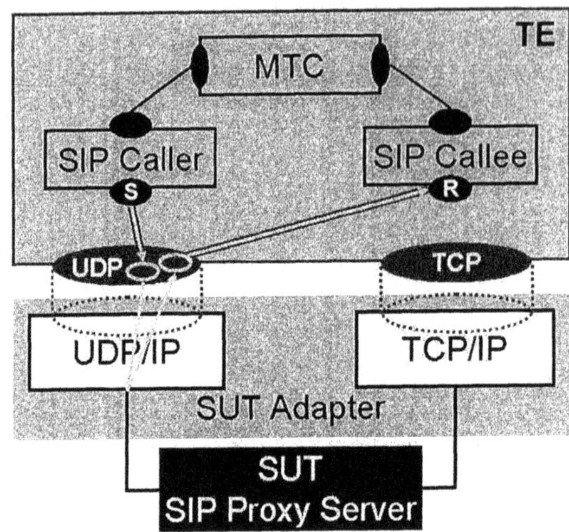

Figure 5. General SIP Proxy Test Architecture for UDP Test.

5. A TTCN-3 NETWORK TESTER APPLICATION EXAMPLE

To illustrate the construction of a TTCN-3 network tester we present a real world IP-based application example. Our example is a tester that checks the ability of a Session Initiation Protocol (SIP) [10] proxy server to build up connections between a calling and a called party. SIP is an IETF signaling protocol for establishing multimedia connections in the internet and future telecommunication networks which may use either on top of UDP/IP or TCP/IP as its transport protocol. Figure 5 displays a general test architecture.

The figure shows that the test system consists of two parallel test components (SIP Caller and Callee) and one coordinating Master Test Component (MTC). The test system contains two TSI ports, i.e., one for the sending and receiving of SIP messages using UDP and one for using TCP.

5.1 TTCN-3 ATS Specification Examples

A TTCN-3 ATS fragment for such a test configuration could be specified as follows:

```
module sipTest {
  testcase UdpTcpTest() runs on MyMtcType system MyTSI {
    var MyPtcType caller = MyPtcType.create;
    var MyPtcType callee = MyPtcType.create;
    map(caller:S, system:UDP); map(callee:R, system:UDP);
    caller.start(callerBehavior(USER1));
    callee.start(calleeBehavior(USER2));
    all component.done;
    unmap(caller:S, system:UDP); unmap(callee:R, system:UDP);
    caller = MyPtcType.create;
    callee = MyPtcType.create;
    map(caller:S, system:TCP); map(callee:R, system:TCP);
    caller.start(callerBehavior(USER1));
    callee.start(calleeBehavior(USER2));
    all component.done;
  }
}
```

First, the MTC creates the SIP caller and callee test components and maps their ports to the UDP test system interface port. In this example it is assumed that the behavioral functions callerBehavior() and calleeBehavior() perform all the necessary actions to assess the SUT. For the TCP tests the same behavior can be reused. PTCs can reuse the component structure while the MTC takes care of the proper test configuration. The SUT Adaptor handles in such a dynamic configuration the protocol and connection management. This split development allows to focus in the specification of test behavior on the coordination and message exchange between the PTCs and ignore for the details of underlying protocol implementations.

TTCN-3 had been designed not only for conformance or functional testing but it should be suitable also for other types of testing like robustness, scalability, interoperability testing, etc. The second scenario is a scalability test where behavior specified for the test case UdpTcpTest() are reused. Here, the SUT is tested to handle an arbitrary number of caller/callee pairs which may use both, UDP and TCP, communication means at the same time.

This scenario is illustrated in the following TTCN-3 ATS fragment:

```
testcase scalabilityTest() runs on MyMtcType system MyTSI {
  var integer i;
  for(i:=1; i < MAXNUMBER; i := i +1) {
    caller[i] = MyPtcType.create;
    callee[i] = MyPtcType.create;
    if(tcpConnection() == true) {
      map(caller[i]:S, system:TCP);
      map(callee[i]:R, system:TCP);
    } else {
      map(caller[i]:S, system:UDP);
      map(callee[i]:R, system:UDP);
    }
    caller[i].start(callerBehavior(USER1 & int2char(i)));
    callee[i].start(calleeBehavior(USER2 & int2char(i)));
    }
}
```

The shown fragment uses component arrays to store references for the PTCs and a function tcpConnection() to decide whether to build up a TCP connection or not for a certain caller/callee pair.

5.2 Implementation of TRI Operations

While the above examples have shown the ability of TTCN-3 to specify dynamic test configurations this section will highlight some implementation issues with respect to TRI. TRI defines two language mappings, a Java and C language mapping [8]. In the following Java will be used as implementation language.

Before the first statement of the MTC will be executed by the TE it will call the **triExecuteTestcase()** operation within the SA, to indicate that the referenced test case with the test system interface port list will be executed. Assuming a static approach to test configuration the communication means (protocol emulation, connections) would be created and parameterized in the implementation of this operation. Since however the SA provides both, UDP and TCP protocols, the scalability scenario introduced above requires initialization of a fixed number of TCP and UDP "connections" to the SUT so that all possible send and receive statements can be implemented. Another approach is to avoid an unnecessary creation of communication means by creating connections depending on the test case to be executed. While the first approach leads to an inefficient tester implementation the later results in a test suite behavior specific test adapter. With the introduction of new test cases the SA would have to be modified.

These problems can be completely avoided by using TRI operations **triMap()** and **triUnmap()**. Connections can be created on demand based on the respective test system interface ports used, thus supporting the newly introduced dynamic test configuration of TTCN-3 in an efficient way. Next to reducing required resources an universal SUT Adapter can be implemented. The following Java code-fragment illustrates this approach:

```
public class MySA implements TriCommunicationSA {
   public TriStatus triExecuteTestcase( TriTestcaseID TCId,
                                        TriPortIdList tsiPorts) {
     // just do nothing
     return new TriStatus (TRI_OK); // Indicate nevertheless OK!
   }
   public TriStatus triMap(   TriPortId compPortId,
                              TriPortId tsiPortId) {
     String portName = tsiPortId.getPortName();
     if(portName.equals("UDP"))
       mapUdpPortAndCreateSocket(compPortId, tsiPortId);
     else
       mapTcpPortAndCreateSocket(compPortId, tsiPortId);
     return new TriStatus (TRI_OK);
   }
   public TriStatus triUnmap( TriPortId compPortId,
                              TriPortId tsiPortId) {
     String portName = tsiPortId.getPortName();
     if(portName.equals("UDP"))
       unmapUdpPortAndFreeSocket(compPortId, tsiPortId);
     else
     // etc ...
   }
   public TriStatus triSend(  TriComponentId componentId,
                              TriPortId      tsiPortId,
                              TriAddress     address,
                              TriMessage     sendMessage) {
     String portName = tsiPortId.getPortName();
     if(portName.equals("UDP")) {
       fetchUdpSocket(componentId).send(sendMessage);
     } else if(portName.equals("TCP")) {
     // etc ...
   }
}
```

This code fragment shows how a test suite behavior independent SA might be implemented. It is by no means complete and should merely illustrate the building and maintaining of communication means (here sockets) solely based on TRI type information, e.g., that port names are obtained in the implementation of the TRI send operation from the source component type. Furthermore it does not address issues with respect to the physical distribution of test components that might be necessary to handle limitation of resources of a single test device.

In addition, it can be concluded from this examples that the resulting SUT Adaptor can not only be used for a SIP test suite but for a multitude of test suites that use UDP and TCP connections as long as the test system interface ports are referenced in the same manner.

6. CONCLUSIONS

We have discussed in this paper the use of the latest version of the TTCN testing language (TTCN-3) and test system implementation concepts defined in the TTCN-3 Runtime Interface (TRI) standard for conventional conformance testing as well as the testing of IP-based applications. We have presented the construction of two different types of TTCN-3 testers, a "classic" conformance tester and a newly defined network tester. For both types of testers we focused on the implementation of TRI operations which manage communication with the SUT, i.e., the SUT Adapter. Our SIP application example has shown that a much more compact and simpler TTCN-3 test system implementation can be achieved for IP-based protocols or applications by applying our network tester approach. Finally, this paper has pointed out the importance and impact of the TRI in the construction of future TTCN-3 testers in general.

ACKNOWLEDGEMENTS

The authors would like to thank all the contributors at the numerous TRI meetings and discussions on the TRI mailing list which have inspired the writing of this paper. At Nokia Stephan thanks Dr. Thomas Deiß for his thorough review and Dr. Colin Willcock, Dr. Stephan Tobies, Jan Spudich, and Martti Söderlund for many discussions about TTCN-3 and tester implementation. Theo thanks at FOKUS Dr. Ina Schieferdecker for pushing the TRI, and at TU Berlin Jacob Wieland, Baltasar Trancon-y-Widemann, and Markus Lepper for intense discussions on TTCN-3 and the TRI.

REFERENCES

[1] International Organization for Standardization, "Information technology - Open Systems Interconnection - Conformance testing methodology and framework - Part 1: General Concepts", ISO/IEC 9646-1, 2nd ed., Geneva, December 1994.

[2] International Organization for Standardization, "Information technology - Open systems interconnection – Conformance testing methodology and framework - Part 3: The Tree and Tabular combined Notation (TTCN)", ISO/IEC 9646-3, 2nd ed., Geneva, November 1998.

[3] P. Cousin, "The European initiative for the development of Infrastructural Tools: the INTOOL programme.", *Proceedings of 10th International Workshop on Testing of Communications Systems*, Cheju Island, Korea, 8-10, September 1997.

[4] European Telecommunications Standards Institute, "Methods for Testing and Specification (MTS); The Tree and Tabular Combined Notation version 3; Part 1: TTCN-3 Core Language", ETSI ES 201 873-1 (v1.0.11), Sophia Antipolis, May 2001.

[5] F. Brady and R.M. Baker, "INTOOL/GCI; Generic Compiler/Interpreter interface; GCI Interface Specification", INTOOL CGI/NPL038 (V2.2), Infrastructural Tools for Information Technology and Telecommunications Conformance Testing, December 1996.

[6] J. Grabowski and D. Hogrefe, "Towards the third edition of TTCN", *Proceedings of 12th International Workshop on Testing of Communication Systems*, Budapest, Hungary, 19-29, September 1999.

[7] J. Grabowski, A. Wiles, C. Willcock, and D. Hogrefe, "On the design of the new testing language TTCN-3", *Proceedings of 13th International Conference on Testing of Communicating Systems (TestCom)*, Ottawa, Canada, 161-76, August 2000.

[8] European Telecommunications Standards Institute, "Methods for Testing and Specification (MTS); The TTCN-3 Runtime Interface (TRI); Concepts and Definition of the TRI", ETSI DTR/MTS-00074, Draft v4.2, September 2001.

[9] G. Holzmann, *Design and validation of computer protocols*, Prentice-Hall, 1991.

[10] M. Handley, H. Schulzrinne, E. Schooler, and J. Rosenberg, "SIP: Session Initiation Protocol", Draft IETF SIP RFC 2543bis-04, July, 2001.

DEFINITION AND UTILISATION OF OMG IDL TO TTCN-3 MAPPINGS

Michael Ebner
Institute for Telematics, University of Lübeck
Ratzeburger Allee 160, D-23538 Lübeck, Germany
Phone: +49 451 500-3721 Fax: +49 451 500-3722
ebner@itm.mu-luebeck.de

Aihong Yin
Fraunhofer Institute for Open Communication Systems (FOKUS)
Kaiserin-Augusta-Allee 31, D-10589 Berlin, Germany
Phone: +49 30 3463-7000 Fax: +49 30 3463-8000
yin@fokus.gmd.de

Mang Li
Department of Computer Science, Ludwig-Maximilians-University Munich
Oettingenstr. 67, D-80538 München, Germany
Phone: +49 89 2178-2164 Fax: +49 89 2178-2262
mang.li@informatik.uni-muenchen.de

Abstract An established middleware technology for Internet-based distributed systems is CORBA, where interfaces are described with IDL. TTCN is a standardised test description language widely used in the telecommunications area. The current version of TTCN, version 3 (TTCN-3), is among others designed to test CORBA-based systems.

This paper presents a definition of the OMG IDL to TTCN-3 mappings, which facilitate the testing of CORBA-based systems. The application of the mappings is shown by an example test for the CORBA Portable Object Adaptor (POA).

Keywords: TTCN-3, CORBA, IDL

1. INTRODUCTION

Nowadays, conformance and functional testing is widely used in the area of telecommunications. Due to the increasing amount of services provided via the

Internet, testing of distributed systems based on the Internet technologies gets more and more important.

The *Common Object Request Broker Architecture* (CORBA) is an established open distributed object-computing infrastructure, standardised by the *Object Management Group* (OMG) (OMG, 2001). The OMG *Interface Definition Language* (IDL) is used to describe object interfaces for CORBA-based systems.

The *Tree and Tabular Combined Notation* (TTCN[1]), a standardised test description language, has been applied to the functional testing of communication protocols for years (ETSI, 2001). The latest widely used version of TTCN is version 2 (TTCN-2). It has been proven that TTCN-2 is generally applicable to the testing of CORBA-based systems (Schieferdecker et al., 1998; Li et al., 1999; Mednonogov, 2000; Mednonogov et al., 2000). In TTCN-2 and its predecessor, the asynchronous communication mechanism on the message-passing basis is the only supported mechanism. Operation invocations, which are primarily used by CORBA applications, are mapped to inter-related messages.

To provide more adequate support for such synchronous communication, new concepts have been developed for version 3 of TTCN (TTCN-3) (Leach, 2000). Among them new constructs for the description of procedure calls and semantics of procedure-based communication ports were added. Following the approach of specification-based testing, as applied in the studies on TTCN-2, some parts of the IDL to TTCN-2 mappings can be reused, others must be changed to reflect the new concepts. This paper presents the recent work of the authors on this aspect (Ebner, 2001a; Ebner, 2001b; Yin, 2001; Yin et al., 2001).

The remainder of this paper is structured as follows. Firstly, the basic concepts of CORBA, IDL and TTCN-3 are introduced. Secondly, the IDL to TTCN-3 mappings are summarized, with the focus on the new rules. Thirdly, the application of the mappings is illustrated by an example test for the CORBA *Portable Object Adaptor* (POA). Finally, some concluding remarks are given.

2. CORBA, IDL AND TTCN-3

This section gives a short introduction on CORBA, IDL and TTCN to motivate the rest of the paper.

2.1 Common Object Request Broker Architecture

The *Common Object Request Broker Architecture* (CORBA) is a standard architecture for distributed object systems. The heart of CORBA is the *Object Request Broker* (ORB) which is the communication infrastructure for the distributed environment. The ORB provides a mechanism for transparently communicating client requests to target object implementations. It simplifies distributed

[1]TTCN (in the context of TTCN-3) is now defined to mean *Testing and Test Control Notation*.

programming by decoupling the client from the details of the method invocations, and hence, makes client requests appear to be local procedure calls. The ORB consists of the ORB core and some interfaces on top of it. The ORB core provides the basic representation of objects and means for the communication of requests. The technology used in the ORB core is hidden by the public interfaces layered on top of it. They are the IDL Stub and Skeletons which present the language mapping and support the static invocation of requests to objects, the *Dynamic Invocation Interface* (DII) and the *Dynamic Skeleton Interface* (DSI) which allow dynamic creation and invocation of requests to objects at runtime, and the *Interface Repository* (IR) that provides storage of object interface definitions which are accessible by applications at run-time (Figure 1).

The *Portable Object Adapter* (POA) is an important component of the CORBA *Application Program Interface* (API) recently specified by the OMG. The POA provides the facility for flexible management of server objects, e.g. creation of object references, activation of objects and dispatching of requests made on the objects, etc. Each POA is associated with a set of policies. The POA policies describe characteristics of the POA and the server objects in the POA. The POA components are described below.

- **Object Id** is a value used by a POA or a user-supplied implementation to identify an object.
- **Servant** is a programming language object or entity that implements requests on one or more objects.
- **Adapter Object Mapping** (AOM) is logically a key-value pair, with the *key* set to `Object Id` and the *value* set to the `address` of the servant. It depends on the `RETAIN` policy.
- **POA Manager** is an object that encapsulates the processing state of one or more POAs.
- **Servant Manager** is an object that supplies a POA with the ability to activate objects on demand when the POA receives a request directed at an inactive object.

2.2 Interface Definition Language

The *Interface Definition Language* (IDL) is a language to *describe* interfaces in an implementation language independent manner and can also be used by other systems than CORBA. It does not support the description of implementation characteristics like behaviour, instances or relationships.

Data Types. IDL supports the most basic data types from C++, but there are no *references* in IDL. Instead, the types `string`, `boolean` and `any` are available. Some data types have a different specification like `char` which is a type of its own in CORBA. The *constructed* types `enum`, `struct`, `array` and `union` are similar to the ones in C++. The *template* type `sequence` is a variable length array of elements of one, but any, IDL type. The type `string` is like `sequence` but it only supports ASCII ISO-Latin characters. Type `any` is like type `Object` in *Java* a placeholder for any possible IDL type.

Modules and Interfaces. The main concept behind IDL consists of interfaces. Each interface may contain constants, types, attributes, exceptions and operations for one object. A module is a method to separate name spaces and may contain any IDL construct. Each IDL construct is automatically *public* according to the object orientated concept. (Multiple-) Inheritance is only permitted for interfaces, not for modules. The inheritance structure may contain loops.

Attributes and Operations. Each client knows the IDL interface specification of each *object* containing all information about the *object.* Attributes are like variable definitions but they behave like operations in CORBA. Each *read-write* attribute gets a *set-* and a *get*-function and each *read-only* attribute gets a *get*-function. The main part of an interface is based on operations. An operation declaration consists of an operation attribute that specifies the invocation semantics, the type of the operation result, the operation name, a parameter list, optional exceptions and optional context expressions.

Exceptions are especially used to handle errors caused by the network environment like connection failures. The context expression allows the client to transfer context specific information, like security context information for the security service.

2.3 Tree and Tabular Combined Notation

The *Tree and Tabular Combined Notation* (TTCN) is the third part of the *Conformance Testing Methodology and Framework* (CTMF) standard for the specification of test suites for conformance testing. In May 2001, the new version of TTCN, called TTCN-3, was finally standardised (ETSI, 2001).

TTCN is designed for functional, black-box testing and to describe *Abstract Test Suites* (ATS) which are independent of a concrete test platform. Therefore, special interfaces defined by TTCN between a *System Under Test* (SUT) and the ATS are required to make a test suite executable. First, there has to be an *Abstract Test System Interface* (ATSI) which defines the sight of the ATS upon the SUT. The access points between ATS and SUT are called *Point of Control and Observation* (PCO). Secondly, there is a *Real Test System Interface* required which maps the ATSI to the SUT (Figure 1).

Test configuration in TTCN is done by the *Main Test Component* (MTC) which controls all other test components called *Parallel Test Components* (PTCs). PTCs

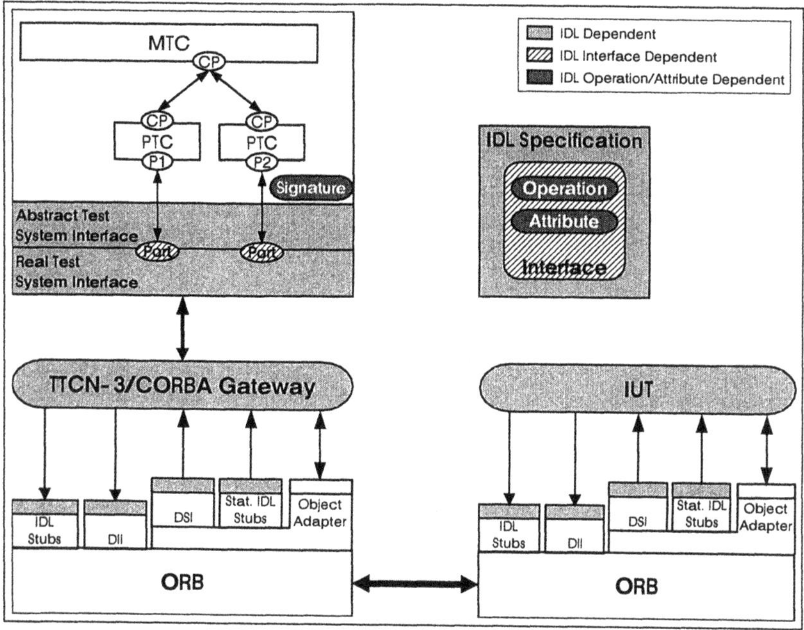

Figure 1. An architecture to use TTCN-3 for testing CORBA-based systems. The upper left corner describes the TTCN-3 part, the upper right corner the interface specifications by IDL, the middle part shows the gateway between TTCN-3 and CORBA and the Implementation Under Test (IUT). The bottom part represents the underlying CORBA system. All parts which depend on the IDL specification are marked (see legend).

can be dynamically created whereas the MTC is created automatically at each test case execution. Test components in TTCN-3 communicate with each other via ports (in TTCN-2 via *Communication Points* (CP)), which are modelled as infinite FIFO queues to store incoming calls. Communication between test components and the test system is also done via ports (in TTCN-2 via PCOs).

TTCN-3 improves concepts of TTCN-2 and introduces new concepts to be a test description language for reactive system tests over a variety of communication platforms such as CORBA -based platforms. An important feature of TTCN-3 is the enhanced communication concept which now supports procedure-based communication to provide synchronous communication, as well as the message-based communication which is asynchronous. In addition, a test execution control part, a module and grouping concept and new data types, are introduced to provide a better control and grouping mechanism.

If TTCN-3 is used for testing systems with interfaces specified by IDL this interface definition can be used as ATSI. Therefore, the mapping suggestion in the next section can be used to generate the *static* ATS parts automatically. This would effect definitions like data types and signatures for procedures. Hence, interface modifications could be seamlessly introduced into the *static* part of TTCN-3 test suites which would improve consistence and allow simplified testing of CORBA-based systems.

3. MAPPING OF OMG IDL TO TTCN-3

The definition of the IDL to TTCN-3 mapping rules is to allow direct use of IDL types and values of the CORBA-based systems in the specification of their tests. The major aspects presented in this section are based on some recent work done by the authors (Ebner, 2001a; Ebner, 2001b; Yin, 2001; Yin et al., 2001).

3.1 Approach

Two different approaches can be followed: either using the *implicit* or the *explicit* mapping. The *implicit* mapping makes use of the *import* mechanism of TTCN-3, denoted by the keywords `language` and `import`. It facilitates the immediate use of data specified in other languages. Therefore, the definition of a specific data interface for each of these languages is required. Currently, ASN.1 data can be used besides the native TTCN-3 types. The data interface for IDL types and values is a topic of on-going research.

The work presented in this paper follows the approach of *explicit* mapping, i.e. IDL data are translated into appropriate TTCN-3 data. And only those TTCN-3 data are further used in the test specification.

3.2 Data Types

Mapping IDL basic data types to TTCN-3 data types is straightforward, because IDL data types are similar to ASN.1 data types which are also used in TTCN-2 (Open Group, 2000; ITU-T, 1997). For example, the *boolean* and *enumeration* types are identical in IDL and TTCN-3. However, TTCN-3 provides more predefined types than TTCN-2, for which a better mapping can be constructed (Table 1). Nevertheless, the `fixed` type and the *constructed* types `union` and `any` require special treatment to get mapped properly. The IDL type `native` is not taken into consideration because of its local semantics.

For the specification of object interfaces IDL type `Object` is used. The interface types for application objects inherit from `Object`. Interface definitions contain structural information which has to be considered in the TTCN-3 configuration architecture and by the TTCN-3/CORBA gateway. Furthermore, object references associated with instances of interface implementations can be passed over operation invocations. Therefore, `Object` is generally mapped to `address` in TTCN-3. In contrary to type `interface`, the IDL type `value` has local operations that are not used outside the object, and are therefore not relevant from the functional testing point of view. However, since the public attributes of `value` instances

Table 1. Mapping list for some data types

OMG IDL	*TTCN-2/ASN.1*	*TTCN-3*
float, double, long double		float
char	GraphicString, IA5String(SIZE(1))	char
wchar	GraphicString, BMPString(SIZE(1))	universal char
string	GraphicString, IA5String	charstring
wstring	GraphicString, BMPString	universal charstring
struct	SEQUENCE	record
sequence (bound)[2]	SEQUENCE SIZE(n) OF	record of (with length restriction)
sequence (unbound)	SEQUENCE OF	record of
Object	IA5String, ObjectInstance	address
exception	SEQUENCE	record

are used to communicate object states, we suggest to map theIDL `value` types to `record` types in TTCN-3. Please refer to the remainder of this section for further details.

Type Extension. To enhance readability and to provide a clear distinction, mapped IDL data types under TTCN-3 get the prefix `CORBA_`. Additionally, to get the same semantic meaning under TTCN-3 as given by IDL, the types get an `extension` attribute containing the source IDL type name. Therefore, a compiler or interpreter can detect the IDL dependency and can react accordingly like executing semantic checks. This includes encoding, too. This feature provides a flexible way of extending the TTCN-3 type system. For instance, the IDL float types `float` and `double` have a range limitation whereas the TTCN-3 `float` type has no such restriction. Thus, a correct mapping would be difficult but the type system extension solves this problem. The same can be done for the integer types. Although TTCN supports range limitation for integers, we suggest to use the `extension` attribute only as the example below illustrates.

```
type integer CORBA_Short with { extension "CORBA v2.4, IDL type: short" };
type float  CORBA_Double with { extension "CORBA v2.4, IDL type: double" };
```

[2]Bound sequences could be matched with arrays inTTCN-3, however, the use of type `record of` with length restriction is preferred to handle bound and unbound sequences equally.

Any Type. In IDL it is possible to express each possible IDL type with the `any` type. There is no corresponding type currently in TTCN-3 available. Therefore, another construct is required. One possible way could be to use a `union` type to store all possible data types. The `union` type comprises all required types, whereas these types have to be known in advance. In order to avoid this restriction a `union` type for all possible types in TTCN-3 used by the IDL mapping rules could be defined. However, it is only possible to use basic data types and well defined constructed types wherefore no generic constructed types for `set`, `record`, `union`, etc. are supported. For instance, it is not possible to provide entries for all possible kinds of type `set` by using a generic `set` type. Hence, the user could define his own *restricted* `any` type in TTCN-3 by using a `union` type containing only all possible types of the concrete application and not all thinkable types. This new `any` type has to be mapped to a full `any` type by the test system. However, this requires a careful handling of `any` types because some type definitions could be missing.

The mapping for TTCN-2 is bound to ASN.1 and therefore, it encounters problems in distinguishing types which are mapped onto the same ASN.1 type (Mednonogov et al., 2000). There is no support of the `any` type given but the use of the design pattern *decorator* is suggested if `any` type is used. Another mapping provides only basic types for the `any` type and leaves structured types open for further study (Li et al., 1999). The use of type extension as described before is not appropriate to solve the `any` type problem, neither. This is because of the TTCN-3 type handling which makes it impossible to handle types which are not known beforehand.

Since data types used by the test system are usually already known at compile time, as it is now the case in TTCN-3, we suggest to use a `union` type for data that are communicated to/over CORBA by the IDL `any` type. The `union` type must cover all data types, either basic or derived, that are translated from the IDL specification used by the test system.

Union Type. In IDL, *unions* are discriminated to determine the actual type. Therefore, a `record` type is used, which contains two members. The first one stores the discriminator information using an enumeration type. And the second member is of the TTCN-3 `union` type, according to the specified IDL `union` members.

Fixed Type. The `fixed` type represents a fixed-point decimal number. There is no corresponding type for `fixed` type in TTCN-3 available. Therefore, a new type has to be created or an existing type has to be used. If we use a `float` with an extension attribute containing the digit and scale the user cannot use this information in his program. Because of the similarities between TTCN-3 and C the solution of the C language mapping of IDL (OMG, 1999, section 1.14) is used. It maps the type `fixed` to a type `struct` which stores the number in a *char* array and the digit and scale number in extra variables. In TTCN-3 it can be realised by a `record` containing a `charstring` to store the number, and two integers for the digit and scale. Hence, the user can access scale and digit, too.

3.3 Modules and Interfaces

IDL uses *modules* as main grouping and scoping units. For this, the *module* concept of TTCN-3 is used.

Interfaces describe objects with all their access methods by using *operations* or *attributes*. Additionally, interfaces can contain local type definitions like *exceptions* and *constants* which can be used by its operations and attributes. Because of lacking an object model in TTCN-3, the group construct is used to retain the scoping information.

Furthermore, for each interface, a procedure-based `port` type is defined for the test specification. It is associated with signatures translated from attributes and operations of the interface (see also section 3.4). Since an interface can be used in operation parameters to pass object references, an `address` type is also declared in the data part.

3.4 Operations, Attributes and Exceptions

Operations, *attributes* and *exceptions* can be mapped well to TTCN-3 because synchronous communication was introduced especially for this purpose.

Exception Declaration. In IDL, exceptions are used in conjunction with operations to handle exceptional conditions during an operation call. Thus, a special *struct*-like `exception` type is provided which has to be associated with each operation that can trigger this exception. TTCN-3 also supports the use of exceptions with procedure calls by binding it to `signature` definitions. However, it provides no special `exception` type. Hence, exceptions are defined as `struct` by using `record`. TTCN-2 has no support of exceptions. Thus, it is realised by using PCOs with asynchronous communication to get exception information from the test system.

Attribute. An attribute is like a *set*- and *get*-operation pair to access a value. If an attribute is marked as `readonly`, the *get*-operation is used only. Therefore, attribute mapping can be done by the operation mapping.

Operation. Apart from attributes, operations are the main part of interface definitions in IDL and are used, for instance, in the CORBA scheme as *procedures* which can be called by clients. Procedure calls in general are supported by

Table 2. Mapping rules for interface elements

OMG IDL		*TTCN-2/ASN.1*	*TTCN-3*
operation		ASP	signature
attribute		ASP pair	signature pair
	readonly	ASP	signature
raise expression		CHOICE	signature exception option
context expression			additional signature parameter
interface	name space		group
	parameter	IA5String	address
	communication	PCO	port

TTCN-3 by means of synchronous communication operations which are used in combination with ports.

IDL supports an optional `oneway` attribute for operations which implies best-effort invocation semantics without a guarantee of delivery but with a most-once invocation semantics. *Message* or *procedure*-based ports could be used for oneway procedures because both would be a valid mapping from IDL perspective. However, the use of *procedure*-based ports for `oneway` procedures is recommended because the IDL specification does not guarantee that oneway calls are non-blocking or asynchronous. Furthermore, CORBA implements oneway procedures by synchronous communication, too.

The parameter attributes `in`, `inout` and `out` describe the transmission direction of parameters and can be mapped directly to the communication parameter attributes in TTCN-3 because they have exactly the same semantics.

A `raise` expression specifies all exceptions which can be thrown by an operation. It can be mapped directly to TTCN-3 because it can be indicated by the procedure signature definition by specifying an exception. Nevertheless, each operation can trigger a standard exception.

A `context` expression provides access to local properties of the called operation. These properties consist of a name and a `string` value. The `context` expression can be matched by redefining the operation with the `context` parameters included in the operation parameters (OMG, 2001, sec. 4.6). This is done in a TTCN-2 mapping introducing an additional array parameter (Mednonogov et al., 2000; Mednonogov, 2000). The additional parameter should be of type `sequence` containing a type `struct` for each context parameter. The `struct` itself contains two variables of type `string` for the context name and value.

4. EXAMPLE

An example for TTCN-3 synchronous communication is explained in this section. It is intended to present the TTCN-3 based ATS for CORBA applications by applying the introduced mapping rules.

4.1 Scenario

In this Section, we consider the functionality of the POA (Section 2.1). Controlling the association between objects and servants for request processing is a key aspect of server application scalability. Depending on the number of objects an application contains, it might want to use a separate servant for each one, use a single servant for all of them, dynamically supply a servant to associate the `Object Id`, or use a combination of these techniques to best manage its resource.

POA policies are objects used to define the characteristics of a POA in server applications. The selected aspects of POA policies are discussed below, which are often used for the design of request processing. A POA with `RETAIN` and `USE_SERVANT_MANAGER` policies (abbr. `POA_Svt_Act`) is created as a child POA of the root POA to present the behaviour of POA policies. The POA `POA_Svt_Act` has an *Adapter Object Mapping* (AOM) and a servant activator which is a type of the servant manager. The POA configuration is illustrated in Figure 2.

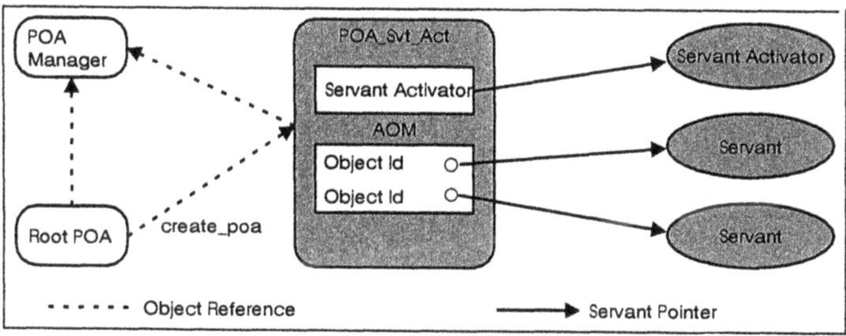

Figure 2. POA Architecture for `POA_Svt_Act`

The servant activator `ServantActivator` is responsible for locating or creating an appropriate servant that corresponds to the `Object Id`. It is used only when an object must be activated during request processing. Therefore, the POA `POA_Svt_Act` has the ability to activate objects on demand.

The behaviour of the POA `POA_Svt_Act` is described in Figure 3, which addresses the case that an object is not active before the request processing. In case the POA `POA_Svt_Act` does not find a servant in the AOM for a given `Object Id`, the servant activator registered with the POA `POA_Svt_Act` is available to determine the servant. It returns the servant that will be used to process the incoming request. The POA `POA_Svt_Act` enters the address of the servant into the AOM so that subsequent requests with the same `Object Id` will be delivered directly to that servant without invoking the servant activator. Finally, the POA performs the request.

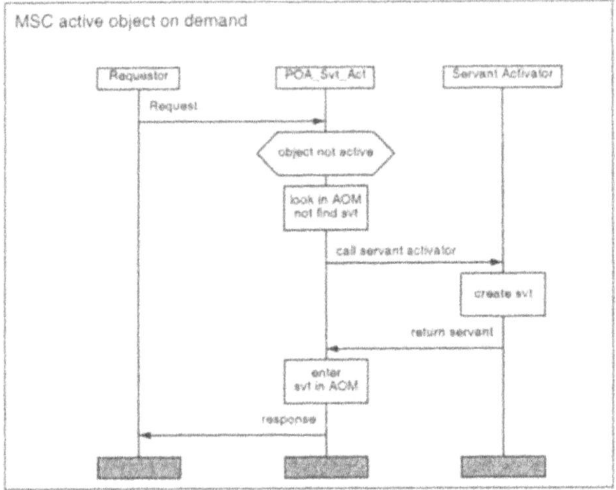

Figure 3. Behaviour of `POA_Svt_Act`

4.2 IDL Specification

The IDL specification below is used to test the selected aspects of the POA `POA_Svt_Act`, which are based on the test sequence diagram (Figure 3). The module `PolicyTest` contains the interfaces `RequestPolicyTest` and `ServantProvider`. The interface `RequestPolicyTest` defines the operations, which can be accessed directly by clients. The interface `ServantProvider` can only be accessed by clients using the object reference. For instance, this object reference is returned by operations that are defined in the interface `RequestPolicyTest` (e.g. `create_objectRef`).

```
module PolicyTest {
  exception WrongPolicy {};
  enum objectState { active, deactive, non_aom };

  interface ServantProvider { long increment(in long m); };

  interface RequestPolicyTest {
    objectState check_objectState( in Object obj );
    Object create_objectRef() raises ( WrongPolicy );
  };
};
```

4.3 TTCN-3 ATS Specification

The specification of the ATS in TTCN-3 can be divided into a *static* part which includes the type definitions and a *dynamic* part which defines the test behaviour.

4.3.1 Static Part. In this part, the IDL data types, operations and interfaces are mapped to TTCN-3 types based on the defined mapping rules.

The Module `PolicyTest` imports definitions from the module `CorbaModule`, which includes the mapping of IDL basic types to TTCN-3 as introduced in Section 3.2. In addition, it contains the derived data type from the IDL specification above.

```
module PolicyTest {
  import all from CorbaModule;

  type record WrongPolicy {} { extension "CORBA v2.4, IDL:exception" };
  type enumerated objectState {active, deactive, non_aom}
        with { extension "CORBA v2.4, IDL::enumerated" };

  // Mapping of IDL interface to TTCN-3 group, port and address
  group CORBA_INTF_RequestPolicyTest {
    // signatures for operations in the IDL interface RequestPolicyTest
    signature check_objectState (in CORBA_Object svtProvider) return objectState;

    signature create_objectRef() return CORBA_Object
       exception( WrongPolicy );
  }
  type port CORBA_RequestPolicyTest procedure {
     out check_objectState, create_objectRef
  };
  type address CORBA_OBJ_RequestPolicyTest;

  // components for MTC and test system interface
  type component MTCType { port CORBA_RequestPolicyTest MTCpco; };
  type component TSIType { port CORBA_RequestPolicyTest SYSpco; };

  // invocation the operation increment
  external function invoke_increment( in CORBA_Object svtProvider,
    in CORBA_Long m) return CORBA_Boolean;
  :
}
```

The IDL module `PolicyTest` is translated into the TTCN-3 module `PolicyTest` based on the mapping rules. For example, the IDL interface `RequestPolicyTest` is mapped to TTCN-3 port type `CORBA_RequestPolicyTest`. It contains the signatures corresponding operations (e.g. `create_objectRef`) defined in the interface `RequestPolicyTest`. The direction `out` indicates that the operation is called by the test system.

Since the operation `increment` of the interface `ServantProvider` cannot be accessed by the client directly, the external function `invoke_increment` was generated in TTCN-3.

4.3.2 Dynamic Part. The dynamic part consists of *test cases* and a *control* part. It is generated manually.

Test Cases. The development of test cases can be done by using test sequence diagrams as shown in Figure 3. They are derived from the textual behavioural description in the IDL specification. The test case `createObjectRef` is used to test whether an object reference can be created with the selected POA.

```
testcase createObjectRef( inout CORBA_Object svtProvider ) {
  map( mtc:MTCpco, system:SYSpco );
  MTCpco.call( activate_object )
  {
    MTCpco.getreply ( create_objectRef ) -> value svtProvider
    {
      MTCpco.call( check_objectState:{ svtProvider } )
      {
        [] MTCpco.getreply ( check_objectState value active ) {
           verdict.set( fail ); stop;
        }
        [] MTCpco.getreply ( check_objectState value inactive ) {
           verdict.set( pass ); stop;
        }
      :
```

First of all, in this test case, the test system performs the call of the remote operation `create_objectRef` defined in the interface `RequestPolicyTest` at the port `MTCpco` in order to create an object reference. Then, the operation `check_objectState` in the interface `RequestPolicyTest` is called by the test system in order to check the state of the created object.

Control Part. In this part, the execution order of test cases is described. The test case `createObjectRef` is used to find out whether an object reference can be created and the state of the object is inactive. If the test cases result is `pass`, the test client makes a request to the created object. This object contains the object reference for the interface `ServantProvider` and operation `increment`. If the request is being fulfilled, the test case `check_createdObj_state` is executed to test whether the created object becomes active.

```
control {
  var boolean is_true;
  var verdicttype theVerdict;
  var CORBA_Object svtProvider := null;

  theVerdict := execute( createObjectRef( svtProvider ), 80E-3 );
  if ( theVerdict == pass ) {
    is_true := invoke_increment( svtProvider, 1 );

    if ( is_true == true ) {
      execute( check_createdObj_state( svtProvider ) );
    }
  }
}
```

5. CONCLUSIONS

Our work presented in this paper is primarily focused on the definition of a set of OMG IDL to TTCN-3 mapping rules, in order to support adequate testing of CORBA-based systems based on their specifications. The first example tests show that the new concepts of TTCN-3, in particular the support of synchronous communication, apply well to these systems.

The defined mapping rules focus on the translation of type and structural information contained in IDL specifications. They can be integrated into the TTCN-3 data concept, e.g. using a specific data interface for IDL. Until this is approved by the TTCN-3 standardisation, the presented mapping rules can be implemented by translators to achieve semi-automated development of test data specifications. To support automated generation of the dynamic part in an ATS, additional formalised behavioural descriptions, e.g. test sequence diagrams, can be considered.

The limitation of the mapping for the IDL `any` type is intensively discussed in the paper. The proposed solution is already applicable for manual or semi-automated translations of IDL data types. It provides input to the consideration of a native TTCN-3 `any` type or the definition of the IDL data interface.

Future work will also address the realisation of the TTCN-3/CORBA gateway. Because of the integrated support of synchronous communication in TTCN-3, its implementation will be simpler than the one for the TTCN-2/CORBA gateway.

References

Ebner, M. (2001a). A Mapping of OMG IDL to TTCN-3. SIIM Technical Report SIIM-TR-A-01-11, Institute for Telematics, Medical University of Lübeck, Germany. Schriftenreihe der Institute für Informatik/Mathematik.

Ebner, M. (2001b). Mapping CORBA IDL to TTCN-3 based on IDL to TTCN-2 mappings. In *Proceedings of the* 11th *GI/ITG Technical Meeting on Formal Description Techniques for Distributed Systems, Bruchsal, Germany, 21.-22. June 2001.* International University in Germany. `http://www.i-u.de/fbt2001/`.

ETSI (2001). Methods for Testing and Specification (MTS) — The Tree and Tabular Combined Notation version 3 — Part 1: TTCN-3 Core Language. European Standard ETSI ES 201 873-1, European Telecommunications Standards Institute, Sophia-Antipolis, France.

ITU-T (1997). Recommendation: Abstract Syntax Notation One (ASN.1): Specification of Basic Notation. International Standard X.680, ITU-T.

Leach, E. (2000). Enhanced Techniques for CORBA Validation CORVAL2 – Validating Multi-Vendor CORBA Conformance and Interoperability in Heterogeneous Environments. D29 – white paper, The Open Group. European Commission Project Number IST-1999-11131.

Li, M., Schieferdecker, I., and Rennoch, A. (1999). Testing the TINA Retailer Reference Points. In 4th *Int. Symposium on Autonomous Decentralized Systems (ISADS'99), Tokyo, Japan, Mar. 1999.*

Mednonogov, A. (2000). Calypso Gateway specification, version 0.07. Technical report, Telecommunications Software and Multimedia Laboratory, Helsinki University of Technology, Finland.

Mednonogov, A., Kari, H., Martikainen, O., and Malinen, J. (2000). Conformance Testing of CORBA Services using Tree and Tabular Combined Notation. In Ural, H., Probert, R., and Bochmann, G., editors, *Proceedings of the IFIP TC6/WG6.1* 13th *International Conference on Testing of Communicating Systems (TestCom 2000), August 29 – September 1, 2000, Ottawa, Canada*, pages 193–208. IFIP – The International Federation for Information Processing, Kluwer Academic Publishers.

OMG (1999). C Language Mapping Specification. OMG Formal Document FORMAL/99-07-35, Object Management Group.

OMG (2001). The Common Object Request Broker — Architecture and Specification. OMG Formal Document FORMAL/2001-02-01, Object Management Group. Version 2.4.2.

Open Group (2000). Inter-Domain Management: Specification & Interaction Translation. Technical Standard C802, Open Group.

Schieferdecker, I., Li, M., and Hoffmann, A. (1998). Conformance Testing of TINA Service Components — The TTCN/CORBA Gateway. In Trigila, S., Mullery, A., Campolargo, M., Vanderstraeten, H., and Mampaey, M., editors, *Proceedings of the* 5th *International Conference on Intelligence and Services in Networks, IS&N'98, Antwerp, Belgium, May 25–28, 1998*, volume 1430 of *Lecture Notes in Computer Science*, pages 393–408. Springer.

Yin, A. (2001). Testing Operation-Based Interfaces — Exemplified for CORBA with ADL and TTCN-3. Diplomarbeit, Telecommunication Network Group, Faculty of Electrical Engineering and Computer Science, Technical University Berlin, Germany.

Yin, A., Schieferdecker, I., and Li, M. (2001). Mapping of IDL to TTCN-3. Technical report, Fraunhofer Institute for Open Communication Systems (FOKUS), Germany.

Author Index

Ahtiainen, Ari, 187
Belinfante, Axel, 219
Besse, Cédric, 169
Binder, Robert V., 75
Bochmann, Gregor v., 373
Boroday, Sergiy, 355
Bredereke, Jan, 79
Cabellos-Aparicio, Albert, 39
Calmet, Jacques, 111
Carapinha, Jorge, 55
Carvalho, Paulo, 55
Castanet, Richard, 249
Cavalli, Ana, 169, 317
Chanson, Samuel T., 151
Dai, Zhen Ru, 407
Domingo-Pascual, Jordi, 39
Ebner, Michael, 443
El-Fakih, Khaled, 373
Feenstra, Jan, 219
Feijs, Loe M. G., 267
Fontes, Francisco, 55
Gehring, Andreas, 17
Goga, Nicolae, 267
Grabowski, Jens, 407
Groz, Roland, 95, 355
Hasegawa, Toru, 21
Heikkilä, Tapio, 209
Horváth, Endre, 235
Jard, Claude, 301
Kato, Toshihiko, 21
Kim, Myungchul, 151, 169
Koné, Ousmane, 129
Kullmann, Peter, 111
Li, Mang, 443
Lima, Solange, 55
Mann, Zoltán Ádàm, 111
Marche, Mikael, 95
Mauw, Sjouke, 267
Neukirchen, Helmut, 407
Ogishi, Tomohiko, 21
Parada, Carlos, 55
Peleska, Jan, 335
Petrenko, Alex, 355
Probert, Robert L., 283
Prokopenko, Svetlana, 317
Quemener, Y.-M., 95, 355
Rößler, Georg, 139
Rouillard, Davy, 249
Sachse, Wolfgang, 201
Schlingloff, Bernd-Holger, 79
Schulz, Stephan, 425
Seol, Soonuk, 151

Serdar, Burak, 391
Solé-Pareta, Josep, 39
Steinert, Thomas, 139
Suzuki, Kenji, 21
Szabó, János Zoltán, 191
Tai, Kuo-Chung, 391
Tenno, Petri, 209
Tretmans, Jan, 267
Väänänen, Jarmo, 209
Vassiliou-Gioles, T., 425
Veciana-Nogués, Carlos, 39
Vries, René G. de, 219
Williams, Alan W., 283
Yevtushenko, Nina, 317, 373
Yin, Aihong, 443
Zaidi, Fatiha, 169

Partners of TestCom 2002

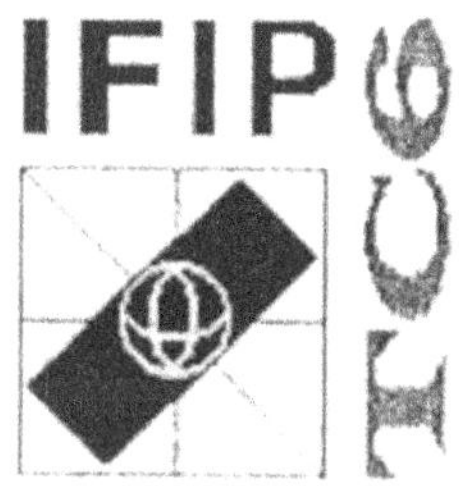

Fraunhofer Institute for Open Communication Systems

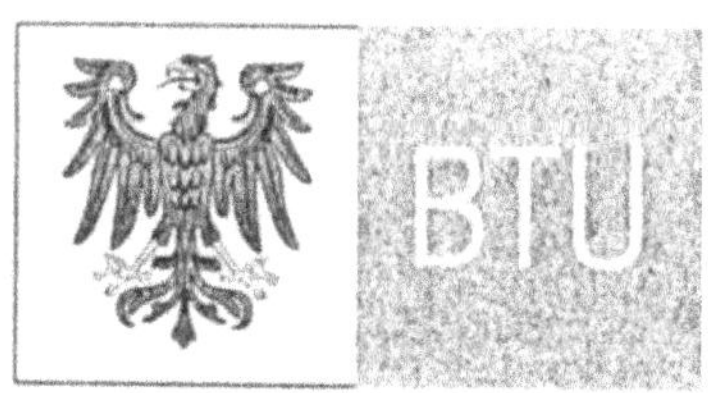

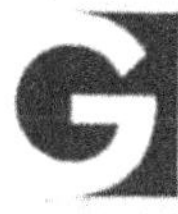

Gesellschaft für Informatik e.V.

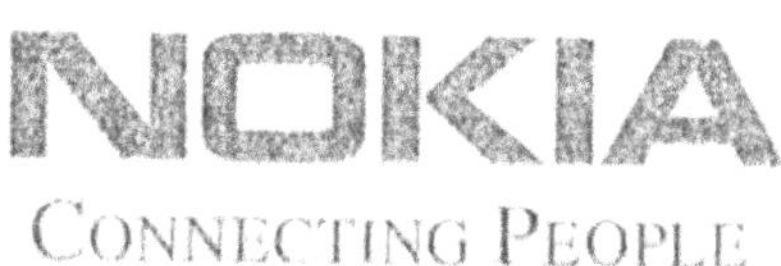

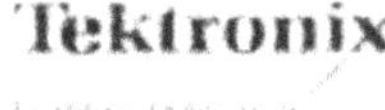

Tektronix Berlin GmbH & Co. KG

<testing_tech>

Testing Technologies

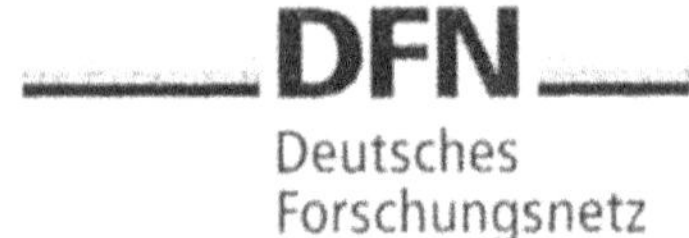

Verein zur Förderung eines Deutschen Forschungsnetzes e.V.

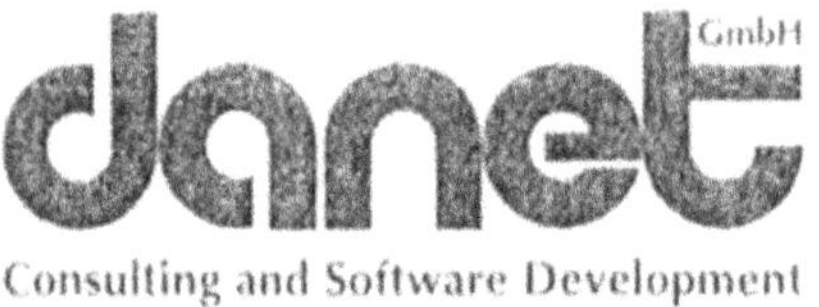

Telelogic

T-Systems

www.ingramcontent.com/pod-product-compliance
Ingram Content Group UK Ltd.
Pitfield, Milton Keynes, MK11 3LW, UK
UKHW022322190726
13856UKWH00001B/160

* 9 7 8 1 4 7 5 7 6 7 0 4 9 *